Clinical topics
in personality disorder

Clinical topics
in personality disorder

Edited by Jaydip Sarkar and Gwen Adshead

RCPsych Publications

Dedication

This book is dedicated to Professors Chris Mace and Sean Spence, who did so much to improve our understanding of disturbed minds, and who combined research enterprise and excellence with warmth and humanity. We thank them and miss them.

RCPsych Publications is an imprint of the Royal College of Psychiatrists,
17 Belgrave Square, London SW1X 8PG
http://www.rcpsych.ac.uk

British Library Cataloguing-in-Publication Data.
A catalogue record for this book is available from the British Library.
ISBN 978 1 908020 39 0

Distributed in North America by Publishers Storage and Shipping Company.

Printed by Bell & Bain Limited, Glasgow, UK.

Contents

Tables

Boxes

Figures

List of contributors

Gwen Adshead Consultant Forensic Psychotherapist, Broadmoor Hospital, Crowthorne, UK

Prija Bajaj Specialist Registrar in Psychiatry, Central and North West London NHS Foundation Trust, London, UK

Penny J. M. Banerjee Consultant Forensic Psychiatrist, East Midlands Centre for Forensic Mental Health, Arnold Lodge, Leicester, UK

Anthony W. Bateman Consultant Psychiatrist and Psychotherapist, Barnet, Enfield and Haringey Mental Health NHS Trust and St Anne's Hospital, London; Visiting Professor, University College London, UK

Kerry Beckley Consultant Clinical Forensic Psychologist, Lincolnshire Partnership Foundation NHS Trust, Lincoln, UK

Nick Benefield Department of Health Advisor on Personality Disorder, and Joint Head of the Department of Health and National Offender Management Service Personality Disorder Policy Team, Department of Health, London, UK

Dawn Bennett Consultant Clinical Psychologist, Lancashire Care NHS Foundation Trust, Blackburn, UK

Paul Brodrick Principal Clinical Psychologist, Bluebird House Secure Adolescent Unit, Southern Health NHS Foundation Trust, Southampton, UK

Andrew Carroll Senior Lecturer in Forensic Psychiatry, Centre for Forensic Behavioural Science, Monash University, Fairfield; Consultant Forensic Psychiatrist, Thomas Embling Hospital, Fairfield, Melbourne, Australia

Ben S. Clark Psychiatrist, c/o Cygnet Hospital Harrow, London, UK

Mike Crawford Professor of Mental Health Research, Centre for Mental Health, Imperial College, London; Honorary Consultant Psychiatrist for Central & North West London NHS Foundation Trust, London, UK

Michael Daffern Associate Professor, School of Psychology and Psychiatry, Monash University, Melbourne, Australia; Principal Consultant, Forensicare, Victoria, Australia; Special Lecturer, Division of Psychiatry, Nottingham University, Nottingham, UK

Quinton Deeley Senior Lecturer in Social Behaviour and Neuro-development, Institute of Psychiatry, King's College London; Honorary Consultant Psychiatrist, South London and Maudsley NHS Trust, London, UK

Mayura Deshpande Consultant Forensic Psychiatrist, Bluebird House Secure Adolescent Unit, Southern Health NHS Foundation Trust, Southampton, UK

Conor Duggan Professor of Forensic Mental Health, Division of Psychiatry, Nottingham University, Nottingham; Honorary Consultant Psychiatrist, Personality Disorder and Secure Women's Services, East Midlands Centre for Forensic Mental Health, Leicester, UK

Sue Evershed Lead Psychologist, Men's Personality Disorder and National Women's Directorate, Rampton Hospital, Retford, UK

Leonard Fagin Honorary Senior Lecturer, Anna Freud Centre, University College, London, UK

Simon Gibbon Consultant Forensic Psychiatrist, East Midlands Centre for Forensic Mental Health, Arnold Lodge, Leicester, UK

Neil Gordon Head of Doctoral Programmes and Masters Programme Lead, Institute of Mental Health, Nottingham, UK

Rex Haigh Consultant Psychiatrist and Clinical Advisor to the Department of Health's Personality Disorder Development Programme 2003–2011

Helen den Hartog Former Service User of the Oxford Therapeutic Community, and a Service User Advisor to the Department of Health's Personality Disorder Development Programme 2003–2011

Kevin Howells Emeritus Professor, School of Community Health Sciences, University of Nottingham, Nottingham, UK

Nick Huband Research Fellow, Division of Psychiatry, Nottinghamshire Healthcare NHS Trust, Nottingham, UK

Ian B. Kerr Consultant Psychiatrist and Psychotherapist, Coathill Hospital, Coatbridge, Scotland; Honorary Research Fellow, School of Health and Related Research, University of Sheffield, Sheffield UK

Gopi Krishnan Consultant Forensic Psychiatrist and Associate Clinical Director, Rampton Hospital, Retford, UK

Rebecca Lawday Lead Psychologist, Secure Women's Services, East Midlands Centre for Forensic Mental Health, Arnold Lodge, Leicester, UK

Chris Mace (deceased) Consultant Psychotherapist, St Michael's Hospital, Warwick; Honorary Senior Lecturer in Psychotherapy, University of Warwick, Coventry, UK

Carlos Mirapeix Psychiatrist and Psychotherapist, Foundation for Personality and Psychotherapy Research, Santander, Cantabria, Spain

Estelle Moore Consultant Clinical and Forensic Psychologist, and Lead Psychologist for the Centralised Groupwork Service, Newbury Therapy Unit, Broadmoor Hospital, Crowthorne, Berkshire UK

Aparna Mordekar Specialty Doctor, Sheffield Health and Social Care NHS Foundation Trust, Sheffield, UK

Jackie Preston Consultant Clinical Psychologist, Bluebird House Secure Adolescent Unit, Southern Health NHS Foundation Trust, Southampton, UK

Jaydip Sarkar Consultant, Department of General and Forensic Psychiatry, Institute of Mental Health, Singapore

Sagari Sarkar Researcher, Department of Forensic and Neuro-developmental Science, Institute of Psychiatry, King's College London, London, UK

Sean A. Spence (deceased) Professor of General Adult Psychiatry, University of Sheffield, Sheffield, UK

Peter Tyrer Professor of Community Psychiatry, Centre for Mental Health, Imperial College, London, UK

Foreword

Effective processes of change generally begin with a trigger event, a period of reaction and uncertainty, and finally a tipping point. This is no less the case in the field of mental health, where major change has frequently come about as a consequence of failures or crisis in service delivery. Too often when this happens the reaction is to seek immediate solutions based on a need to be seen to act. However, this encourages an oversimplification of complex problems and a tendency to deny uncertainty and the limits of existing knowledge. The result can be decision-making driven by the immediate reaction to events and the need to resolve public and political anxieties. The best evidence base has not always been the key determinant of policy established in this way and any impact on outcomes for either public or patients has not always been that expected.

It is rewarding, therefore, to find that in one area of policy, the national concern about dangerous offenders has generated a momentum in research, practice and training and has resulted in a positive tipping point for policy-based practice on learning.

The long history of public prejudice, clinical ambivalence and the associated exclusion of patients with personality disorder from health and social care treatment services has been a troubling one. Too often our lack of knowledge and skills has been concealed by an underdeveloped judgement on the treatability of patients. Mainstream psychiatry has struggled with the absence of appropriate practice skills for complex psychological conditions and, although work on improving the treatment of severe and moderate mental illnesses has made significant progress in the past half-century, interventions for personality disorders have been harder to crack. The development of social therapies, in particular therapeutic communities, has been one of the few areas of optimism. However, this has been undermined by the difficulty of research into complex dynamic relational models of treatment and the sheer complexity of cases and measurable outcomes. In consequence, there has been a widespread need for improved practice skills underpinned by sound research.

In the UK, the establishment of the joint Department of Health and Ministry of Justice Dangerous and Severe Personality Disorder (DSPD) Programme, with all its imperfections, generated major growth points in professional awareness, government investment, policy attention, service and workforce development as well as practice and research interest in the significance of personality disorders in mental health and offending behaviours. This programme facilitated the establishment of new pilot services in prisons, secure psychiatric hospitals and community-based forensic settings. Pilot services have provided a test bed for innovative models of practice from which new insights and approaches are being developed and researched. Early intervention programmes, where the emergence of personality disorder in adolescents has seen families and communities struggling to access appropriate services, are now being rolled out. Mainstream mental health services have begun to grapple with the significance and ownership of personality disorder in their caseloads and to respond with new specialist services in the community.

The National Institute for Health and Clinical Excellence (NICE) has developed guidance on borderline and antisocial personality disorders. The need for more consistent and longer-term interventions has resulted in a new pathway strategy for offenders with personality disorder, training and workforce developments alongside policy, commissioning and practice guidance, and a growth in research activities. All are important indicators that a new period in understanding has been reached.

These different aspects of work on personality disorder represent a cross-governmental approach and a recognition of the importance of a biopsychosocial paradigm to understanding the spectrum of complex psychological disorders in which comorbidity remains central in our developing understanding in this field. A wide range of services and professions across health, social care, criminal justice, the independent sector and academia have all contributed to a developing body of knowledge and understanding from which we cannot now retreat.

The authors included in this book represent many of the current leaders in National Health Service clinical practice and academic research in the field of personality disorder in the UK. They bring research, clinical experience and conceptual focus to a variety of the health and social care settings where personality disorder is a primary concern. They present the latest findings and current thinking on personality disorder primarily in the implementation of community and secure psychiatric services. A major area of concern remains the evidence on which practice can be strengthened and how this important work can be broadened to support greater collaboration with practitioners and researchers in the criminal justice field, where the prevalence of personality disorder means that its significance to effective intervention is vital.

The overarching messages that stand out from this book provide a framework for future work in this field. Personality disorder is now better understood than at any other time in the history of UK mental health services. A psychologically informed approach is essential in working jointly with populations shared across a number of different public services. Effective treatment is possible but many unresolved challenges remain. These include the need to identify different service populations who require adaptation and variation in the structure and emphasis of treatment models. The identification and measurement of outcomes to satisfy political, clinical and patient expectations remains elusive but is no longer unachievable. All these elements provide an exciting position from which the future of working with personality disorder can be launched.

The collective impact of all this work suggests that at this tipping point, new and exciting areas of practice, research and policy development can be launched. It is therefore important that developing experience and evidence from the field is disseminated to those seeking to improve services and further research into effective interventions.

The learning and challenges raised by this collection of chapters provide a major contribution to our current practice in the field and to the prioritising of future policy and research. If we are able to ensure that the wide spectrum of those working in the fields of justice, care and treatment better understand the basis of their human business and the causes of troubling behaviour, it will both change their practice and contribute to improvement in our investigation of what works and why.

Nick Benefield
Department of Health Advisor on Personality Disorder
and Joint Head of the Department of Health and
National Offender Management Service Personality Disorder Policy Team

Part 1

The nature of the problem

CHAPTER 1

The nature of personality disorder

Gwen Adshead and Jaydip Sarkar

Summary   The lack of a medically grounded approach to personality disorder and its management has led to its comparative neglect as a topic by many clinicians in the UK. In this article we present evidence that personality disorders are, like other mental disorders, the social manifestations of a pathological process. This process presents with characteristic clinical features that are developmental in nature. These cause disturbances in arousal, affect and reality testing that have an impact on interpersonal social functioning. Personality disorder may therefore be conceived of primarily as a socioemotional disability, not dissimilar to Axis I conditions.

The term 'personality' derives from the Greek word *persona* or mask. It refers both to an individual's attitudes and ways of thinking, feeling and behaving, and to the social ways in which individuals interact with their environment. At an individual level, personality is not a single unitary entity, but a way to organise a number of different capacities that underpin one's sense of self (Allport, 1961). At a social level, an individual personality profile allows one to be recognised over time by others, and is a powerful regulator of social relationships, which, as we are group animals, are crucial for our survival.

In evolutionary terms, personality is best understood as a regulation of biopsychosocial factors in the service of good-quality survival of the individual within the particular constraints of their habitat and environment (Box 1.1).

Theories of personality

In Ancient Greece, physicians attributed individual differences in personality to imbalances of bodily fluids or humors; other popular theories have included the influence of the stars' positions at birth, body build and skull shape (Knutson & Heinz, 2004). In the 20th century, research into personality moved to the level of the psychological, although still influenced by dominant social assumptions such as gender or racial difference. Freud

> **Box 1.1**   The function of the personality
>
> Personality function involves regulation of:
> - individual levels of arousal, impulsivity and emotions
> - self-directness and self-soothing in response to survival challenges of stress and change
> - reality testing
> - maintaining an integrated sense of self over time
> - social cooperativeness through verbal and non-verbal communications and predictability of behaviour

emphasised the role of innate drives, an early account of what we might now understand as the genetic basis of stress responses. He is also attributed as being the first to describe the concept of 'defences' against stress and their effect on the expression of adult personality. Later theorists, such as Klein and Bowlby (in somewhat different ways), emphasised the importance of the interaction between the child's innate individual features and the environment in the development of normal personality functioning.

In the 1960s, Allport highlighted the role of 'traits' in the makeup of personality, which he defined as the 'dynamic organization [...] of those psychophysical systems that determine characteristics of behaviour and thought' (Allport, 1961: p. 28). Factor analysis enabled the description of personality in terms of dimensions such as dominance and affiliation (Freedman *et al*, 1951).

Like Allport, some theorists see the self as an organising principle of a number of personality traits, some of which are inherited, and some of which develop in relation to early social experience with others. Others see the self as the subjective experience of personal identity (the 'I' of experience) and the personality as the objective aspect (the 'me' that others experience). More recent concepts of personality link it with related concepts such as the self and personal identity (McAdams, 1992).

Personality and its disorders

The concepts of self, person and identity raise many complex questions for psychiatrists. Space does not permit an analysis of all of these, but an important one is the question of change and stability of the personality. Within general medicine, changes in function are usually associated with pathology. But, in relation to personality function, it is not clear to what extent change can be expected over time or in response to different situations, nor whether such changes indicate pathology or are flexible responses to different demands. Similarly, personality disorder is defined in ICD-10

(World Health Organization, 1992) and DSM-IV-TR (American Psychiatric Association, 2000) as 'enduring' characteristics from early childhood; yet changes in personality after brain trauma have been recognised since the 19th century, and DSM-IV-TR recognises acquired personality disorder after exposure to traumatic stressors. If personality disorder can be acquired as a result of psychological or neurological change, then it can be the result of pathology, and not a permanent feature of a person.

Second, in everyday life, it is obvious that there are discrepancies between how people see themselves and how others see them: but it is not so clear what the discrepancies mean. This has implications for how disorders of personality are detected and assessed. Consider this example: three people experience a man as bullying, two see him as assertive and he sees himself as threatened. Each of these perspectives has some validity, which suggests that assessment of personality, or any presumed disorder of personality, requires not only self-report data but also other-report data. However, unlike other domains of medicine, where informants may have objective and valid information about a patient's symptoms, it is by no means clear whether informants can provide information that is not confounded by their personal experience of the patient and their interpersonal relationship.

Third, and related, individual emotional experience is probably not purely individual, or at least not purely internal. An individual who experiences a strong emotion is able to transmit that experience to others (and *vice versa*), probably through the operation of mirror neurons (Gallese, 2001), which fire when another's emotional experience is witnessed. The closer the emotional tie, the more pronounced the experience: we do feel the pain of others, especially those with whom we are in close relationships (Singer *et al*, 2004). Caregivers of infants, both human and non-human, regulate the stress responses of those infants through attachment relationships. This means that a well-functioning personality has to regulate and respond to another's feelings, not just to their own experience. Some disorders of personality have a greater impact on social relations than others, especially in relationships that involve the attachment system, such as parenting and intimate relationships.

The diagnosis of personality disorder

If personality is a property of human organisms, then there is no particular reason to suppose that it cannot become dysfunctional. The difficulty is with the conceptualisation of that dysfunction. If 'personality' is conceived as a limited number of traits in each individual, which are largely genetically driven, then a limited number of categories of disorder may seem appropriate. This categorical approach to diagnosis underpins the ICD and the DSM systems, both of which distinguish personality disorders from other psychiatric disorders. The principal features of personality disorders in both systems are summarised in Box 1.2.

Box 1.2   Principal features of ICD-10 and DSM-IV-TR classification

Personality disorders are disorders that:

- begin early in development and last a lifetime
- tend to be inflexible and pervasive across different domains of functioning
- lead to clinically significant distress or impairment
- are not due to another mental disorder or direct physiological effects of a substance or medical condition
- deviate markedly from the expectation of the person's culture

(World Health Organization, 1992; American Psychiatric Association, 2000)

There are a number of criticisms of the international classificatory systems. First, they do not address the primary aspects of personality pathology, namely social relationships with others. Second, a dimensional (rather than categorical) account of personality and its disorders might offer improved descriptions of the social and interpersonal dysfunctional aspects of personality disorder. On this account, personality disorder reflects the abnormal functioning of normal dimensions at different times and in different settings: individuals can develop degrees of severity of personality disorder (e.g. Yang *et al*, 2010) or their personalities might become disordered for a period, then recover. Third, as has already been described above, there is now considerable evidence that personality disorder is not enduring (Seivewright *et al*, 2002, 2004; Shea *et al*, 2002).

Signs and symptoms of personality disorder

Like any other mental disorder, personality disorders have signs and symptoms. These constitute the three major components described in Box 1.3.

At a general level, patients with personality disorders across all clusters find it hard to make and maintain relationships in any social domain.

Box 1.3   Major components of clinical features in personality disorder

- An intrapersonal component: marked individual dysregulation of arousal, impulse and affect systems in response to stress; individuals typically present as either hyperaroused or hypoaroused in unpredictable ways
- An interpersonal component: dysfunctional interpersonal attachment patterns that reduce healthy functioning and are a further source of stress; these may take the form of getting too close or being detached and uninvolved
- A social component: dysfunctions in social behaviours which bring individuals with personality disorders into conflict with others and sometimes into contact with statutory agencies such as mental health or criminal justice systems

> **Box 1.4**   DSM-IV clusters of personality disorders
>
> Cluster A : Odd or eccentric behaviours (schizoid, paranoid and schizotypal)
>
> Cluster B: Flamboyant to dramatic behaviours (antisocial, borderline, narcissistic and histrionic)
>
> Cluster C: Fearful and anxious behaviours (avoidant, dependent and obsessive–compulsive)

The more severe the personality disorder, the more socially isolated the individual is likely to be (Yang *et al*, 2010). In broad terms, those with personality disorder demonstrate three distinct patterns of social engagement (or lack of it) with others. Although these patterns do not neatly map onto DSM clusters A, B and C (Box 1.4), people with cluster A disorders tend to move away from social attachments, either by taking up a frightened position with regard to others, or by flight into safety through isolation. Conversely, people with cluster C disorders move towards others as sources of support and dependence, and even if those sources of support become persecutory, individuals are relatively unable to disengage and assert themselves. Finally, people with cluster B disorders often tend to move against others. Ironically, to move against others, they have to first move towards them. Hence, their interactions are characterised by an ambivalence to social encounters that is most visible in those with borderline and narcissistic personality disorders.

Thus, a man with a mild degree of a cluster A (schizoid) disorder may still be able to form relationships in the workplace, or have some degree of emotional attachment to a friend or family member. A woman with a moderate degree of cluster B borderline personality disorder is unlikely to be able to maintain emotionally intimate relationships with sexual partners, and may have complex relationships with carers, but may still be able to maintain work relationships. These two individuals will be quite unlike a man with a severe degree of cluster B antisocial personality disorder, who is unlikely to have ever been able to connect to any social group for work or social purposes, and close emotional relationships will be unknown to him (and he may indeed treat them with contempt). His chances of being both a criminal rule breaker and an exploiter of the vulnerable are much higher than for individuals with other types of personality disorder.

The symptoms of personality disorder are listed in Box 1.5. Symptoms of negative affect vary according to cluster, but include anxiety, irritability, low mood, intense distress, feelings of rage, fear of abandonment, the perception that others are threatening or attacking the individual, and dissociative experiences associated with stress. Individuals with emotionally impulsive borderline personality disorder frequently describe brief periods of pseudo-hallucinations that almost invariably take the form of voices telling them

Box 1.5 Symptom subtypes in personality disorders

Arousal Over- or underarousal, often self-medicated with drugs or alcohol; enhanced tendency to dissociate in cluster B; emotional indifference

Affect Anger; suspicion; fearfulness; detachment; coldness or restricted emotion; resentfulness; anxiety about new activities; irritability; low mood; intense distress; feelings of rage and fear of abandonment; fear that others are threatening or attacking them; rapidly shifting emotions

Cognition Poor reality testing in terms of dissociation; brief psychotic episodes; odd beliefs and magical thinking; cognitive distortions; preoccupations and ruminations in cluster C

Somatic self-identity Somatic disorders, ranging from preoccupations with the somatic self to attacks on the physical body in the form of self-harm

Psychological self-identity Disorders of sense of self; lack of sense of agency; exaggerated sense of self-importance; belief that the self is in danger from others; difficulty in distinguishing self from others

to harm themselves or others. People with antisocial personality disorder may report little distress, but complain of persecutory anxiety or anger with others whom they perceive to have let them down. They may also enjoy feelings of contempt for other people's distress, excitement in controlling others and hostility towards dependence and neediness.

The signs of personality disorder (Box 1.6) are manifested in disturbances of social relationships, i.e. at the interpersonal level, at the boundary between the individual and their social world. The signs include repeated behaviours that are socially rejecting, self-destructive or result in social exclusion, and more elaborate and enduring dysfunctional relationship styles. However, behaviours alone cannot determine the presence of a personality disorder; there must also be evidence of disturbance of affect and arousal regulation. It is also important to consider behaviours that do not attract attention, but are still pathological, such as social withdrawal.

In a particular subgroup of people who behave antisocially, lack of response to other's distress is noted to be a distinguishing feature (Cleckley, 1964). Later researchers, principally Robert Hare, have confirmed the existence of a subgroup of individuals (mainly in the cluster B antisocial subgroup) who have both a pronounced lack of empathy for others and display predatory or cruel behaviours towards others. It has been suggested that these individuals do not recognise facial signals of distress in others and do not detect emotional tone, probably as a result of amygdala dysfunction (Blair, 2003). In the most severe cases, this lack of response can be associated with extremes of cruelty and violence to others, and is captured by the clinical concept of 'psychopathy' (Hare, 1991).

Although the international classificatory systems have yet to accept psychopathy as a 'disorder', its assessment is standard in most forensic

---

Box 1.6 Signs of personality disorder

Note: not all will be present in all disorders, nor do signs alone confirm the diagnosis

- Self-harming and suicidal behaviours
- Substance and alcohol misuse, dependence
- Eating disorders
- Unstable relationships and social isolation
- Persistent complaining and vexatious litigation
- Deceptive behaviour, such as duping, conning and factitious illnesses
- Attacks on attachment figures (partners, children, care staff, etc.)
- Persistent rule-breaking, violent attacks on others

---

psychiatric settings. The standard measure of psychopathy is useful for distinguishing 'milder' from more 'severe' or 'extreme' forms of antisocial personality disorder. However, clinicians not working with forensic patients are unlikely to see such individuals.

On the basis of the above, it may be argued that dysfunctional social relationships are a diagnostic feature of personality disorders that distinguish them from mental illnesses. The counterargument is that many serious mental disorders (especially chronic psychotic disorders and mood disorders) also have profound effects on social relationships. Social isolation is a common problem for many service users with severe mental illness and it is usually caused by relationship breakdown occasioned by aspects of the illness. The difference may be in degree, and the types of relationship breakdown, rather than an absolute difference.

Social difficulties in relationships with mental health professionals

These interpersonal and social difficulties are also inevitably manifest in relationships with healthcare professionals. Patients with personality disorder generally do not take on the conventional 'sick role', in which the patient is compliant, obedient and grateful. For these reasons, attempts to care for such patients on the basis of conventional therapeutic relationships are unlikely to succeed, and staff need particular competencies to provide a service for such individuals (Home Office & Department of Health, 2005).

Individuals in the different clusters have different approaches to help-seeking from mental health professionals (Tyrer *et al*, 2003). Those in clusters A and C and the more antisocial individuals may rebuff help, or (in the case of antisocial people) denigrate caregivers and therapies. Cluster C patients with dependent personality disorders, however, commonly form submissive, clinging relationships with clinicians rather than rebuffing help. In contrast, people with more borderline personality pathology have highly ambivalent attachment patterns, which mean that they may seek and then reject help. They are likely to be fearful of asking for help, and this fear can cause increasing arousal and ultimately hostility towards those they are approaching for help. There is evidence that help-seeking and care-seeking behaviours (including engagement in and adherence to therapy) are influenced by attachment experiences in childhood (Henderson, 1974; Dozier *et al*, 2001). This suggests that there is a link between personality disorder and attachment history.

Prevalence and incidence

Prevalence data are similar worldwide and recent figures from the World Health Organization show no important or consistent differences across countries (Huang *et al*, 2009). In the UK, the prevalence of any personality disorder is about 4% overall (Coid *et al*, 2006) – considerably higher than the prevalence of psychotic disorders.

In primary care, the prevalence of personality disorder is around 10–12%, and it consists mainly of patients with depressive and somatising symptoms. However, the prevalence of personality disorder in general psychiatric out-patients is 33%, rising to about 40% in eating disorder services and 60% in substance misuse services (Herzog *et al*, 1992; Sanderson *et al*, 1994; Rounsaville *et al*, 1998; Moran *et al*, 2000; Torgersen *et al*, 2001).

In forensic services and prisons, the prevalence of personality disorder is 70%, and the principal subtypes are antisocial, borderline and narcissistic (Singleton *et al*, 1998). Prisoners' problems include lack of empathy, social hostility and contempt for weakness, as well as affect dysregulation. In specialist forensic personality disorder treatment settings, virtually all patients have comorbid psychiatric disorders such as substance misuse or depression, and most fulfil criteria for several personality disorders (Duggan *et al*, 2007).

Prevalence data can be misleading because of selection bias. Services for behavioural conditions such as eating disorder, substance misuse or antisocial behaviour are likely to be 'selecting' for comorbid personality disorders that manifest in the particular behaviour. It is important for clinicians not to generalise about personality disorders as a whole on the basis only of the group they see in their service settings.

Pathogenesis

Social dysfunction in adulthood (including both self-harm and antisocial behaviour) is more likely when genetic vulnerability for arousal and affect dysregulation interacts with environmental adversity and negative life experiences during early development (National Scientific Council on the Developing Child, 2010). Genetic studies suggest that personality disorder is strongly heritable (Jang *et al*, 1996); one model hypothesises a vulnerability to the replication of genes for proteins that are relevant to neurophysiological processes such as arousal, response times and homeostatic mechanisms. However, it is also clear, from both retrospective and prospective studies, that early childhood adversity is highly relevant to the development of psychological signs and symptoms of personality disorder (Kessler *et al*, 2010). Physical abuse and neglect appear to increase the risk of developing all types of psychiatric morbidity, especially substance misuse. Sexual abuse appears specifically to increase the risk of developing depression and borderline personality disorder.

There are three major theoretical approaches to explaining how early childhood relationships and maltreatment result in the adult interpersonal dysfunction found in personality disorder.

Approach 1: The impact of external events on neurobiological development and gene–environment interaction

Humans are unique among animals in their long period of total dependence on others for survival after birth. The key outcome of an optimal experience of care and nurture is the development of the neuroarchitecture that is necessary for two essential capacities: first, the activation and regulation of affects in the task of self-survival; and second, the regulation of affects in social relationships to produce positive environments.

Being raised in a hostile or abusive environment is posited to increase the risk of developing personality disorder because of the direct effect of chronic stress on the developing cytoarchitecture of the autonomic nervous system, limbic system, amygdala and the right orbitofrontal cortex (Schore, 2001). A distressed infant experiences high degrees of arousal, mediated by the sympathetic division of the autonomic nervous system. Being a catabolic system, the autonomic nervous system makes available large amounts of energy to prepare the infant for a self-preservative action repertoire of 'fight or flight'. The infant experiences the peripheral and central effects of noradrenaline (e.g. more rapid heart and pulse rate, increased blood pressure, dilated pupils), which are uncomfortable. The amygdala is activated by a whole range of stimuli that represent unexpected or unfamiliar/novel events, which may be negatively (fear/threat) or positively (reward/pleasure) valenced. During periods of high stress, the amygdala and limbic system are activated, leading to enhanced learning of fear and stress cues, both external (loud voice, pain, etc.) and internal (rapid heart beat, dryness of mouth, etc.) (Makino *et al*, 1994), i.e. there is hypersensitisation to effects of stress. When soothed by the carer, the infant's parasympathetic system, which has opposite effects, is activated and restores homeostasis. The autonomic system then returns to its normal rate and rhythm (Sarkar & Adshead, 2006).

The basic task of child care consists in responding sensitively to episodes of interactive signals produced by the autonomic nervous system in both infant and carer. These episodes emerge when the infant reaches about 2 months of age, and they are highly arousing, affect-laden and short interpersonal events that expose the infant to high levels of cognitive and social information (Feldman *et al*, 1999). As the infant grows, it is the memory of the relationship, rather than the particular caregiver, that becomes the (accessory) affect regulator, allowing attachment to develop with others on the basis of this template.

A good-quality affect regulatory system, based on secure bonding between carer and infant, leads to optimal maturation of the right hemisphere of the brain at a critical period during the first 2–3 years of life (Schore, 2003). The right orbitofrontal cortex (ROFC) acts as a regulator and modulator both of amygdala responses to fear and distress and of autonomic nervous system response (LeDoux, 1996; National Scientific Council on the Developing Child & National Forum on Early Childhood Policy and Programs, 2011). Any measurable damage to cytoarchitecture of the developing ROFC results in failure to develop a top-down regulatory system (Taylor *et al*, 1997; Schore, 2003).

Any adverse experience during childhood risks some degree of ROFC neuronal disorganisation and is likely to lead to impaired emotional regulation throughout the individual's lifetime. This in turn affects the ability to optimally organise an integrated sense of self (Sarkar & Adshead, 2006). The degree of disorganisation arises from an interaction between genetic vulnerability and the degree, nature and duration of the environmental insult (National Scientific Council on the Developing Child, 2010). For example, monkeys with a genetic marker for reduced serotonin metabolism are more at risk of developing impulsive behaviours that increase the likelihood of social exclusion and early death. This risk is greatly enhanced if these genetically vulnerable monkeys are exposed to poor maternal rearing (Suomi, 1999, 2003). Among boys, it has been shown that genetically determined low monoamine oxidase A (MAOA) activity, leading to dysregulation of the 5-HT system, moderates the association between childhood maltreatment and later vulnerability to the effects of environmental stress, thus causing mental health problems (Kim-Cohen *et al*, 2006).

Such data suggest an evolutionary aspect to personality development. Individuals who exhibit antisocial behaviour are moving away from the more adaptive species-preservative behaviour seen in higher mammals towards a more ancient self-preservative reptilian behaviour. As the name suggests, species-preservative behaviour has evolved to improve the chances of survival of a species (Henry & Wang, 1998). When trauma results in a stressful loss of control, the self-preservative fight/flight catecholamine coping response takes priority. Problems arise when this becomes the default response to a wide range of events, people and circumstances.

Approach 2: Theories that address social attachment over time

Longitudinal studies of attachment styles suggest that individuals with insecure attachment to caregivers in childhood tend to grow up into adults who form insecure attachments with peers and who become insecure parents to their own offspring (Grossman *et al*, 2000; Waters *et al*, 2000). Although there is some flexibility in the system, the more insecure the attachment organisation in childhood, the more likely the individual is to remain insecure in adulthood.

Many of the features of insecure attachment in adulthood resemble the signs and symptoms of personality disorder, and it has been suggested that insecure attachment should be seen as a dimension of personality disorder (Livesley, 1998).There have been numerous studies of attachment patterns in people with personality disorders, all of which indicate that such individuals show higher rates of insecure attachment than the general population (Cassidy & Shaver, 2008). Specifically, the pathology of borderline personality disorder is associated with a subtype of insecure attachment called preoccupied or enmeshed attachment, whereby the individual is highly ambivalent about those to whom they are attached (either in a passive or angry way, or both). Individuals who display antisocial violent behaviour towards others are more likely to exhibit a dismissing attachment pattern, in which weakness or vulnerability are denied and attachment to others is seen as unnecessary or contemptible (Pfafflin & Adshead, 2003; van IJzendoorn & Bakermans-Kranenburg, 2009).

Approach 3: Theories of personality disorder as persistence of childhood thinking/feeling patterns

A number of different theorists have suggested that it is maladaptive for immature patterns of thought, belief or value to persist into adulthood, especially those immature cognitions and emotions that have occurred in response to childhood stress (Young, 2002). Work in the field of post-traumatic stress disorders suggest that in response to high arousal and distress, cognitions, images and emotions can remain stored in situationally accessible memory (Brewin *et al*, 1996). Other theorists have emphasised the importance of thoughts, feelings and beliefs as organised 'defences' against distress, and suggested that personality disorder may be best understood as a collection of immature defences (Vaillant, 1993, 1994; Bond, 2004; Cramer, 2006).

Psychological defences (Box 1.7) are those personality traits, cognitions and beliefs that help an individual regulate their own sense of distress. Defences have conscious and unconscious aspects, both of which are

---

Box 1.7 Examples of psychological defences in everyday use

- Mature: humour, altruism, sublimation, suppression
- Neurotic: idealisation, intellectualisation
- Immature: denial, displacement, dissociation, somatisation

mediated through memory, and which may be expressed physically. Defences develop in childhood but are used continually throughout life. Every single person uses a mixture of mature, neurotic and immature defences, and optimal social and personal functioning is associated with maximal use of mature and minimal use of immature defences.

Longitudinal studies have shown that people can and do change the characteristic pattern of defences that they use, particularly at times of stress (Vaillant, 1993; Soldz & Vaillant, 1998). Most people utilise immature defences under stress, but most healthy people go back to using mature defences when the stress is over. In adulthood, persistent use of immature defences in general social relationships leads to problems (Vaillant, 1993; Kernberg & Caligor, 2005).

Studies of people with personality disorder indicate that they almost exclusively use immature defences, and do not use mature defences (Vaillant, 1994). However, there is no specific pattern of defences that maps onto any specific personality disorder diagnosis. There may be an interaction with attachment style, in that insecure and disorganised attachment strategies may in turn affect the profile of defences that an individual will preferentially use at times of stress. Most psychological therapies for personality disorder address the cognitive and emotional aspects of psychological defences. There is evidence that individuals can learn to use more mature defences, and thereby improve their psychosocial function (Vaillant, 1997; Bond, 2004).

Course of the disorder

Personality disorders are long-term, chronic disorders, with varying degrees of severity (Tyrer & Johnson, 1996; Yang *et al*, 2010). Some forms have a relapsing and remitting nature, depending environmental factors and comorbidity. There is evidence that a proportion of individuals gradually experience remission of the disorder over time (Paris, 2003). Given the link with affect and arousal regulation, one would expect patients with personality disorder to exhibit more signs and symptoms when they are distressed, aroused or depressed. This may explain why psychotropic mood-stabilising or sedating medication is helpful for some individuals with personality disorder.

A rule of thumb is that symptoms of personality disorder will be exacerbated during periods of stress, particularly if the stress is linked to relationships with partners, parents or dependants. As a result, people with personality disorders may behave in socially alienating ways at times of stress – ironically, at the time of their greatest need. Patients with the disorder may consequently be excluded from help or they may reject help, without realising that they are doing so. Appropriate clinical skills are therefore of paramount importance in terms of acknowledging such features as signs of a disorder rather than an expressed view that the person is rejecting services or trying to manipulate professionals.

Severe personality disorder

Personality disorders have not typically been graded in terms of severity, partly because of the tradition of using categorical descriptions. However, it has long been recognised that not all personality disorders cause the same degree of dysfunction. Millon (1981) suggests that borderline, paranoid and schizotypal personality disorders are the most severe types within a social system, because these personality styles characteristically produce significant social incompetence and isolation. Blackburn (2000) suggests that individuals with dependent, histrionic, narcissistic and antisocial personality disorders are deemed to be the least severely disordered in terms of social adaptation. However, if severity is defined by the degree of disorganisation caused by a personality disorder within a society, then antisocial and narcissistic personality disorders may both be defined as 'severe'. Here the meaning of the word 'severe' depends on whether one understands it in terms of individual social adaptation or the impact of the individual on a social group.

Severity of personality disorder implies something quite different if the categorical approach of the international classificatory systems is employed. There is some disagreement between the ICD and DSM systems on the types and number of personality disorders that they respectively recognise as existing. It has been suggested that the threshold for making a diagnosis of personality disorder is lower in ICD-10 (Tyrer & Johnson, 1996), although DSM-IV recognises eleven different types of the disorder, compared with the eight endorsed by ICD-10. The two systems also differ in their respective recommended guidelines for diagnosing personality disorder. The DSM-IV is a more rigid system that advocates a checklist approach to diagnosis, in that a specific number of observable behaviours have to be present for a diagnosis (even though the preamble to DSM-IV warns against a 'cook book' approach). The ICD-10, a trait-based system, allows the clinician a greater degree of flexibility in establishing a diagnosis.

Tyrer & Johnson (1996) suggest a five-point rating of severity: 0, 'no personality disorder'; 1, 'personality difficulty' (any subthreshold criterion of a personality disorder); 2, 'simple personality disorder' (one or more personality disorders within the same cluster); 3, 'complex personality disorder' (personality abnormalities spanning more than one cluster as diagnosed by the international classificatory systems); and 4, 'severe personality disorder' (two or more personality disorders in more than one DSM cluster with one being antisocial personality disorder). A recent study using this rating found different prevalences of personality disorders of different severity: the most severe cases were seen in specialist services and milder conditions were seen in primary care (Yang *et al*, 2010).

Severity could be defined in terms of the harm done to others, even if this would apply only to small subgroup of people with personality disorders. In 1999, a Royal College of Psychiatrists' working party reviewed the diagnosis of psychopathic and antisocial personality disorders (Royal College of

Psychiatrists, 1999), and proposed an additional category, defined as those who manifest 'gross societal disturbance'. A 'gross' disturbance was defined as having one cluster B diagnosis and a personality disorder in at least one other cluster also. No detailed rationale was provided for such a grouping, nor did the document explain further what might constitute 'gross societal disturbance'. However, that same year the UK Home Office and the Department of Health identified a subgroup of offenders with personality disorders who were violent and defined them as having 'dangerous and severe personality disorder' or DSPD (Home Office & Department of Health, 1999). The DSPD condition, perhaps extrapolating from the recommendations of the College, was defined as the presence of (a) two or more personality disorders, (b) a Psychopathy Checklist score (Hare, 1991) of over 30, and (c) a functional link between the disorder and the violence. The link between severity of personality disorder and severity of risk to others is made quite explicit. This makes sense for a public protection agenda, but has clinical limitations. One objection is that there are many individuals who are dangerous to others as a result of having a single personality disorder, but who do not fulfil criteria (a) or (b). The most obvious group in this category are perpetrators of child and partner abuse.

If personality disorder were to be rated in terms of severity, then this would make it more like depressive disorders and intellectual disability, and less like schizophrenia and bipolar affective disorders, which are described in terms of categorical types rather than dimensional severity. One advantage of a severity rating is that it might help determine workforce competencies and other resource allocation requirements. It might also lay the foundation for research into prognosis and outcomes. For example, several new community services for personality disorder have taken a 'complex needs' approach to determining the service configuration and skills mix appropriate for each individual. They categorise a personality disorder as severe if the individual's problems involve several areas of care. Thus, a patient might have attachment difficulties and also require containment in a secure unit. Such patients typically fulfil criteria for several personality disorders and also have comorbid Axis I conditions.

Personality disorder and mental illness

It is commonly argued that personality disorder is not a mental illness, and/or that it is qualitatively different from mental disorders such as schizophrenia. One argument seems to be principally that people with personality disorders do not lose their capacity for reality testing (e.g. do not have symptoms such as hallucinations and delusions). However, there are a number of counterarguments to this. First, loss of reality testing is not the sole test of whether someone has a mental illness or not. Addiction disorders and neurotic disorders such as depression are still classified as mental illnesses. Further, the presence of psychotic symptoms does not determine mental illness status, since psychotic symptoms occur in many physical disorders, such as delirium or the encephalitides. Finally, even if one does use psychotic symptoms as a defining diagnostic test for mental illness, there is plenty of evidence that some types of personality disorder do involve psychotic symptoms, albeit usually of brief duration.

There are other good reasons to think that personality disorder has more in common with the Axis I conditions than traditionally supposed. First, it has an aetiology that brings about pathology and, like many medical conditions, it afflicts only a minority of the population, who are consequently quantitatively different from the norm. Second, personality disorder produces a pattern of symptoms and signs that are common to a group, and make group members resemble each other. There is evidence of abnormal brain structure and function in personality disorders, and overlap of psychopathology between Axis I and II disorders in terms of cognitive/perceptual organisation, impulse control, affect regulation and anxiety modulation (see Chapter 10, this volume).

Third, there is the issue of comorbidity or co-occurrence of Axis I and Axis II disorders, which suggests at least a close relationship between the disorders. For example, at least one cluster A disorder (schizotypal personality disorder) lies on a continuum with schizophrenia; cluster B disorders, especially borderline and antisocial personality disorders, co-occur with substance misuse (Knutson & Heinz, 2004); and cluster C disorders preferentially co-occur with increased rates of somatoform disorders (Tyrer et al, 1997). People with either cluster B or C disorders have a higher risk of comorbidity with all types of Axis I disorders (Dolan-Sewell et al, 2001). Conversely, the coexistence of personality disorder with an Axis I disorder can lead to poorer outcomes (Newton-Howes et al, 2006). In one study of patients with mental disorders managed by community teams, 40% fulfilled criteria for at least one personality disorder (Newton-Howes et al, 2010). There seems to be an interaction between two or more mental health conditions such that there is an additive (if not multiplicative) effect in terms of 'load' of clinical symptomatology and socioclinical outcomes.

In contrast to the expanding evidence base that there is at least a complex relationship between Axis I and Axis II disorders, there is no new evidence in support of the assertion that (a) personality disorder is fundamentally different from mental illness, or (b) that Axis I and Axis II disorders are alternatives that cannot coexist. Although the multiaxial nature of the DSM should make it obvious that disorders can coexist, it is still common to hear clinicians refer to these conditions as if they were alternatives.

Conclusion

There is a great deal more to know about personality disorder. At present, there is still theoretical debate about how to classify it, which in turn makes consensus on how best to assess and diagnose it difficult to achieve. Intriguing ethical questions arise as we rethink old ideas about the disorder: if it is an acquired disorder, how can we justify not providing services for its treatment? Should we concentrate resources on that very small group of individuals with the most severe form that makes them dangerous to others, even if they are probably the least treatable group? Or should we focus resources on the larger, much more treatable group, where the benefits of treatment have been proven in terms of cost-offset (Dolan *et al*, 1996)? Or should we concentrate resources on the prevention of the development of personality disorders? We can currently do little to alter genetic vulnerability, but we could offer treatment to parents who frighten and maltreat their children, and spend more money on improving the environments in which vulnerable children grow up. These, and other questions, were unthinkable 20 years ago: who knows what we will think about personality disorder 20 years from now?

References

Allport, G. W. (1961) *Pattern and Growth in Personality*. Rinehart & Winston.

American Psychiatric Association (2000) *Diagnostic and Statistical Manual of Mental Disorders (4th edn, Text Revision) (DSM-IV-TR)*. APA.

Blackburn, R. (2000) Treatment or incapacitation? Implications of research on personality disorders for the management of dangerous offenders. *Legal and Criminological Psychology*, 5, 1–21.

Blair, R. J. R. (2003) Neurobiological basis of psychopathy. *British Journal of Psychiatry*, 182, 5–7.

Bond, M. (2004) Empirical studies of defence style. *Harvard Review of Psychiatry*, 12, 263–278.

Brewin, C. R., Dalgleish, T. & Joseph, S. (1996) A dual representation theory of post-traumatic stress disorder. *Psychology Review*, 103, 670–686.

Cassidy, J. & Shaver, P. (2008) *Handbook of Attachment (2nd edn)*. Guilford Press.

Cleckley, H. (1964) *The Mask of Sanity (4th edn)*. C. V. Mosby.

Coid, J., Yang, M., Tyrer, P., et al (2006) Prevalence and correlates of personality disorder in Great Britain. *British Journal of Psychiatry*, 188, 423–431.

Cramer, P. (2006) *Protecting the Self: Defense Mechanisms in Action*. Guilford Press.

Dolan, B. M., Warren, F. M., Menzies, D., et al (1996) Cost-offset following specialist treatment of severe personality disorders. *Psychiatric Bulletin*, 20, 413–417.

Dolan-Sewell, R. T., Krueger, R. F. & Shea M. T. (2001) Co-occurrence with syndrome disorders. In *Handbook of Personality Disorders: Theory, Research and Treatment* (ed. W. J. Livesley), pp. 84–103. Guilford Press.

Dozier, M., Lomax, L., Tyrrell, C. L., et al (2001) The challenge of treatment for clients with a dismissing states of mind. *Attachment and Human Development*, 3, 62–76.

Duggan, C., Mason, L., Banerjee, P., et al (2007) Value of standard personality assessments in informing clinical decision-making in a medium secure unit. *British Journal of Psychiatry*, 190 (suppl 49), s15–s19.

Feldman, R., Greenbaum, C. W. & Yirmiya, N. (1999) Mother–infant affect synchrony as an antecedent of the emergence of self-control. *Developmental Psychology*, 35, 223–231.

Freedman, H. B., Leary, T. F., Ossorio, A. G., et al (1951) The interpersonal dimension of personality. *Journal of Personality*, 20, 143–161.

Gallese, V. (2001) The 'shared manifold' hypothesis: from mirror neurons to empathy. *Journal of Consciousness Studies*, 8, 33–50.

Grossman, K. E., Grossman, K. & Waters, E. (2000) *Attachment from Infancy to Adulthood: The Major Longitudinal Studies*. Guilford Press.

Hare, R. D. (1991) *The Hare Psychopathy Checklist – Revised*. Multi-Health Systems.

Henderson, S. (1974) Care eliciting behaviour in man. *Journal of Nervous and Mental Disease*, **159**, 172–181.

Henry, J. P. & Wang, S. (1998) Effects of early stress on adult affiliative behaviour. *Psychoneuroendocrinology*, **23**, 863–875.

Herzog, D., Keller, M., Lavori, P., *et al* (1992) The prevalence of personality disorders in 210 women with eating disorders. *Journal of Clinical Psychiatry*, **53**, 147–152.

Home Office & Department of Health (1999) *Managing Dangerous People with Severe Personality Disorder: Proposals for Policy Development*. Home Office & Department of Health.

Home Office & Department of Health (2005) *Personality Disorder Capacity Plans*. Home Office & Department of Health.

Huang, Y., Kotov, R., de Girolamo, G., *et al* (2009) DSM-IV personality disorders in the WHO World Mental Health Surveys. *British Journal of Psychiatry*, **195**, 46–53.

Jang, K. L., Livesley, W. J., Vernon, P. A., *et al* (1996) Heritability of personality disorder traits: a twin study. *Acta Psychiatrica Scandinavica*, **94**, 438–444.

Kernberg, O. F. & Caligor, E. (2005) A psychoanalytic theory of personality disorders. In *Major Theories of Personality Disorder* (2nd edn) (eds M. F. Lenzenweger & J. F. Clarkin), pp. 114–156. Guilford Press.

Kessler, R. C., McLaughlin, K. A., Greif Green, J., *et al* (2010) Childhood adversities and adult psychopathology in the WHO World Mental Health Surveys. *British Journal of Psychiatry*, **197**, 378–385.

Kim-Cohen, J., Caspi, A., Taylor, A., *et al* (2006) MAOA, maltreatment and gene-environment interaction predicting children's mental health: new evidence and a meta-analysis. *Molecular Psychiatry*, **11**, 903–913.

Knutson, B. & Heinz, A. (2004) Psychobiology of personality disorders. In *Textbook of Biological Psychiatry* (ed. J. Panksepp), pp. 145–166. Wiley-Liss.

LeDoux, J. (1996) *The Emotional Brain: The Mysterious Underpinnings of Emotional Life*. Simon & Schuster.

Livesley, J. (1998) Suggestions for a framework for empirically based classification of personality disorder. *Canadian Journal of Psychiatry*, **43**, 137–147.

Makino, S., Gold, P. W. & Shulkin, J. (1994) Corticosterone effects on corticotrophin-releasing hormone mRNA in the central nucleus of the amygdala and the parvocellular region of the paraventricular nucleus of the hypothalamus. *Brain Research*, **640**, 105–112.

McAdams, D. (1992) The five factor model of personality: a critical appraisal. *Journal of Personality*, **60**, 329–361.

Millon, T. (1981) *Disorders of Personality: DSM III Axis II*. John Wiley & Sons.

Moran, P., Jenkins, R., Tylee, A., *et al* (2000) The prevalence of personality disorder among primary care attenders. *Acta Psychiatrica Scandinavica*, **102**, 52–57.

National Scientific Council on the Developing Child (2010) *Early Experiences Can Alter Gene Expression and Affect Long Term Development: Working Paper No 10*. Center on the Developing Child, Harvard University.

National Scientific Council on the Developing Child & National Forum on Early Childhood Policy and Programs (2011) *Building the Brain's "Air Traffic Control" System: How Early Experiences Shape the Development of Executive Function: Working Paper No 11*. Center on the Developing Child, Harvard University.

Newton-Howes, G., Tyrer, P. & Johnson, T. (2006) Personality disorder and outcome of depression: meta-analysis of published studies. *British Journal of Psychiatry*, **188**, 13–20.

Newton-Howes, G., Tyrer, P., Anagnostakis, K., *et al* (2010) The prevalence of personality disorder, its co-morbidity with mental state disorders and its clinical significance in community mental health teams. *Social Psychiatry and Psychiatric Epidemiology*, **45**, 453–460.

Paris, J. (2003) *Personality Disorders Over Time: Precursors, Course and Outcome*. American Psychiatric Press.

Pfafflin, F. & Adshead, G. (2003) *A Matter Of Security: Attachment Theory in Forensic Psychiatry and Psychotherapy*. Jessica Kingsley.

Rounsaville, B., Kranzler, H., Ball, S., *et al* (1998) Personality disorders in substance abusers: relation to substance use. *Journal of Nervous and Mental Disease*, **186**, 87–95.

Royal College of Psychiatrists (1999) *Offenders with Personality Disorder (Council Report CR71)*. Gaskell.

Sanderson, W., Wetzler, S., Beck, A., *et al* (1994) Prevalence of personality disorders among patients with anxiety disorders. *Psychiatry Research*, **51**, 167–174.

Sarkar, J. & Adshead, G. (2006) Personality disorders as disorganisation of attachment and affect regulation. *Advances in Psychiatric Treatment*, **12**, 297–305.

Schore, A. (2001) The effect of early relational trauma on right brain development, affect regulation and infant mental health. *Infant Mental Health Journal*, **22**, 201–249.

Schore, A. (2003) *Affect Dysregulation and Disorders of the Self*. W. W. Norton.

Seivewright, H., Tyrer, P. & Johnson, T. (2002) Changes in personality status in neurotic disorder. *Lancet*, **359**, 2253–2254.

Seivewright, H., Tyrer, P. & Johnson, T. (2004) Persistent social dysfunction in anxious and depressed patients with personality disorder. *Acta Psychiatrica Scandinavica*, **109**, 104–109.

Shea, M., Stout, R., Gunderson, J., *et al* (2002) Short-term diagnostic stability of schizotypal, borderline, avoidant and obsessive-compulsive personality disorders. *American Journal of Psychiatry*, **159**, 2036–2041.

Singer, T., Seymour, B., O'Doherty, J., *et al* (2004) Empathy for pain involves the affective but not sensory components of pain. *Science*, **303**, 1157–1162.

Singleton, N., Gatwood, R. & Meltzer, H. (1998) *Psychiatric Morbidity among Prisoners in England and Wales*. TSO (The Stationery Office).

Soldz, S. & Vaillant, G. (1998) A 50-year longitudinal study of defense use among inner city men: a validation of the DSM-IV defense axis. *Journal of Nervous and Mental Disease*, **186**, 104–111.

Suomi, S. (1999) Attachment in rhesus monkeys. In *Handbook of Attachment* (eds J. Cassidy & P. Shaver), pp. 181–197. Guilford Press.

Suomi, S. J. (2003) Gene–environment interactions and the neurobiology of social conflict. *Annals of the New York Academy of Science*, **1008**, 132–139.

Taylor, G. J., Bagby, M. & Parker, J. D. (1997) *Disorders of Affect Regulation*. Cambridge University Press.

Torgersen, S., Kringlen, E. & Cramer, V. (2001) The prevalence of personality disorders in a community sample. *Archives of General Psychiatry*, **58**, 590–596.

Tyrer, P. & Johnson, T. (1996) Establishing the severity of personality disorder. *American Journal of Psychiatry*, **153**, 1593–1597.

Tyrer, P., Gunderson, J. G., Lyons, M., *et al* (1997) Extent of comorbidity between mental state and personality disorders. *Journal of Personality Disorders* 11: 242–59.

Tyrer, P., Milchard, S., Methuen, C., *et al* (2003) Treatment rejecting and treatment seeking personality disorders: Type R and Type S. *Journal of Personality Disorders*, **17**, 263–268.

Vaillant, G. (1993) *The Wisdom of the Ego*. Harvard University Press.

Vaillant, G. (1994) Ego mechanisms of defence and personality psychopathology. *Journal of Abnormal Psychology*, **103**, 44–50.

Vaillant, L. M. (1997) *Changing Character: Short Term Anxiety Regulating Psychotherapy for Affects, Attachment and Defenses*. Basic Books.

van IJzendoorn, M. & Bakermans-Kranenburg, M. (2009) The first 10 000 Adult Attachment Interviews: distribution of adult attachment representations in clinical and non-clinical groups. *Attachment & Human Development*, **11**, 223–263.

Waters, E., Merrick, S., Treboux, D., *et al* (2000) Attachment security in infancy and early adulthood: a twenty-year longitudinal study. *Child Development*, **71**, 684–689.

World Health Organization (1992) *The International Statistical Classification of Diseases and Related Health Problems, Tenth Revision (ICD-10)*. WHO.

Yang, M., Coid, J. & Tyrer, P. (2010) Personality pathology recorded by severity: national survey. *British Journal of Psychiatry*, **197**, 193–199.

Young, J. E. (2002) Schema-focused therapy for personality disorders. In *Cognitive Behavior Therapy: A Guide for the Practicing Clinician* (vol. 1) (ed. G. Simos), pp. 201–22. Brunner Routledge.

CHAPTER 2

Differences between psychopathy and other personality disorders: evidence from neuroimaging

Sagari Sarkar, Ben S. Clark and Quinton Deeley

Summary The ICD-10 and DSM-IV-TR diagnostic guidelines do not list psychopathy as a distinct psychiatric entity. However, there are significant overlaps between psychopathy and DSM-IV-TR cluster B personality disorders. Neuro-imaging studies implicate deficits in the structure and function of frontal and limbic regions in this group of personality disorders, while highlighting both distinctions and overlaps between syndromes. In this chapter, these data are reviewed, and implications for diagnosis and clinical practice are discussed.

In his influential book *The Mask of Sanity*, Hervey Cleckley presented a series of vignettes which distilled typical features of large numbers of individuals with psychopathy whom he had interviewed (Cleckley, 1941). He described them as charming, callous and superficial, commenting that their lack of conscience or genuine emotion was camouflaged by the 'mask' of a healthy, functional individual. People with psychopathy commit a large amount and wide variety of violent and non-violent crimes, and are resistant to attempts at rehabilitation (Reid & Gacono, 2000). The definition of psychopathy has changed little since Cleckley's time, and the aetiology of the condition remains unknown.

Psychopathy shares general features with personality disorders listed in DSM-IV-TR (American Psychiatric Association, 2000), even though it is not included among them. Personality disorders comprise a group of disorders that usually result in impaired interpersonal functioning. Individuals exhibit enduring patterns of cognition, emotion and behaviour that deviate markedly from cultural expectations. The three clusters of personality disorders listed in DSM-IV-TR (American Psychiatric Association, 2000) fall under the headings 'odd–eccentric' (cluster A), 'emotional–dramatic' (cluster B) and 'anxious–fearful' (cluster C), and each contains further subtypes.

Reclassification of psychopathy

Psychopathy as a distinct psychiatric condition disappeared from diagnostic classifications with the publication of DSM-III (American Psychiatric Association, 1980). In DSM-IV-TR, psychopathy is called antisocial personality disorder and in ICD-10 (World Health Organization, 2004) it is dissocial personality disorder. However, although both antisocial and dissocial personality disorders include several traits reflecting psychopathic personality (for example, lack of guilt/remorse, impulsivity), it is possible to meet the diagnostic criteria for these disorders solely on the basis of the behavioural manifestations of antisocial behaviour (for example, violation of social norms, irresponsibility, criminality). Hence, the emotional dysfunction at the core of Cleckley's notion of 'the psychopath' is not essential for antisocial or dissocial personality disorder, even if it is present in some cases. The Psychopathy Checklist (PCL; Hare, 1980) and the later Psychopathy Checklist – Revised (PCL-R; Hare, 1991, 2003) were therefore designed to operationalise Cleckley's psychopathy construct to provide a formal diagnostic instrument for the disorder. The PCL-R is considered by many to be the gold-standard instrument for this disorder (Morana *et al*, 2005).

Assessment of psychopathy and personality disorder

The PCL-R consists of 20 items falling broadly into two dimensions: Factor 1 items are predominantly emotional or interpersonal traits such as deception, remorselessness, shallow affect and callousness, whereas Factor 2 items assess behavioural manifestations of the disorder, such as criminality, violence and dysfunctional lifestyle (Box 2.1). Characteristics from both factors are needed for a diagnosis of psychopathy to be made. Although many consider the first dimension to differentiate psychopathy from other personality disorders (Kiehl, 2006), there is considerable overlap between a number of these traits, not only between psychopathy and antisocial/dissocial personality disorder, but also between psychopathy and other DSM-IV cluster B disorders (Table 2.1), including borderline, histrionic and narcissistic personality disorders. This supports the view that psychopathy comprises a 'higher-order' collection of disordered personality traits from many categories (Blackburn, 2005).

Psychopathy

Recent epidemiological studies of psychopathy report that it occurs in about 0.6% of the general population (Coid *et al*, 2009*a*) and 7.7% of male prisoners (Coid *et al*, 2009*b*) in the UK. Psychopathic traits may occur in children, remaining relatively stable throughout adolescence and into adulthood (Frick *et al*, 2003*a*; Loney *et al*, 2007; Lynam *et al*, 2007). Even early in life, psychopathic traits (named 'callous–unemotional'

Box 2.1   The 20 items of the Psychopathy Checklist – Revised (PCL-R)

Factor 1

Interpersonal

- Glibness – superficial charm
- Grandiose sense of self-worth
- Pathological lying
- Conning – manipulative

Affective

- Lack of remorse or guilt
- Shallow affect
- Callous – lack of empathy
- Failure to accept responsibility

Factor 2

Lifestyle

- Need for stimulation
- Parasitic lifestyle
- Lack of realistic, long-term goals
- Impulsivity
- Irresponsibility

Antisocial

- Poor behavioural control
- Early behavioural problems
- Juvenile delinquency
- Revocation of conditional release
- Criminal versatility

Additional items: 'Promiscuous sexual behaviour' and 'Many short-term marital relationships' do not load onto these two factors but contribute to an individual's score on this instrument.

(Hare, 2003)

---

traits when present in children) distinguish these youngsters from other children with conduct disorder with regard to the onset and severity of their antisocial behaviour and the risk of associated harm. Children with both conduct disorder and callous–unemotional traits present with more

Table 2.1   Common traits between cluster B personality disorders (DSM-IV-TR) and psychopathy (PCL-R)

Subtype	DSM-IV-TR trait	PCL-R trait
Antisocial personality disorder	Engagement in illegal acts Deceitfulness, conning Impulsivity, failure to plan ahead Lack of remorse	Criminal versatility Pathological lying, conning Impulsivity, lack of goals Lack of remorse or guilt
Borderline personality disorder	Unstable interpersonal relationships Impulsive sexual behaviour Difficulty controlling anger	Many short-term marital relationships Promiscuous sexual behaviour Poor behavioural controls
Histrionic personality disorder	Shallow emotions	Shallow affect
Narcissistic personality disorder	Exploits others for own gain Lacks empathy Grandiose sense of self-importance	Manipulative Callous, lack of empathy Grandiose sense of self-worth

PCL-R, Psychopathy Checklist – Revised.

severe behavioural problems (Dolan, 2004; Frick *et al*, 2005), have a greater likelihood of their antisocial behaviour persisting into adulthood and manifesting as antisocial personality disorder and psychopathy (Frick *et al*, 2003*b*; Lynam *et al*, 2007), and have a higher risk of future substance use disorders and other adverse outcomes (Lynam & Gudonis, 2005).

Studies also suggest that conduct disorder with callous–unemotional traits has a stronger genetic basis than conduct disorder alone (Viding *et al*, 2005), with unique risk factors and a significantly greater heritability rate (Frick & Dickens, 2006). Hence, psychopathy has been viewed as an early-onset developmental disorder, with specific genetic and neurocognitive constraints (Blair *et al*, 2005). Nevertheless, many authors also emphasise the importance of not applying the term 'psychopath' to children, both to avoid stigma and because decisions about individuals based on the construct are speculative owing to limitations in the evidence base (Johnstone & Cooke, 2007).

Psychopathy and its relation to antisocial personality disorder

As noted earlier, severe emotional dysfunction (for example, lack of guilt or victim empathy) is necessary for a diagnosis of psychopathy, but not for antisocial personality disorder. Psychopathy is also distinguished by high levels of both reactive (elicited by frustration) and instrumental (goal-directed) violence (Blair, 2001). Further, prevalence rates differ between antisocial personality disorder and psychopathy, suggesting that the diagnoses are not equivalent. In the UK, rates of antisocial personality disorder are estimated at up to 3% in the general population (Coid, 2003) and up to 80% among prisoners (Hare, 2003). This compares with less than 1% for psychopathy in the general population (Coid *et al*, 2009*a*) and just under 8% among prisoners (Coid *et al*, 2009*b*).

Although most adult offenders with psychopathy meet criteria for antisocial personality disorder, only about 30% of those with antisocial personality disorder meet criteria for psychopathy (Hart & Hare, 1997). This has led to the view that psychopathy should be regarded as a particularly severe subtype of antisocial personality disorder (Dolan & Doyle, 2007).

Borderline personality disorder

Borderline personality disorder is characterised by instability in inter-personal relationships, self-image and emotion regulation, and marked impulsivity. Individuals with borderline personality disorder are at a greater risk of self-injurious behaviour and suicide compared with the general population (Oumaya *et al*, 2008). The incidence of borderline personality disorder in the general population ranges from 0.7 to 2% (Torgersen *et al*, 2001; Coid, 2003) to over 20% in psychiatric settings (American Psychiatric Association, 2000). In contrast to antisocial personality disorder and psychopathy, it is diagnosed more frequently in women – although this may reflect gender bias in diagnosis and not true gender distribution (Chanen, 2006). The self-harming behaviour of individuals with borderline personality disorder contrasts with the outwardly directed aggression characteristic of antisocial personality disorder and psychopathy.

Narcissistic personality disorder

Narcissistic traits include grandiosity, need for admiration and lack of empathy. Estimated rates of narcissistic personality disorder in the general population range from 0.8 to 4% (Torgersen et al, 2001; Kay, 2008), and may decline with increasing age in adulthood (Stinson et al, 2008). Narcissistic personality disorder is commonly comorbid with antisocial personality disorder (Stuart et al, 1998). Like borderline personality disorder, it is associated with an elevated risk of suicide (Ronningstam et al, 2008). Neural correlates of narcissistic personality disorder are unknown, although the neural correlates of particular traits (for example, lack of empathy) are being investigated in relation to psychopathy (see below).

Histrionic personality disorder

Histrionic traits include excessive emotionality, attention-seeking and a seductive demeanour. The general population prevalence of histrionic personality disorder is around 2%, with no gender difference in rates (Grant et al, 2004). Neural correlates of histrionic personality disorder have not been investigated.

Neuroimaging correlates of psychopathy

A number of neural regions are thought to underlie the core deficits seen in psychopathy, in particular the amygdala and prefrontal cortex. The functional significance of these and other key regions will be outlined here, followed by a brief overview of relevant neuroimaging findings.

Amygdala

Emotional dysfunction

Research into the neurobiological basis of emotional dysfunction in psychopathy has focused on the amygdala because of its role in the emotion processing (particularly of fearful expressions) and emotion learning. For example, patients with amygdala lesions have deficits in the recognition of fearful expressions (Adolphs et al, 1999). Further, in healthy individuals the amygdala is more active during processing of fear and disgust than of happy and neutral expressions (Costafreda et al, 2008). Also, the amygdala is critically involved in stimulus-reinforcer association learning (Rolls, 2000), which contributes to moral socialisation – for example, by learning to avoid antisocial behaviour because of its association with emotionally negative outcomes. In particular, the psychologist James Blair hypothesised that, in healthy individuals, distress cues (such as facial and vocal expressions of fear) function as aversive unconditioned stimuli that elicit empathic responses (feeling the distress of others) (Blair, 1995; Blair *et al*, 2005). In this view, amygdala dysfunction in the 'at-risk' child with callous–unemotional traits and in the adult with psychopathy results in insensitivity to distress cues and failure to learn to avoid behaviour that engenders distress in others.

Processing distress cues

Several lines of evidence now support the view that children with callous–unemotional traits and adults with psychopathy have deficits in processing distress cues, in association with abnormalities of the amygdala. For example, a meta-analysis has shown that relative to control groups, anti-social populations show significant deficits in recognising fearful, sad and surprised expressions, with a significantly greater deficit in fear recognition relative to other expressions (Marsh & Blair, 2008). Individuals with psychopathy show reduced potentiation of the eye blink startle reflex by visual threat primes (Patrick *et al*, 1993), which is related to amygdala function. They also show reduced autonomic responsiveness to distress cues (for example, a crying face), but not to threatening or neutral images (Blair *et al*, 1997). These selective deficits in autonomic responses to facial distress cues are likely to be related to amygdala dysfunction. For example, adolescents with conduct disorder and callous–unemotional traits show reduced amygdala responses to fearful expressions relative to controls (Marsh *et al*, 2008; Jones *et al*, 2009). Also, compared with controls, adults with psychopathy show an atypical pattern of greater visual cortical (fusiform gyrus) activity in response to neutral expressions and reduced activity in response to fearful expressions. This may indicate reduced feedback modulation of the fusiform gyrus by the amygdala during fear processing, and contribute to deficits in the recognition of and affective responsiveness to fearful expressions (Deeley *et al*, 2006).

Reduced amygdala activation was also found in adults scoring high on the PCL-R during moral decision-making tasks (Glenn *et al*, 2009).

Structure and function of the amygdala

At a structural level, morphological differences have been found in the amygdala of individuals with psychopathy (Yang *et al*, 2009). In addition, volumes were correlated negatively with both total and two-factor PCL-R scores, especially Factor 1.

Thus, people with psychopathy show evidence of abnormalities of amygdala structure and function that are related both to clinical features and to the underlying information processing deficits – such as impaired emotion recognition, empathy and associative learning – which may help explain them.

Emotion processing and learning

It should also be emphasised that in addition to findings of abnormalities in the processing of distress cues and in the structure and function of the amygdala, there is increasing evidence of abnormalities in distributed brain systems involved in emotion processing and learning. For example, significant differences are seen between healthy individuals and those with psychopathy during fear conditioning. In fear conditioning paradigms, a previously neutral stimulus is paired with an aversive cue (unconditioned stimulus) so that the neutral stimulus will also become aversive. While acquiring this association, people with psychopathy show significantly less activity of the amygdala, orbitofrontal cortex, anterior cingulate cortex and insula than healthy controls; they also fail to show conditioned skin conductance response to presentations of the neutral stimulus (Birbaumer *et al*, 2005).

Another study employing an affective memory task reported reduced affect-related activity in the amygdala/hippocampal formation, para-hippocampal gyrus, ventral striatum and in the anterior and posterior cingulate gyri in criminals with psychopathy compared with controls (Kiehl *et al*, 2001). The criminals also showed evidence of overactivation in the bilateral frontotemporal cortices when processing affective stimuli.

Hence, individuals with psychopathy show differences in distributed brain systems involved in emotion processing and memory in two kinds of emotion learning task. Widespread neurobiological differences in respond-ing to and learning about emotive stimuli may contribute to the deficient affective experience and fearlessness of individuals with psychopathy. These differences may be in addition to more specific deficits in processing and learning from distress cues that may account for impairments in empathy and the use of instrumental aggression.

Prefrontal cortex

The importance of the frontal lobes to social behaviour was first recognised in the 19th century following the case of Phineas Gage, in whom frontal lobe damage resulted in profound personality change marked by inappropriate social behaviour (Harlow, 1869). A 'frontal lobe' syndrome was subsequently described on the basis of clinical observation of the behaviour of patients with frontal lobe lesions (Lishman, 1998). Characteristic features included apathy, emotional lability, lack of social awareness, unconcern for social rules, impulsiveness and frustrative aggression (more commonly known as reactive aggression). This has led to the suggestion that related traits in psychopathy and other personality disorders may also result from frontal lobe abnormalities (Damasio, 2000).

Subsequent advances in neuroimaging have allowed the neuro-psychological, symptom and trait associations of frontal regions in clinical populations to be defined with increasing precision. Key regions include the prefrontal cortex (frontal regions anterior to the motor cortices) and its subdivisions (anterior portions of the dorsolateral and medial cortices, and the orbital cortex). The ventromedial prefrontal cortex is a term used to refer to the orbitofrontal and/or the ventral portion of the medial wall of the frontal lobe (Stuss & Levine, 2002). Lesion-deficit studies demonstrate that damage to the ventromedial prefrontal cortex in particular is associated with an increased risk of reactive aggression (Blair & Cipolotti, 2000). Furthermore, a recent study showed ventromedial prefrontal cortex damage to be associated with deficits in moral judgement. Vignettes detailing failed attempts at harming others were judged as more morally permissible by patients with ventromedial prefrontal cortex lesions compared with controls without such lesions (Young et al, 2010).

Some studies have examined the prefrontal or frontal cortex as a whole, rather than its subdivisions. Two of these have reported reduced prefrontal (Yang et al, 2005) or frontal (Muller et al, 2008) grey matter volume in adults with psychopathy. Higher total as well as subfactor psychopathy scores (arrogant/deceptive, affective and impulsive/unstable) have been associated with low prefrontal grey matter volume (Yang et al, 2005). Further, cortical blood perfusion measured with single photon emission computed tomography (SPECT) was found to be inversely related to PCL subscores in the frontal and temporal lobes of violent offenders (Factor 1, 'disturbed interpersonal attitudes') (Soderstrom et al, 2002). Hence, there is evidence of reduced prefrontal volume and abnormal frontal and temporal blood flow in individuals with psychopathy relative to controls.

Other studies have revealed more specific associations between psychopathic traits and subregions of the prefrontal cortex. In particular, the association between ventromedial prefrontal cortex damage and reactive aggression in patients with brain injury is mirrored by impairments of ventromedial prefrontal cortex structure and function in individuals with psychopathy, among other abnormalities. For example, one study revealed reduced grey matter volume in the orbitofrontal cortex, frontopolar cortex and postcentral gyri in men with antisocial personality disorder relative to controls, with individuals with psychopathy showing the smallest volumes in these areas (Tiihonen et al, 2008).

A study of children with callous–unemotional traits and conduct disorder reported increased grey matter concentration in the medial orbitofrontal cortex and anterior cingulate cortex (De Brito et al, 2009). Given evidence that callous–unemotional traits in childhood may contribute to the development of adult psychopathy (Lynam et al, 2007), these findings may indicate an early developmental origin of prefrontal abnormalities in individuals at risk of adult psychopathy.

Neuropsychological deficits

These findings raise the question of how abnormalities of prefrontal cortical structure and function contribute to emotional dysfunction and/

or antisocial behaviour. Neuropsychological studies attempt to identify impairments in information processing linked to abnormal brain structure and function that contribute to clinical phenotypes. Here, we consider two models of neuropsychological deficits in psychopathy linked to ventromedial prefrontal cortex dysfunction, tested by reversal learning and gambling tasks respectively. In individuals with psychopathy, both tasks may show differences in affective learning associated with ventromedial prefrontal cortex dysfunction that contributes to recidivism and insensitivity to risk and punishment.

Reversal learning

On tests of reversal learning, individuals are required to alter a dominant rewarded response when task contingency is reversed (a previously rewarded response is now punished). Impaired reversal learning performance by individuals with ventromedial prefrontal cortex damage highlights involvement of this region in this task (Fellows & Farah, 2003). Individuals with psychopathy show greater response perseveration and, during functional magnetic resonance imaging (fMRI), display aberrant activation of the ventromedial prefrontal cortex during the reversal phase (Budhani *et al*, 2007; Finger *et al*, 2008). Increased activity of the ventromedial prefrontal cortex in response to punished error may underpin an inability to respond appropriately to aversive reinforcement in order to regulate behaviour (Rolls *et al*, 1994).

Gambling tasks

Ventromedial prefrontal cortex dysfunction in psychopathy is also suggested by response patterns on the Iowa Gambling Task that resemble those of patients with orbitofrontal cortex damage (Bechara *et al*, 1994; Mitchell *et al*, 2002; van Honk *et al*, 2002). This task requires individuals to choose cards from four decks of playing cards in order to receive rewards (financial gain) and avoid punishment (financial loss). The four decks are unequally weighted for losses and gains, with two decks consistently producing both high rewards and high losses and the other two small rewards and small losses. Over time, healthy individuals choose the latter two packs to produce a net gain. By contrast, individuals with ventromedial prefrontal cortex lesions show no bias towards these safer packs, demonstrating this region's importance in this type of decision-making (Bechara *et al*, 1994). Studies have shown that individuals with subclinical psychopathy (van Honk *et al*, 2002), children with callous–unemotional traits (Blair, 2001) and adults with psychopathy (Mitchell *et al*, 2002) perform similarly to patients with ventromedial prefrontal cortex lesions on gambling tasks.

Frustration/aggression

Ventromedial prefrontal cortex dysfunction is also associated with an increased risk of reactive aggression in both individuals with brain injury and individuals with psychopathy (Blair & Cipolotti, 2000). Possible

29

explanations of this association include increased frustration due to perseveration of unsuccessful responses or recurrent social conflict because of a more general inability to suppress impulses and desires (including aggressive impulses when challenged or threatened).

Disconnectivity between prefrontal cortex and limbic regions in psychopathy

Evidence suggests that abnormalities in the structure and function of the prefrontal cortex and limbic regions in children with callous–unemotional traits and/or individuals with psychopathy should not be viewed in isolation from one another. For example, an fMRI study reported reduced connectivity between the amygdala and prefrontal areas in adolescents with conduct disorder compared with controls, when watching displays of deliberately inflicted pain (Decety *et al*, 2009).

A study using diffusion tensor imaging (DTI) found that individuals with psychopathy showed reduced fractional anisotropy – a measure of tract microstructural integrity – of the uncinate fasciculus (Craig *et al*, 2009). This white matter pathway connects the limbic and ventral frontal brain regions. A measure of anatomical difference in the uncinate fasciculus was also inversely correlated with PCL Factor 2 scores (antisocial behaviour). These findings imply that reduced communication between limbic (emotion processing) and frontal (executive) regions may contribute to the behavioural problems of people with antisocial personality disorder.

Individuals with psychopathy show evidence of structural and functional abnormalities of the ventromedial prefrontal cortex, amygdala and other components of distributed networks involved in recognising and responding to distress cues, more general emotion processing and learning, behavioural regulation and decision-making.

Neuroimaging correlates of personality disorders

Few studies of cluster B personality disorders relate to antisocial and borderline personality disorder. Here we outline their results.

Antisocial personality disorder

As in psychopathy, structural and functional abnormalities of the prefrontal cortex have been found in antisocial personality disorder. Prefrontal grey matter volume has been found to be reduced in adults (Raine *et al*, 2000) and children (Huebner *et al*, 2008) with antisocial personality compared with healthy controls. Medial frontal cortical thinning has been recorded in antisocial personality disorder (Narayan *et al*, 2007). Reduced anterior cingulate cortex activation is seen in children with the disorder while viewing negative affective stimuli (Sterzer *et al*, 2005; Stadler *et al*, 2007). Positron emission tomography (PET) studies have reported reduced metabolism in prefrontal areas in violent individuals (Goyer *et al*, 1994; Volkow *et al*, 1995).

Reduced volume of the temporal regions is seen in adults (Barkataki *et al*, 2006) and children (see Sterzer & Stadler, 2009) with antisocial personality disorder, including reduced amygdala volume (Sterzer *et al*, 2007) and additional hippocampal reduction, with both volumes inversely related to severity of conduct disorder (Huebner *et al*, 2008). Reduced amygdala function has been reported in children with conduct disorder presented with negative emotional visual stimuli (Sterzer *et al*, 2005), although increased activation was also found (Herpertz *et al*, 2008).

Enhanced activation of the amygdala, plus striatal and temporal areas, was found in a sample of boys with conduct disorder while viewing scenes showing others experiencing pain (Decety *et al*, 2009). Increased signals in these areas were not evident in the control sample, even though both groups displayed similar activation increases within the pain matrix comprising the anterior insula, medial cingulate cortex, somatosensory cortex and periaqueductal grey. The study also reported reduced functional connectivity between amygdala and prefrontal regions in the conduct disorder group. However, comparisons of findings across ages should be made with caution.

Neuroimaging data indicate that prefrontal and temporal regions show reduced grey matter in antisocial personality disorder, and this may relate to functional deficits additionally seen in these regions. However, studies are not consistent in their methods of allocating or defining clinical groups, making it difficult to draw reliable conclusions from studies of antisocial personality disorder and psychopathy, and when comparing these groups. For example, some studies (such as Barkataki *et al*, 2006) did not administer the PCL or an equivalent measure, so they may, in fact, be examining psychopathy and not antisocial personality disorder alone.

Borderline personality disorder

Neuropsychological assessments of individuals with borderline personality disorder have reported deficits in tasks reliant on frontal and temporal brain areas (Swirsky-Sacchetti *et al*, 1993), such as executive function and memory tasks. Emotion processing deficits are also seen in borderline personality disorder, with impaired recognition of emotional faces (Levine *et al*, 1997) and impairments of emotion recognition when integrating facial expressions and prosody (Minzenberg *et al*, 2006). The increased startle response to aversive stimuli in borderline personality disorder (Hazlett *et al*, 2007) contrasts with the pattern found in psychopathy (Patrick *et al*, 1993).

Structural abnormalities

Structural anomalies found in borderline personality disorder predominantly involve frontal and limbic regions. Significant frontal volume reductions have been found in the whole frontal lobe (Lyoo *et al*, 1998), the cingulate cortex (Hazlett *et al*, 2005) and the orbitofrontal cortex (Chanen *et al*, 2008). Significant reductions in anterior cingulate cortex (Minzenberg *et al*, 2008) and cingulate gyrus (Soloff *et al*, 2008) grey matter concentration have also been reported.

A number of MRI studies report structural differences of the amygdala in people with borderline personality disorder compared with healthy controls. However, the direction of these differences varies between studies, with reduced volume (Weniger *et al*, 2009), increased (Minzenberg *et al*, 2008) and decreased (Soloff *et al*, 2008) grey matter concentration, and no volumetric difference (New *et al*, 2007) being variously reported. Lack of consistency among these findings may arise from methodological differences between studies, including use of mixed- *v*. single-gender cohorts (for discussion of further limitations see Minzenberg *et al*, 2008).

Structural abnormalities of the hippocampus are also seen in borderline personality disorder, with individuals showing reduced hippocampal volume (Zetzsche *et al*, 2007; Weniger *et al*, 2009) and reduced grey matter concentration (Soloff *et al*, 2008) compared with healthy controls. Other medial temporal and limbic structural findings include reduced grey matter concentration in the parahippocampal gyrus and uncus (Soloff *et al*, 2008). These findings suggest that common traits of borderline personality disorder and psychopathy (such as impulsivity, poor behavioural control) may be due to similar patterns of frontal and limbic abnormality (Blair *et al*, 2005).

Differences between activity in frontal and limbic areas

Functional studies also find activity in frontal and limbic areas to differ in people with borderline personality disorder compared with healthy controls. For example, anterior cingulate cortex hypoactivation is seen during emotion processing (Wingenfeld *et al*, 2009). Coupled with fMRI findings of increased amygdala activation during emotion processing (Herpertz *et al*, 2001; Donegan *et al*, 2003; Koenigsberg *et al*, 2009), these results support frontolimbic deficit theories of borderline personality disorder. These propose that amygdala hyperactivation and anterior cingulate cortex hypoactivation in response to emotional stimuli produce heightened emotional arousal in combination with a reduced ability to inhibit and regulate emotional expression (Wingenfeld *et al*, 2009). These linked processes could account for the increased intensity of affective experience shown by individuals with borderline personality disorder.

Clinical implications

From this discussion it can be seen not only that psychopathy and each of the cluster B personality disorders share certain traits, but also that there is some overlap in brain anomalies found in the three conditions for which neuroimaging data exist (antisocial and borderline personality disorders and psychopathy). Shared features of borderline personality disorder and psychopathy may reflect similar cognitive and neural mechanisms. For example, 'emotion' executive dysfunction associated with prefrontal structural and functional abnormalities may contribute to impulsivity, disinhibition and increased risk of reactive aggression (although other factors may influence whether aggression is directed to the self or others). Conversely, the increased affective intensity of borderline personality disorder, in contrast to the reduced affective experience of individuals with psychopathy, may reflect respective differences in amygdala reactivity. However, it should be noted that clinical features such as 'reactive aggression', 'disinhibition' and 'affective intensity' are not caused by single brain structures acting in isolation. This raises the possibility that the relative contribution of a given structure (such as the orbitofrontal cortex or amygdala) to a clinical feature (for example, reactive aggression) may vary depending on the characteristics of other components of relevant brain systems (such as the anterior cingulate cortex).

Future research

In general, psychiatric research is increasingly focused on understanding reciprocal influences within and between the levels at which people are constituted (for example, genes, cells, brain systems, social environment), and may ultimately reveal a range of mechanisms by which clinical features such as reactive aggression or impulsivity are produced.

Despite the volume of imaging data related to psychopathy and other personality disorders, there still remains a great deal to be learnt about the neurobiology of these complex disorders. Identification of neural mechanisms underlying their clinical features may enable improved understanding of diagnosis, aetiology, treatment and prognosis. Future research would benefit from the establishment of common technical parameters, study populations and clinical definitions, to facilitate comparisons between studies. The distinct, yet overlapping, nature of these diagnoses from a neurobiological as well as a clinical perspective further supports the view that personality disorders may be better classified using dimensional rather than categorical methods.

References

Adolphs, R., Tranel, D., Hamann, S., et al (1999) Recognition of facial emotion in nine individuals with bilateral amygdala damage. *Neuropsychologia*, **37**, 1111–1117.

American Psychiatric Association (1980) *Diagnostic and Statistical Manual for Mental Disorders (3rd edn) (DSM-III)*. APA.

American Psychiatric Association (2000) *Diagnostic and Statistical Manual for Mental Disorders, Fourth Edition (Text Revision) (DSM-IVTR)*. APA.

Barkataki, I., Kumari, V., Das, M., et al (2006) Volumetric structural brain abnormalities in men with schizophrenia or antisocial personality disorder. *Behavioural Brain Research*, **169**, 239–247.

Bechara, A., Damasio, A. R., Damasio, H., *et al* (1994) Insensitivity to future consequences following damage to human prefrontal cortex. *Cognition*, **50**, 7–15.

Birbaumer, N., Veit, R., Lotze, M., *et al* (2005) Deficient fear conditioning in psychopathy: a functional magnetic resonance imaging study. *Archives of General Psychiatry*, **62**, 799–805.

Blackburn, R. (2005) Psychopathy as a personality construct. In *Handbook of Personology and Psychopathology* (eds S. Strack & T. Millon), pp. 271–291. John & Wiley & Sons.

Blair, R. J. (1995) A cognitive developmental approach to morality: investigating the psychopath. *Cognition*, **57**, 1–29.

Blair, R. J. (2001) Neurocognitive models of aggression, the antisocial personality disorders, and psychopathy. *Journal of Neurology, Neurosurgery and Psychiatry*, **71**, 727–731.

Blair, R. J. & Cipolotti, L. (2000) Impaired social response reversal: a case of 'acquired sociopathy'. *Brain*, **123**, 1122–1141.

Blair, R. J., Jones, L., Clark, F., *et al* (1997) The psychopathic individual: a lack of responsiveness to distress cues? *Psychophysiology*, **34**, 192–198.

Blair, J., Mitchell, D., Mitchell, D. R., *et al* (2005) *The Psychopath: Emotion and the Brain*. Blackwell Publishing.

Budhani, S., Marsh, A. A., Pine, D., *et al* (2007) Neural correlates of response reversal: considering acquisition. *Neuroimage*, **34**, 1754–1765.

Chanen, A. M. (2006) Borderline personality disorder: sex differences. In *Mood and Anxiety Disorders in Women* (eds D. J. Castle, J. Kulkarni & K. M. Abel), pp. 20–38. Cambridge University Press.

Chanen, A. M., Velakoulis, D., Carison, K., *et al* (2008) Orbitofrontal, amygdala and hippocampal volumes in teenagers with first-presentation borderline personality disorder. *Psychiatry Research*, **163**, 116–125.

Cleckley, H. M. (1941) *The Mask of Sanity*. Mosby Medical Library.

Coid, J. (2003) Epidemiology, public health and the problem of personality disorder. *British Journal of Psychiatry*, **182**, s3–s10.

Coid, J., Yang, M., Ullrich, S., *et al* (2009*a*) Prevalence and correlates of psychopathic traits in the household population of Great Britain. *International Journal of Law and Psychiatry*, **32**, 65–73.

Coid, J., Yang, M., Ullrich, S., *et al* (2009*b*) Psychopathy among prisoners in England and Wales. *International Journal of Law and Psychiatry*, **32**, 134–141.

Costafreda, S. G., Brammer, M. J., David, A. S., *et al* (2008) Predictors of amygdala activation during the processing of emotional stimuli: a meta-analysis of 385 PET and fMRI studies. *Brain Research Reviews*, **58**, 57–70.

Craig, M. C., Catani, M., Deeley, Q., *et al* (2009) Altered connections on the road to psychopathy. *Molecular Psychiatry*, **14**, 946–953.

Damasio, A. R. (2000) A neural basis for sociopathy. *Archives of General Psychiatry*, **57**, 128–129.

De Brito, S. A., Mechelli, A., Wilke, M., *et al* (2009) Size matters: increased grey matter in boys with conduct problems and callous–unemotional traits. *Brain*, **132**, 843–852.

Decety, J., Michalska, K. J., Akitsuki, Y., *et al* (2009) Atypical empathic responses in adolescents with aggressive conduct disorder: a functional MRI investigation. *Biological Psychology*, **80**, 203–211.

Deeley, Q., Daly, E., Surguladze, S., *et al* (2006) Facial emotion processing in criminal psychopathy: preliminary functional magnetic resonance imaging study. *British Journal of Psychiatry*, **189**, 533–539.

Dolan, M. (2004) Psychopathic personality in young people. *Advances in Psychiatric Treatment*, **10**, 466–473.

Dolan, M. & Doyle, M. (2007) Psychopathy: diagnosis and implications for treatment. *Psychiatry*, **6**, 404–408.

Donegan, N. H., Sanislow, C. A., Blumberg, H. P., *et al* (2003) Amygdala hyperreactivity in borderline personality disorder: implications for emotional dysregulation. *Biological Psychiatry*, **54**, 1284–1293.

Fellows, L. K. & Farah, M. J. (2003) Ventromedial frontal cortex mediates affective shifting in humans: evidence from a reversal learning paradigm. *Brain*, **126**, 1830–1837.

Finger, E. C., Marsh, A. A., Mitchell, D. G., *et al* (2008) Abnormal ventromedial prefrontal cortex function in children with psychopathic traits during reversal learning. *Archives of General Psychiatry*, **65**, 586–594.

Frick, P. J. & Dickens, C. (2006) Current perspectives on conduct disorder. *Current Psychiatric Reports*, **8**, 59–72.

Frick, P. J., Cornell, A. H., Barry, C. T., *et al* (2003a) Callous–unemotional traits and conduct problems in the prediction of conduct problem severity, aggression, and self-report of delinquency. *Journal of Abnormal Child Psychology*, **31**, 457–470.

Frick, P. J., Kimonis, E. R., Dandreaux, D. M., *et al* (2003b) The 4 year stability of psychopathic traits in non-referred youth. *Behavioral Sciences and the Law*, **21**, 713–736.

Frick, P. J., Stickle, T. R., Dandreaux, D. M., *et al* (2005) Callous–unemotional traits in predicting the severity and stability of conduct problems and delinquency. *Journal of Abnormal Child Psychology*, **33**, 471–487.

Glenn, A. L., Raine, A. & Schug, R. A. (2009) The neural correlates of moral decision-making in psychopathy. *Molecular Psychiatry*, **14**, 5–6.

Goyer, P. F., Andreason, P. J., Semple, W. E., *et al* (1994) Positron-emission tomography and personality disorders. *Neuropsychopharmacology*, **10**, 21–28.

Grant, B. F., Hasin, D. S., Stinson, F. S., *et al* (2004) Prevalence, correlates, and disability of personality disorders in the United States: results from the National Epidemiologic Survey on alcohol and related conditions. *Journal of Clinical Psychiatry*, **65**, 948–958.

Hare, R. D. (1980) A research scale for the assessment of psychopathy in criminal populations. *Personality and Individual Differences*, **1**, 111–119.

Hare, R. D. (1991) *The Hare Psychopathy Checklist – Revised*. Multi-Health Systems.

Hare, R. D. (2003) *Manual for the Revised Psychopathy Checklist (2nd edn)*. Multi-Health Systems.

Harlow, J. M. (1869) Recovery from the passage of an iron bar through the head. Reprint: Harlow, J. M. & Miller, E. (1993) *History of Psychiatry*, **4**, 274–281.

Hart, S. D. & Hare, R. D. (1997) *Psychopathy: Assessment and Association with Criminal Conduct*. John Wiley & Sons.

Hazlett, E. A., New, A. S., Newmark, R., *et al* (2005) Reduced anterior and posterior cingulate gray matter in borderline personality disorder. *Biological Psychiatry*, **58**, 614–623.

Hazlett, E. A., Speiser, L. J., Goodman, M., *et al* (2007) Exaggerated affect-modulated startle during unpleasant stimuli in borderline personality disorder. *Biological Psychiatry*, **62**, 250–255.

Herpertz, S. C., Dietrich, T. M., Wenning, B., *et al* (2001) Evidence of abnormal amygdala functioning in borderline personality disorder: a functional MRI study. *Biological Psychiatry*, **50**, 292–298.

Herpertz, S. C., Huebner, T., Marx, I., *et al* (2008) Emotional processing in male adolescents with childhood-onset conduct disorder. *Journal of Child Psychology and Psychiatry and Allied Disciplines*, **49**, 781–791.

Huebner, T., Vloet, T. D., Marx, I., *et al* (2008) Morphometric brain abnormalities in boys with conduct disorder. *Journal of the American Academy of Child and Adolescent Psychiatry* 47, **540–7.**

Johnstone, L. & Cooke, D. J. (2007) Psychopathy and young offenders. *Psychiatry*, **6**, 429–432.

Jones, A. P., Laurens, K. R., Herba, C. M., *et al* (2009) Amygdala hypoactivity to fearful faces in boys with conduct problems and callous–unemotional traits. *American Journal of Psychiatry*, **166**, 95–102.

Kay, J. (2008) Toward a clinically more useful model for diagnosing narcissistic personality disorder. *American Journal of Psychiatry*, **168**, 1379–1382.

Kiehl, K. A. (2006) A cognitive neuroscience perspective on psychopathy: evidence for paralimbic system dysfunction. *Psychiatry Research*, **142**, 107–128.

Kiehl, K. A., Smith, A. M., Hare, R. D., *et al* (2001) Limbic abnormalities in affective processing by criminal psychopaths as revealed by functional magnetic resonance imaging. *Biological Psychiatry*, **50**, 677–684.

Koenigsberg, H. W., Siever, L. J., Lee, H., *et al* (2009) Neural correlates of emotion processing in borderline personality disorder. *Psychiatry Research*, **172**, 192–199.

Levine, D., Marziali, E. & Hood, J. (1997) Emotion processing in borderline personality disorders. *Journal of Nervous and Mental Disease*, **185**, 240–246.

Lishman, W. A. (1998) *Organic Psychiatry: The Psychological Consequences of Cerebral Disorder (3rd edn)*. Blackwell Science.

Loney, B. R., Taylor, J., Butler, M. A., *et al* (2007) Adolescent psychopathy features: 6-year temporal stability and the prediction of externalizing symptoms during the transition to adulthood. *Aggressive Behavior*, **33**, 242–252.

Lynam, D. R. & Gudonis, L. (2005) The development of psychopathy. *Annual Review of Clinical Psychology*, **1**, 381–407.

Lynam, D. R., Caspi, A., Moffitt, T. E., *et al* (2007) Longitudinal evidence that psychopathy scores in early adolescence predict adult psychopathy. *Journal of Abnormal Psychology*, **116**, 155–165.

Lyoo, I. K., Han, M. H. & Cho, D. Y. (1998) A brain MRI study in subjects with borderline personality disorder. *Journal of Affective Disorders*, **50**, 235–243.

Marsh, A. A. & Blair, R. J. R. (2008) Deficits in facial affect recognition among antisocial populations: a meta-analysis. *Neuroscience and Biobehavioral Reviews*, **32**, 454–465.

Marsh, A. A., Finger, E. C., Mitchell, D. G., *et al* (2008) Reduced amygdala response to fearful expressions in children and adolescents with callous–unemotional traits and disruptive behavior disorders. *American Journal of Psychiatry*, **165**, 712–720.

Minzenberg, M. J., Poole, J. H. & Vinogradov, S. (2006) Social-emotion recognition in borderline personality disorder. *Comprehensive Psychiatry*, **47**, 468–474.

Minzenberg, M. J., Fan, J., New, A. S., *et al* (2008) Frontolimbic structural changes in borderline personality disorder. *Journal of Psychiatric Research*, **42**, 727–733.

Mitchell, D. G., Colledge, E., Leonard, A., *et al* (2002) Risky decisions and response reversal: is there evidence of orbitofrontal cortex dysfunction in psychopathic individuals? *Neuropsychologia*, **40**, 2013–2022.

Morana, H. C., Arboleda-Florez, J. & Camara, F. P. (2005) Identifying the cutoff score for the PCL-R scale (Psychopathy Checklist-Revised) in a Brazilian forensic population. *Forensic Science International*, **147**, 1–8.

Muller, J. L., Ganssbauer, S., Sommer, M., *et al* (2008) Gray matter changes in right superior temporal gyrus in criminal psychopaths: evidence from voxel-based morphometry. *Psychiatry Research*, **163**, 213–222.

Narayan, V. M., Narr, K. L., Kumari, V., *et al* (2007) Regional cortical thinning in subjects with violent antisocial personality disorder or schizophrenia. *American Journal of Psychiatry*, **164**, 1418–1427.

New, A. S., Hazlett, E. A., Buchsbaum, M. S., *et al* (2007) Amygdala-prefrontal disconnection in borderline personality disorder. *Neuropsychopharmacology*, **32**, 1629–1640.

Oumaya, M., Friedman, S., Pham, A., *et al* (2008) Borderline personality disorder, self-mutilation and suicide: literature review. *L'Encéphale*, **34**, 452–458.

Patrick, C. J., Bradley, M. M. & Lang, P. J. (1993) Emotion in the criminal psychopath: startle reflex modulation. *Journal of Abnormal Psychology*, **102**, 82–92.

Raine, A., Lencz, T., Bihrle, S., *et al* (2000) Reduced prefrontal gray matter volume and reduced autonomic activity in antisocial personality disorder. *Archives of General Psychiatry*, **57**, 119–127.

Reid, W. H. & Gacono, C. (2000) Treatment of antisocial personality, psychopathy, and other characterologic antisocial syndromes. *Behavioral Sciences and the Law*, **18**, 647–662.

Rolls, E. T. (2000) Precis of the brain and emotion. *Behavioral and Brain Sciences*, **23**, 177–191.

Rolls, E. T., Hornak, J., Wade, D., *et al* (1994) Emotion-related learning in patients with social and emotional changes associated with frontal lobe damage. *Journal of Neurology, Neurosurgery and Psychiatry*, **57**, 1518–1524.

Ronningstam, E., Weinberger, I. & Maltsberger, J. T. (2008) Eleven deaths of Mr. K.: contributing factors to suicide in narcissistic personalities. *Psychiatry*, **71**, 169–182.

Soderstrom, H., Hultin, L., Tullberg, M., *et al* (2002) Reduced frontotemporal perfusion in psychopathic personality. *Psychiatry Research*, **114**, 81–94.

Soloff, P., Nutche, J., Goradia, D., *et al* (2008) Structural brain abnormalities in borderline personality disorder: a voxel-based morphometry study. *Psychiatry Research*, **164**, 223–236.

Stadler, C., Sterzer, P., Schmeck, K., *et al* (2007) Reduced anterior cingulate activation in aggressive children and adolescents during affective stimulation: association with temperament traits. *Journal of Psychiatric Research*, **41**, 410–417.

Sterzer, P. & Stadler, C. (2009) Neuroimaging of aggressive and violent behaviour in children and adolescents. *Frontiers in Behavioural Neuroscience*, **3**, 35.

Sterzer, P., Stadler, C., Krebs, A., *et al* (2005) Abnormal neural responses to emotional visual stimuli in adolescents with conduct disorder. *Biological Psychiatry*, **57**, 7–15.

Sterzer, P., Stadler, C., Poustka, F., *et al* (2007) A structural neural deficit in adolescents with conduct disorder and its association with lack of empathy. *Neuroimage*, **37**, 335–342.

Stinson, F. S., Dawson, D. A., Goldstein, R. B., *et al* (2008) Prevalence, correlates, disability, and comorbidity of DSM-IV Narcissistic Personality Disorder: results from the Wave 2 National Epidemiologic Survey on alcohol and related conditions. *Journal of Clinical Psychiatry*, **69**, 1033–1045.

Stuart, S., Pfohl, B., Battaglia, M., *et al* (1998) The cooccurrence of DSM-III-R personality disorders. *Journal of Personality Disorder*, **12**, 302–315.

Stuss, D. T. & Levine, B. (2002) Adult clinical neuropsychology: lessons from studies of the frontal lobes. *Annual Review of Psychology*, **53**, 401–433.

Swirsky-Sacchetti, T., Gorton, G., Samuel, S., *et al* (1993) Neuropsychological function in borderline personality disorder. *Journal of Clinical Psychology*, **49**, 385–396.

Tiihonen, J., Rossi, R., Laakso, M. P., *et al* (2008) Brain anatomy of persistent violent offenders: more rather than less. *Psychiatry Research*, **163**, 201–122.

Torgersen, S., Kringlen, E. & Cramer, V. (2001) The prevalence of personality disorder in a community sample. *Archives of General Psychiatry*, **58**, 590–596.

van Honk, J., Hermans, E. J., Putman, P., *et al* (2002) Defective somatic markers in sub-clinical psychopathy. *Neuroreport*, **13**, 1025–1027.

Viding, E., Blair, R. J., Moffitt, T. E., *et al* (2005) Evidence for substantial genetic risk for psychopathy in 7-year-olds. *Journal of Child Psychology and Psychiatry and Allied Disciplines*, **46**, 592–597.

Volkow, N. D., Tancredi, L. R., Grant, C., *et al* (1995) Brain glucose metabolism in violent psychiatric patients: a preliminary study. *Psychiatry Research: Neuroimaging*, **61**, 243–253.

Weniger, G., Lange, C., Sachsse, U., *et al* (2009) Reduced amygdala and hippocampus size in trauma-exposed women with borderline personality disorder and without post-traumatic stress disorder. *Journal of Psychiatry and Neuroscience*, **34**, 383–388.

Wingenfeld, K., Rullkoetter, N., Mensebach, C., *et al* (2009) Neural correlates of the individual emotional Stroop in borderline personality disorder. *Psychoneuroendocrinology*, **34**, 571–586.

World Health Organization (2004) *International Statistical Classification of Diseases and Related Health Problems, Tenth Revision (ICD-10)*. WHO.

Yang, Y., Raine, A., Lencz, T., *et al* (2005) Volume reduction in prefrontal gray matter in unsuccessful criminal psychopaths. *Biological Psychiatry*, **57**, 1103–1108.

Yang, Y., Raine, A., Narr, K. L., *et al* (2009) Localization of deformations within the amygdala in individuals with psychopathy. *Archives of General Psychiatry*, **66**, 986–994.

Young, L., Bechara, A., Tranel, D., *et al* (2010) Damage to ventromedial prefrontal cortex impairs judgment of harmful intent. *Neuron*, **65**, 845–851.

Zetzsche, T., Preuss, U. W., Frodl, T., *et al* (2007) Hippocampal volume reduction and history of aggressive behaviour in patients with borderline personality disorder. *Psychiatry Research*, **154**, 157–170.

CHAPTER 3

Challenges in the treatment of dangerous and severe personality disorder

Kevin Howells, Gopi Krishnan and Michael Daffern

Summary   Dangerous and severe personality disorder (DSPD) services have a relatively short history, are currently under review and may be reconfigured in the next few years. Despite such uncertainties, implementation of therapeutic programmes for patients and prisoners in this category is likely to remain a high priority. We describe the background to the DSPD initiative in England and consider issues that arose in planning and delivering treatment services. Two bodies of evidence are particularly relevant: previous research into personality disorder and its treatment, which we suggest is, as yet, of limited value, and research into the outcomes of offender treatment programmes. The latter is clearly relevant but greater consideration of adapting programmes for the patient population and of breadth of treatment is required in the DSPD setting. The important task is to integrate components for the treatment of personality disorder and offending behaviour in a holistic manner. We describe further challenges in delivering treatment and suggest that ongoing evaluation of treatments is critical in this area of practice, given the impoverished knowledge base.

In the past, personality disorder has been the Cinderella of Cinderella health services. Many psychiatrists have considered personality disorder to be untreatable, some doubting the legitimacy of treating it within the health system. The issue of how to treat and manage (predominantly) men with severe personality or psychopathic disorder who also pose a risk to the public has been even more contentious. This latter group was traditionally managed within the criminal justice system, but the problem of defining which agencies should be responsible for them was brought into sharp focus during the acrimonious public debate following the conviction of Michael Stone for the murder of a mother and child in 1998. Although Stone was considered to have a personality disorder, psychiatrists dealing with him did not consider the disorder treatable and hence he could not be detained under the Mental Health Act 1983. In February 1999, the UK Government announced proposals to introduce the Dangerous and Severe

Personality Disorder (DSPD) pilot programme, the legal provision for which would be embedded within a new legislative framework.

The DSPD programme was originally described as 'the third way' to deal with a group of individuals who, over many years, were at the boundary between the health and criminal justice systems. Four sites in high-security (two in health settings – Rampton and Broadmoor Hospitals – and two in the prison estate – HMP Frankland and HMP Whitemoor) were established. A number of units in medium-security and community settings were also set up. These various units were intended to pilot the provision of DSPD services in England, with the objectives of developing an evidence base with regard to this hitherto neglected population, researching effective treatments and thus potentially contributing to improved public protection.

It must be emphasised that DSPD is not a clinical category or classification. The working definition of DSPD (Department of Health *et al*, 2004) is a determination that:

- an individual presents a significant risk (of serious physical or psychological harm from which it would be difficult or impossible for the victim to recover)
- an individual presents with a significant disorder of personality
- the risk presented is functionally linked to the personality disorder (see discussion below).

The criteria for admission to a DSPD unit are listed in Box 3.1. At the time of writing, what were DSPD services are being decommissioned, although high-security personality disorder services are likely to continue for the foreseeable future. It appears probable that services will be increasingly based on the criminal justice system, with high secure health facilities such as Rampton hospital continuing to have a role in treating those people who cannot be managed in other personality disorder services. The admission criteria for admission to future services and facilities remain to be specified.

There is a wide range of theoretical approaches for understanding personality disorder and its causation and a correspondingly wide range of potential therapies. Psychodynamic (including psychoanalytic), behavioural, cognitive, interpersonal and social theories have all been advanced (for an

---

Box 3.1 DSPD units: admission criteria

A score of 30 or above on the Revised Psychopathy Checklist (PCL-R; Hare, 1991);
or
a PCL-R score of 25–29 plus at least one DSM-IV personality disorder diagnosis other than antisocial personality disorder;
or
two or more DSM-IV personality disorder diagnoses

overview see Alwin *et al*, 2006). How personality disorder is to be treated will depend on how it is defined and understood. Personality disorders are increasingly seen as statistical extremes in the distribution of normal personality traits (the continuum model), but they are also identified in terms of individual dysfunction. This dysfunction has been viewed as arising from impairment of the organisational, integrative and self-regulatory processes required to achieve evolutionary tasks of: (a) stability of the self system; (b) satisfactory interpersonal functioning (e.g., meeting needs for intimacy, affiliation and attachment); and (c) social integration in the form of prosocial and cooperative behaviour (Livesley, 2001, 2007). Personality dysfunction and statistical deviation from the norm may be independent dimensions. Depending on the situation and the individual's role, personality may be highly abnormal in the statistical sense without being dysfunctional (Alwin *et al*, 2006).

Prevalence studies indicate that personality disorders are very common in adult prisoners, juveniles in prison and in mentally disordered offenders, with antisocial personality disorder being the most common category (Fazel & Danesh, 2002). As yet we have few published data on the prevalence of the criteria defining DSPD in the prison population. There is evidence that offenders with personality disorders have a higher risk for violent crime (Powis, 2002), particularly when the disorder is of a psychopathic type (Hemphill *et al*, 1998). Evidence linking personality disorder to violent offending, including sexual offending, is crucial, given the requirement for DSPD admission that there be a functional link. The notion of a functional link is increasingly seen as far from straightforward, with some theoreticians suggesting that a clear-cut and substantive link between personality disorder and serious offending has still to be established (Duggan & Howard, 2009).

It is not at all clear how the functional link can be determined for the individual offender/patient, beyond establishing that the person belongs to two populations that overlap, namely those with personality disorders and those who engage in serious violent offending. Demonstrating the presence of a functional link would require one of two sorts of clinical evidence: either evidence that manipulation (e.g., treatment) of the personality disorder led to a reduction in violent offending, or evidence that for the individual the two phenomena systematically covary over time in a way that suggests functional causation, that is, that periods of personality disorder are followed by (cause) periods in which offending is elevated. As we shall discuss below, evidence that treatment for personality disorder will reduce offending is not yet available. Indeed, one of the major purposes of the DSPD initiative was to determine whether such reduction is possible. The second (covariation) type of evidence is also impossible to obtain, for the reason that, by definition, personality disorders are stable aspects of the individual, not expected to show marked temporal variation. Whereas it would be possible to demonstrate a functional link by temporal covariation between, say, substance misuse and offending, it is not possible

> **Box 3.2** Minimum risk assessments required on admission to a DSPD unit
>
> Violence:
>
> - Violence Risk Scale (VRS; Wong & Gordon, 1999)
> - Historical, Clinical and Risk Management (HCR-20) scale (Webster *et al*, 1997)
>
> Sexual offending:
>
> - Risk Matrix 2000 (Thornton *et al*, 2003)
> - Static 99 (Nunes *et al*, 2002)
> - Structured Assessment of Risk and Needs (SARN; Thornton, 2002)
>
> Personality disorder:
>
> - The Revised Psychopathy Checklist (PCL-R; Hare, 1991)
> - Psychopathy Checklist – Screening Version (PCL-SV; Hart *et al*, 1995)
> - International Personality Disorder Examination (IPDE; World Health Organization, 1997).

for personality disorder. Substance misuse is typically episodic, and periods of misuse could be compared with periods of no use to determine whether criminal behaviour is lower in the latter. If personality disorders turn out to be less stable than has previously been assumed, then covariation evidence may indeed be useful.

Assessment

There is a consensus that structured assessments are required, both for the personality disorder component (Tyrer *et al*, 2007; Banerjee *et al*, 2009; National Collaborating Centre for Mental Health, 2009) and the risk/ offending behaviour component of DSPD. All individuals admitted to the four high secure DSPD services complete the structured assessments listed in Box 3.2. These relate more to the presence or absence of risk and personality disorder (admission criteria) than to the assessment of clinical therapeutic needs. Therefore they would need to be, and are, followed by more detailed clinical assessments that allow for a full formulation of all of the patient's mental health and social problems, not just those specifically related to their crime, and for subsequent identification of specific treatment targets. Such assessments need to cover behavioural, cognitive, affective, interpersonal and self-regulatory domains. The crucial role of case formulation has been emphasised by clinicians in DSPD services (Jones, 2010) and in a report on personality disorder (Alwin *et al*, 2006: p. 32):

> 'The provision of effective treatment for individuals with personality disorder requires the ability to place their experiences in a contextual and explanatory framework that can help to raise that person's own awareness of their behaviours, thoughts and emotions [...] Formulation is necessary [and]

41

goes beyond diagnosis through the generation of a working model based on an assessment of the range of personality traits presented.'

Treatment of personality disorders

People with personality disorders have received a wide range of pharmaco-logical and psychosocial treatments. Some of the latter are listed in Box 3.3. Although the evidence base is not large, there are indications that some psychotherapeutic interventions may be effective (Bateman & Fonagy, 1999; Perry *et al*, 1999; Leichsenring & Leibing, 2003; Verheul *et al*, 2003; Chapter 13, this volume). However, it remains to be determined whether any one approach is more effective than another or whether it is the non-specific aspects of a treatment (e.g., structure, specification of targets for change and forming a therapeutic relationship) that produce the treatment effect. Although many of these therapies have some evidential support for other mental disorders, and even for personality disorders, there is virtually no evidence of their effectiveness with individuals who combine severe personality disorder with high-risk forms of violence (Warren *et al*, 2003; McMurran, 2008; National Collaborating Centre for Mental Health, 2009; Tennant & Howells, 2010). The challenges for DSPD services are two-fold: to adapt such interventions for the distinctive characteristics of people with DSPD (see, as an example, the discussion of low treatment readiness below) and to prioritise research and evaluation into the effectiveness of these programmes in a DSPD context (also discussed below).

For the purposes of the present chapter, the literature cited above is of limited relevance, for two reasons. First, previous outcome studies have looked at a restricted set of personality disorders, most commonly border-line personality disorder. Offenders with borderline personality disorder do form a significant proportion of those admitted to DSPD units (Sheldon & Krishnan, 2009). Given the emphasis on psychopathy in DSPD admission criteria, it is likely that antisocial personality disorder will predominate, with other DSM-IV (American Psychiatric Association, 1994) Cluster B disorders, including borderline personality disorder, also evident (Sheldon

---

Box 3.3 Examples of therapies for personality disorders

Dialectical behaviour therapy

Cognitive–behavioural therapy (including schema therapy)

Emotion regulation therapies (e.g. anger management)

Cognitive analytic therapy

Therapeutic communities

Livesley's eclectic/pragmatic approach

& Krishnan, 2009). The therapy outcome data for antisocial personality disorder and psychopathic disorder are sparse indeed (D'Silva *et al*, 2004; National Collaborating Centre for Mental Health, 2009) with some evidence of adverse treatment outcomes (Harris *et al*, 1994).

Second, the outcome studies that do exist rarely address the needs of forensic or high-risk populations of a DSPD type, who are likely to reject rather than seek treatment (Tyrer *et al*, 2003) and to manifest their disorder in particularly antisocial ways. At present, it is reasonable to conclude that we do not know which treatments, if any, for personality disorder will prove to be effective for the DSPD population (Warren *et al*, 2003; National Collaborating Centre for Mental Health, 2009; Howells *et al*, 2011). Nevertheless, some interventions (e.g., cognitive–behavioural therapy, dialectical behaviour therapy, psychodynamic therapy) have sufficient initial credibility in related populations to warrant implementing exploratory therapeutic programmes so that their effectiveness can be evaluated (see below).

Livesley (2001, 2007) has argued for an integrated and multifaceted approach to treating personality disorder in people with DSPD. Integration has three components: (a) an eclectic use of diverse models and therapeutic strategies, based on their demonstrated effectiveness; (b) delivering treatments in an integrated way; (c) focusing treatment efforts to produce integration and coherence of personality functioning. In Livesley's model, the breakdown of integrative functioning and of a coherent sense of identity is central to personality disorders. Livesley's approach might be characterised as pragmatic eclecticism, selecting different treatments to target specific components of personality disorder, while also addressing the overall integration of the components themselves. Integration of the different treatments is achieved through non-specific aspects, of which the therapeutic alliance, promotion of motivation and the structured nature of the treatments are particularly important. It will be apparent from this brief account of Livesley's model that achieving integration will be even more important, and challenging, in a DSPD context, given that offending behaviour will also require integration within the general treatment framework. If his model is correct, it would suggest that the separate therapeutic programmes that tend to characterise correctional offender rehabilitation would be deficient in a DSPD context.

Treatment of high-risk offending behaviours

There are some fascinating contrasts to be made between therapeutic approaches to personality disorder and therapeutic approaches to high-risk offending behaviours. As already mentioned, therapies for personality disorder have had a wide range of theoretical orientations, with no one orientation yet demonstrated to be superior. They are more likely to be delivered in mental health settings (although two of the four current DSPD units in England and Wales are based in prisons and a move to services based in the criminal justice system is currently being planned). There appears as yet to be little consensus among researchers and clinicians as to what types of programme and programme features are likely to be associated with good outcomes.

The development of offending behaviour programmes, on the other hand, has created what appears to be a current consensus, based on the 'what works' literature (McGuire, 1995, 2002, 2008), that cognitive–behavioural treatments are the most effective and such treatments and programmes dominate the offender treatment and rehabilitation scene internationally (Box 3.4). The variation between offending behaviour programmes is more one of type of offending or type of 'criminogenic need' being targeted (sex offending, violent behaviour, anger problems, cognitive and problem-solving deficits, substance misuse) rather than of fundamental theoretical orientation. In the main, offender treatment theorists and clinicians are confident that programme features associated with good outcomes have been identified, including the principles of risk, need, responsivity, professional discretion and programme integrity (Andrews & Bonta, 2006), and that the task has become one of ensuring that such principles do govern programme design and implementation.

These principles have only recently begun to influence forensic mental health services (Howells *et al*, 2004), where a different culture appears to have existed, apparently uncomfortable with and even inimical to 'correctional' ways of working. Arguably, DSPD is the area of forensic mental health services in which most progress has been made in building offending behaviour programme principles into the service, even though DSPD integrated treatment approaches are still at an early stage of development. Certainly, risk and needs assessment are a major component of the

---

Box 3.4 What works: principles identified in the literature on offender programmes

Risk principle: the intensity of treatment offered should be proportional to the risk of future serious offending

Needs principle: effective treatment targets 'criminogenic needs', that is, factors shown to predict future offending

Responsivity principle: the manner of delivery of the programme should be consistent with the characteristics and abilities of the group being treated

Professional discretion: professional over-ride is necessary in some treatment decisions

Programme integrity: the extent to which the programme is conducted in practice as intended in theory and design

(McGuire, 1995, 2002, 2008)

assessment programme in DSPD services, just as they are in correctional programmes. It should be noted, however, that the risk principle in offender rehabilitation relates to treatment 'dosage'; that is, ensuring that those posing higher risk receive more intensive treatment. Those admitted to DSPD services are already shown to pose a high risk; therefore, the focus of risk assessment needs to be the identification of dynamic risk factors that need to be addressed as treatment targets.

The challenge of treating people with DSPD is that both a personality disorder and an offending behaviour focus are required. Individuals need to change not only dysfunctional aspects of their personality, but also the dynamic needs that lead them to offend: their so-called criminogenic needs. Addressing both personality disorder and offending behaviour raises serious issues of how the different theoretical models underlying personality disorder and offending can be made compatible, for the benefit of both staff and the offender/patient. How, for example, could a psychodynamic view of personality disorder be married with a cognitive–behavioural view of offending behaviour?

Offending behaviour treatments in DSPD or similar units should, in principle, focus on the same criminogenic needs as would programmes with any other high-risk offenders in the criminal justice system (National Collaborating Centre for Mental Health, 2009). Such programmes would typically include sexual offending, anger and violence, substance misuse, and cognitive skills and problem-solving. The Chromis programme (HM Prison Service, 2005) and the Violence Reduction Program (Wong, 2004) are two credible and sophisticated programmes of this sort undergoing trial in DSPD services. For a clinical account of typical therapeutic programmes, see those described in Tennant & Howells (2010). For opposing views of programme effectiveness see Tyrer *et al* (2010) and Howells *et al* (2011).

The exact nature of the previous offences committed by people admitted to DSPD units is beginning to be determined. Severe sexual and violent offending appear to be common, both as index offences and as previous behaviour (Sheldon & Krishnan, 2009). In planning treatments for such offending, it would be foolish to ignore the considerable scientific literature that now exists in relation to understanding and treating these forms of behaviour (Marshall *et al*, 1999; Polaschek & Collie, 2004; McGuire, 2008). A sceptic might make the rejoinder that such knowledge and treatments are based on 'mentally normal' offenders and are hence not relevant to mentally disordered offenders, particularly those with personality disorders. This argument is unconvincing for several reasons. First, it is probable that many of the thousands of offenders who have been treated in such programmes would indeed meet the criteria for personality disorder were they to be assessed. We know that personality disorders are very common in offender groups, but that formal screening for them is rare. Second, what evidence is available suggests that the criminogenic needs (dynamic risk factors) of 'mentally normal' and mentally disordered offenders are largely the same (Bonta *et al*, 1998). This provides a prima facie case for delivering offender

45

programmes for sexual and violent offending (and programmes addressing other criminogenic factors, such as substance misuse and poor cognitive skills) to people with DSPD.

The essential requirement, of course, is that the responsivity principle is observed (Andrews & Bonta, 2006), that is, that the style of delivery of these programmes, and to a degree their content, are modified to make them suitable for participants who have personality disorders, in the same way that offender programmes would have to be modified for people with intellectual difficulties or distinctive ethnic or cultural needs (Day, 2003). Understanding the difficulties that people with DSPD are likely to experience in completing offending behaviour programmes and then modifying the programmes to accommodate their needs are important tasks for the future (Tennant & Howells, 2010).

Despite the dissemination of 'what works' offender treatment programmes around the world, in recent years critiques have begun to emerge that might suggest a need to broaden and refine the approach. Such critiques are very pertinent to the development of DSPD treatments in that the new approaches advocated require intensive, individually focused therapeutic efforts which are difficult to deliver in typical offender programmes within the criminal justice system. The approaches are feasible in DSPD settings, as these environments generally have the requisite high levels of clinical and staffing resources and were designed for intensive and prolonged treatment. In one such critique, Thomas-Peter (2006) points to the dangers in 'what works' programmes of narrowness of therapeutic expertise, the fragmentation of knowledge and the 'disaggregation' of the individual into a series of unconnected problems. From this perspective, a more integrated and holistic approach to offender treatment is required.

Although such criticisms would not be accepted by all advocates of offender programmes, the difficulty of 'disaggregating' participants in therapy and the necessity to address their criminogenic attributes and any other clinical needs in a holistic way is being increasingly recognised. Ward & Brown's critique of the offender treatment literature from the 'good lives' perspective points in the same direction (Ward & Brown, 2004; Ward & Maruna, 2007). The question of how programmes addressing the criminogenic and non-criminogenic problems of offenders should be sequenced is an important one.

Challenges in the implementation of treatment for DSPD or similar groups in the future

It is common in new initiatives such as the DSPD programmes, or any reconfigured services for this population in the future, to witness a gap between theories and expectations before implementation and the harsh realities of the implementation phase. In this section we wish to address some of the challenges that inhabit the gap.

The reluctant patient

Low engagement in therapeutic programmes and failure to complete them are vital issues in the treatment and rehabilitation of offenders, of mentally disordered offenders and of patients admitted to DSPD services. Non-completion of therapy is particularly evident in individuals with personality disorder (McMurran *et al*, 2010). The potential consequences of low engagement are many and include diminished staff morale, poor institutional support for programmes and poor treatment outcomes.

There have been many attempts to explain low engagement. Low motivation, resistance and low responsivity are terms sometimes used to explain it but all of these are problematic. In recent years, we have seen the suggestion in the literature that such concepts be subsumed under the term (low) treatment readiness (Ward *et al*, 2004; Day *et al*, 2010). For a review of the applicability of the concept of low treatment readiness to offenders with personality disorders see Day *et al* (2010). Clinical observation suggests that these individuals are very commonly 'unready' for treatment, in part because of their internal characteristics (beliefs, emotional reactions, identities and behavioural deficits that undermine engagement and the forming of a therapeutic alliance) and in part because of external, situational influences, such as perceived coercion into treatment. Some preliminary work on treatment readiness in a DSPD population (Sheldon *et al*, 2010) has begun to define the nature of treatment readiness in this group, indicating that not all patients are poorly engaged and that the great majority complete the therapeutic programmes they are offered. In this study, negative cognitive beliefs about the self (low self-efficacy) and about the programmes and staff (low trust) characterised those who failed to complete.

It follows that the assessment and modification (when low) of readiness should be a vital task in services for people with DSPD. Clinical evaluation of readiness is particularly relevant at three points: at the point of referral, when the patient/offender is being assessed for suitability for admission; shortly after admission, when there is a clinical need to understand the person's perceptions of and expectations about treatment; and as part of treatment planning and monitoring.

Maintaining staff morale and a positive therapeutic environment

Preserving a cohesive and optimistic therapeutic environment can be challenged by the aggression, self-harm and sexually abusive behaviour that is sometimes shown by in-patients or prisoners with psychopathic and personality disorders in DSPD and similar units. These behaviours can disrupt achievement of therapeutic objectives. There is the risk that perpetrators will be denied access to certain programmes or therapeutic activities or that other patients may be reluctant to attend programmes with them because of a fear of victimisation. Staff resources can be directed away from the provision of therapy to the management of disruptive patients. A tense and hostile therapeutic milieu is to be avoided because it is likely to distract patients from treatment tasks and to erode staff persistence, confidence and optimism about therapeutic programmes.

In DSPD units, or similar units in the future, structure is required to ensure that patients experience a sense of predictability about the environment and of safety and support while participating in the lengthy therapeutic process. The demands and stresses of living in long-term detention are many, even in the best planned of units, particularly for patients who have limited coping resources. Providing a structured and safe environment has to be balanced with ensuring that it is not so contrived that any therapeutic gains cannot be generalised to more normal settings. Thus, measurement and monitoring of the therapeutic environment is as important as conventional monitoring of the patient's progress. In recent years, promising methods have become available for assessing whether environments are therapeutic, as perceived by both patients and staff (Howells *et al*, 2009).

'Does it work?'

Three relatively independent types of evaluation are critical in relation to treatment programmes for DSPD: evaluation of regime, evaluation of specific component treatments and evaluation of programme quality. The first is predicated on the fact that DSPD services are more than the sum of particular treatment programmes. As discussed above, patients in DSPD units live in a structured and highly regulated institutional environment, in most cases for several years at least. The therapeutic climate of DSPD units is likely to vary, as are ways of relating to patients and managing their behaviour. The aggregate of all these general and specific programme factors constitutes the regime and it is important to establish whether that regime is more effective in bringing about change, both clinical and criminogenic, than another regime. An important evaluation, for example, though not one that would be easy to conduct, is whether forensic hospital DSPD regimes are more effective than prison-based ones. There would be major obstacles to randomisation of allocation to hospitals *v.* prisons. A regime evaluation would require measurement of the non-specific aspects of therapeutic environments such as the therapeutic climate (Campling *et al*, 2004; Howells *et al*, 2009) and would need to include important longer-term outcomes such as effective resettlement and recidivism reduction.

An evaluation of component treatments is a different matter. The question here is whether a particular treatment (e.g., dialectical behaviour therapy) is more effective than no treatment or an alternative treatment. Given that patients with DSPD are likely to receive multiple, sequential interventions, it will be difficult to test whether any one treatment affects long-term outcomes such as resettlement and reconviction, as the study would be confounded by the other treatments received.

Randomised controlled trials (RCTs) are clearly relevant to both types of evaluation mentioned above. Although the importance of RCTs is widely supported, and their absence in relation to personality disorder, particularly personality disorder associated with violent offending, widely lamented, the fact that RCTs are not the only method for gaining knowledge about treatment effectiveness is increasingly acknowledged (Bloom *et al*, 2003; Davies *et al*, 2007). Sophisticated methods now exist for controlled evaluations of single cases in the form of 'single-case designs' (Bloom *et al*, 2003). The traditional bugbears of single-case methods have been, first, their perceived vulnerability to threats to internal validity, that is, to the possibility that the treatment effect observed in a particular patient (e.g., improvement in control of aggression) may be attributable to factors other than the treatment itself. Second, they appear also vulnerable to a major threat to external validity in the form of uncertain generalisability of findings from the individual to a larger group of patients. Both of these potential weaknesses are addressed to some extent in contemporary versions of single-case methodology (Bloom *et al*, 2003). Davies *et al* (2007) have suggested that the conditions prevailing in DSPD services are particularly suited to the requirements of single-case methods, particularly the need for prolonged pre-treatment baselines and for intensive observation through baseline, intervention and follow-up phases.

The third type of treatment evaluation is that of the quality of the programme. Quality control of treatment programmes – accreditation, programme checklists, integrity checks and so on – is common in offender treatment programmes in criminal justice systems. In England and Wales, Canada and New Zealand, for example, offender programmes must pass rigorous standards, typically in the form of accreditation requirements. Systematic evaluation of programmes against such criteria is less common in forensic mental health settings, for a variety of reasons (Howells *et al*, 2004). One reason for the difference is likely to be that forensic mental health professionals, because of the limited knowledge base in the literature, are less sure of which critical programme features are associated with good outcomes, whereas offender programme professionals have a stronger sense of 'what works' in offender rehabilitation (McGuire, 2002; Hollin & Palmer, 2006).

Evaluation of treatment is likely to remain a priority within the reconfigured DSPD treatment services. For a more detailed discussion of evaluation issues in DSPD and similar populations, the reader should consult a review by Langton (2007).

The above challenges are only a few of those met by mental health professionals and managers in DSPD services. Managing expectations of referring agencies, government departments and the broader community and ensuring that staff with appropriate training and expertise can be recruited and retained are also formidable tasks, though they are tasks that are now being addressed nationally (Personality Disorder Institute, 2009). As people with DSPD begin to move through the forensic mental health and criminal justice systems, attention will be increasingly and inevitably focused on effectively managing the transition from high secure to medium secure and ultimately to community services (Duggan, 2007; Tetley *et al*, 2011).

The development of DSPD services was a response to the realisation that the needs of this important group of people were not well understood and that suitable therapeutic services were lacking. The early years of DSPD services have seen the evolution of clinical expertise and 'know how' (Tennant & Howells, 2010; Howells *et al*, 2011). The dissemination and broader application of such expertise to the larger group of people who meet the current criteria for DSPD (or any similar criteria to come) but are not offered services is an important priority for the future.

In conclusion, the DSPD initiative has been a controversial one throughout its relatively brief history and a marked diversity of views continues to exist as to its achievements and future shape and direction. Tyrer *et al* (2010) have expressed the most sceptical view in the recent literature, while Howells *et al* (2011) have pointed to the lessons learned in practice in treating this group of people and to the evolving scientific and clinical understanding of high-risk offenders with personality disorders and of their treatment needs. Future services, whose nature is currently under discussion and review, will need to take heed of what has been learned and to build constructively on research and clinical findings and evolving clinical expertise.

References

Alwin, N., Blackburn, R., Davidson, K., *et al* (2006) *Understanding Personality Disorder: A Report by the British Psychological Society*. British Psychological Society.

American Psychiatric Association (1994) *Diagnostic and Statistical Manual of Mental Disorders (4th edn) (DSM-IV)*. APA.

Andrews, D. A. & Bonta, J. (2006) *Psychology of Criminal Conduct* (4th edn). Anderson Publishing.

Banerjee, P. J. M., Gibbon, S. & Huband, N. (2009) Assessment of personality disorder. *Advances in Psychiatric Treatment*, **15**, 389–397.

Bateman, A. & Fonagy, P. (1999) Effectiveness of partial hospitalization in the treatment of borderline personality disorder: a randomized controlled trial. *American Journal of Psychiatry*, **156**, 1563–1569.

Bloom, M., Fischer, J. & Orme, J. G. (2003) *Evaluating Practice: Guidelines for the Accountable Professional (4th edn)*. Allyn & Bacon.

Bonta, J., Hanson, K. & Law, M. (1998) The prediction of criminal and violent recidivism among mentally disordered offenders: a meta-analysis. *Psychological Bulletin*, **123**, 123–142.

Campling, P., Davis, S. & Farquharson, G. (eds) (2004) *From Toxic Institutions to Therapeutic Environments: Residential Settings in Mental Health Services*. Gaskell.

Davies, J., Howells, K. & Jones, L. (2007) Evaluating innovative treatments in forensic mental health: a role for single-case methodology? *Journal of Forensic Psychiatry and Psychology*, **18**, 353–367.

Day, A. (2003) Reducing the risk of re-offending among Australian indigenous offenders. What works for whom? *Journal of Offender Rehabilitation*, **37**(2), 1–16.

Day, A., Casey, S., Ward, T., *et al* (2010) *Transitions to Better Lives: Offender Readiness and Rehabilitation*. Willan publishers.

Department of Health, Home Office & HM Prison Service (2004) *Dangerous and Severe Personality Disorder (DSPD) High Security Services: Planning and Delivery Guide*. Home Office.

D'Silva, K., Duggan. C. & McCarthy, L. (2004) Does treatment really make psychopaths worse? A review of the evidence. *Journal of Personality Disorders*, **18**, 163–177.

Duggan, C. (2007) To move or not to move – that's the question! Some reflections on the transfer of DSPD patients in the face of uncertainty. *Psychology, Crime and Law*, **13**, 113–122.

Duggan, C., & Howard, R. C. (2009) The 'functional link' between personality disorder and violence: a critical appraisal. In *Personality, Personality Disorder and Risk of Violence* (eds M. McMurran & R. Howard), pp. 19–37. John Wiley & Sons.

Fazel, S. & Danesh, J. (2002) Serious mental disorder in 23000 prisoners. A systematic review of 62 surveys. *Lancet*, **359**, 545–550.

Hare, R. (1991) *Manual for the Hare Psychopathy Checklist – Revised*. Multi-Health Systems.

Harris, G., Rice, M. & Cormier, C. (1994) Psychopaths: is the therapeutic community therapeutic? *Therapeutic Community*, **15**, 283–299.

Hart, S., Cox, D. & Hare, R. (1995) *The Hare PCL:SV Psychopathy Checklist: Screening Version*. Multi-Health Systems.

Hemphill, J., Hare, R. & Wong, S. (1998) Psychopathy and recidivism: a review. *Legal and Criminological Psychology*, **3**, 139–170.

HM Prison Service (2005) *Chromis Manuals*. Offending Behaviour Programme Unit.

Hollin, C. R. & Palmer, E. J. (2006) Offending behaviour programmes: controversies and resolutions. In *Offending Behaviour Programmes. Development, Application, and Controversies* (eds C. R. Hollin & E. J. Palmer, pp. 247–278. John Wiley & Sons.

Howells, K., Day, A. & Thomas-Peter, B. (2004) Treating violence: forensic mental health and criminological models compared. *Journal of Forensic Psychiatry and Psychology*, **15**, 391–406.

Howells, K., Tonkin, M., Milburn, C., *et al* (2009) The EssenCES measure of social climate: a preliminary validation and normative data in UK high secure hospital settings. *Criminal Behaviour and Mental Health*, **19**, 308–320.

Howells, K., Jones, L., Harris, M., *et al* (2011) The baby, the bathwater and the bath itself: a response to Tyrer *et al.*'s review of the successes and failures of dangerous and severe personality disorder. *Medicine, Science and the Law*, **51**: 129–133.

Jones, L. (2010) Case formulation with personality disordered offenders. In *Using Time, Not Doing Time: Practitioner Perspectives on Personality Disorder and Risk* (eds A. Tennant & K. Howells), pp. 45–62. Wiley-Blackwell.

Langton, C. M. (2007) Assessment implications of 'What Works' research for Dangerous and Severe Personality Disorders service evaluations. *Psychology, Crime and Law*, **13**, 97–112.

Leichsenring, F. & Leibing, E. (2003) The effectiveness of psychodynamic therapy and cognitive behaviour therapy in the treatment of personality disorders: a meta-analysis. *American Journal of Psychiatry*, **160**, 1223–1232.

Livesley, W. J. (2001) Commentary on reconceptualizing personality disorder categories using trait dimensions. *Journal of Personality*, **69**, 277–286.

Livesley, W. J. (2007) The relevance of an integrated approach to the treatment of personality disordered offenders. *Psychology, Crime and Law*, **13**, 27–46.

Marshall, W. L., Anderson, D. & Fernandez, Y. (1999) *Cognitive Behavioural Treatment of Sex Offenders*. John Wiley & Sons.

McGuire, J. (ed.) (1995) *What Works: Reducing Reoffending*. John Wiley & Sons.

McGuire, J. (ed.) (2002) *Offender rehabilitation and Treatment: Effective Programmes and Policies to Reduce Re-Offending*. John Wiley & Sons.

McGuire, J. (2008) A review of effective interventions for reducing aggression and violence. *Philosophical Transactions of the Royal Society B: Biological Sciences*, **363**, 2577–2597.

McMurran, M. (2008) Personality disorders. In *The Handbook of Forensic Mental Health* (eds K. Soothill, P. Rogers & M. Dolan), pp. 375–399. Willan Publishing.

McMurran, M., Huband, N. & Overton, E. (2010) Non-completion of personality disorder treatments: A systematic review of correlates, consequences, and interventions. *Clinical Psychology Review*, **30**, 277–287.

National Collaborating Centre for Mental Health (2009) *Antisocial Personality Disorder: The NICE Guideline on Treatment, Management and Prevention (NICE Clinical Guideline 77)*. British Psychological Society & Royal College of Psychiatrists.

Nunes, K. L., Firestone, P., Bradford, J. L., *et al* (2002) A comparison of modified versions of the Static-99 and the Sex Offender Risk Appraisal Guide (SORAG). *Sexual Abuse: A Journal of Research and Treatment*, **14**, 253–269.

Perry, J. C., Banon, E. & Ianni, F. (1999) Effectiveness of psychotherapy for personality disorders. *American Journal of Psychiatry*, **156**, 1312–1321.

Personality Disorder Institute (2009) Implementation of the Knowledge and Understanding Framework. Personality Disorder Institute (http://www.personalitydisorder.org.uk/2009/11/kuf-implementation).

Polaschek, D. L. L. & Collie, R. M. (2004) Rehabilitating serious violent adult offenders: an empirical and theoretical stocktake. *Psychology, Crime and Law*, **3**, 321–334.

Powis, B. (2002) *Offenders' Risk of Serious Harm. A Literature Review (Occasional Paper 81)*. Home Office.

Sheldon, K. & Krishnan, G. (2009) Clinical and risk characteristics of patients admitted to a secure hospital-based dangerous and severe personality disorder unit. *British Journal of Forensic Practice*, **11**(3), 19–27.

Sheldon, K., Howells, K. & Patel, G. (2010) An empirical evaluation of reasons for non-completion of treatment in a dangerous and severe personality disorder unit. *Criminal Behaviour and Mental Health*, **20**, 129–143.

Tennant, A. & Howells, K. (eds) (2010) *Using Time, Not Doing Time: Practitioner Perspectives on Personality Disorder and Risk*. Wiley-Blackwell.

Tetley, A. C., Evershed, S. & Krishnan, G. (2011) The transition from high secure, to medium secure, services for people with personality disorder: patients and clinicians experiences. *Journal of Forensic Psychiatry and Psychology*, **22**, 321–339.

Thomas-Peter, B. A. (2006) The modern context of psychology in corrections: influences, limitations and values of 'what works'. In *Psychological Research in Prisons* (ed. G. J. Towl), pp. 24–39. BPS Blackwell.

Thornton, D. (2002) Constructing and testing a framework for dynamic risk assessment. *Sexual Abuse: A Journal of Research and Treatment*, **14**, 139–153.

Thornton, D., Mann, R., Webster, S., *et al* (2003) Understanding and managing sexually coercive behaviour. *Annals of the New York Academy of Science*, **989**, 225–235.

Tyrer, P., Mitchard, S., Methuen, C., *et al* (2003) Treatment rejecting and treatment seeking personality disorders: Type R and Type S. *Journal of Personality Disorders*, **17**, 263–268.

Tyrer, P., Coombs, N., Ibrahimi, F., *et al* (2007) Critical developments in the assessment of personality disorder. *British Journal of Psychiatry*, **190** (suppl. 49), s51–s59.

Tyrer, P., Duggan, C., Cooper, S., *et al* (2010) The successes and failures of the DSPD experiment: the assessment and management of severe personality disorder. *Medicine, Science and the Law*, **50**, 95–99.

Verheul, R., Van Den Bosch, L. M. C., Koeter, M. W. J., *et al* (2003) Dialectical behaviour therapy for women with borderline personality disorder: 12-month, randomised clinical trial in The Netherlands. *British Journal of Psychiatry*, **182**, 135–140.

Ward, T. & Brown, M. (2004) The good lives model and conceptual issues in offender rehabilitation. *Psychology, Crime & Law*, **10**, 243–257.

Ward, T. & Maruna, S. (2007) *Rehabilitation*. Routledge.

Ward, T., Day, A., Howells, K., *et al* (2004) The multifactor offender readiness model. *Aggression and Violent Behavior*, **9**, 645–673.

Warren, F., Preedy-Fayers, K., McGauley, G., *et al* (2003) *Review of Treatments for Severe Personality Disorder*. Home Office.

Webster, C. D., Douglas, K. S., Eaves, D., *et al* (1997) *HCR-20: Assessing Risk for Violence (Version 2)*. Simon Fraser University, Forensic Psychiatric Services Commission of British Columbia.

Wong, S. (2004) *The Violence Reduction Program*. Correctional Services Canada.

Wong, S. C. P. & Gordon, A. (1999) *Manual for the Violence Risk Scale (Version 2)*. Regional Psychiatric Centre (Prairies) & University of Saskatchewan.

World Health Organization (1997) *International Personality Disorder Examination (IPDE Manual)*. American Psychiatric Publishing.

CHAPTER 4

Are you looking at me? Understanding and managing paranoid personality disorder

Andrew Carroll

Summary Paranoid personality disorder is a neglected topic in clinical psychiatry, and is often the subject of diagnostic confusion and therapeutic pessimism. This chapter presents a summary of the key diagnostic issues relating to paranoid personality disorder and describes various psychological and social processes mooted to be central to the genesis of paranoid thinking and behaviours. The evidence relating to paranoid personality disorder and risk of violence is summarised and clinically useful guidance for the safe treatment of people with the disorder is outlined.

Trust is central to the relationship between doctor and patient. An important skill in psychiatry, therefore, is the ability to relate to and effectively treat patients in whom the capacity for trust is diminished as a consequence of psychopathology. The focus of this chapter is paranoid personality disorder, a condition in which mistrust of other people is the cardinal feature. It is not an uncommon disorder, with a prevalence in community samples of around 1.3% (Torgersen, 2005), rising to up to 10% in psychiatric out-patient samples (Bernstein *et al*, 1993). Despite this, the research base on the disorder remains relatively sparse (Bernstein & Useda, 2007).

Diagnosis

Clarifying the diagnosis of a patient with paranoid thinking is an essential first step to management, with ramifications for prognosis, treatment and medico-legal issues such as involuntary treatment or criminal responsibility. The DSM-IV-TR criteria for paranoid personality disorder (American Psychiatric Association, 2000) have been criticised for underrepresenting the typical affective and interpersonal features of the disorder, features that give a richer sense of the typical presentation (Bernstein & Useda, 2007) (Box 4.1).

Box 4.1   Paranoid personality disorder: DSM v. Bernstein & Useda

Summarised DSM-IV-TR criteria (American Psychiatric Association, 2000)

- Extreme distrust of others from an early age
- Bearing persistent grudges
- Preoccupation with suspicions that others want to harm or deceive them
- Belief that sexual partners are unfaithful
- Reluctance to confide for fear of malicious use of information given
- Perception of innocent incidents as threatening

Primary traits identified by Bernstein & Useda (2007)

- Mistrust/suspiciousness
- Antagonism/aggressiveness
- Introversion/excessive autonomy
- Hypersensitivity
- Hypervigilance
- Rigidity

As with all personality disorders, diagnosis is dependent on longitudinal evidence that maladaptive features of feeling, thinking and behaving are enduring over time. Collateral data are thus essential to demonstrate that the features are not confined to particular situations (such as clinical encounters) and that they have been in evidence since adolescence or early adulthood. The most likely differential diagnoses (Box 4.2) are discussed in the remainder of this section.

Box 4.2   The most likely differential diagnoses

- Normality
- Other personality disorders
  - Schizoid
  - Schizotypal
  - Avoidant
  - Narcissistic
  - Antisocial
  - Comorbidity
- Anxiety disorders
  - Social phobia
  - Social anxiety
  - Panic disorder
- Depression
- Delusional disorder
- Other psychotic illnesses
  - Schizophrenia
  - Chronic organic psychoses
  - Substance-induced psychoses
  - Brief reactive psychoses

Normality

A normal response to unusual circumstances should always be considered as part of the differential diagnosis of a patient with features suggestive of paranoid personality disorder. Features of personality disorders in general can be considered as extreme, maladaptive variants of normal traits (Widiger & Frances, 2002). Dimensional rather than categorical analysis seems especially applicable to paranoid thinking: 'one person's paranoia is another's due caution, and one person's trust is another's gullibility [...] normal development entails learning that "not everyone who seems trustworthy is trustworthy" ' (Blaney, 1999: p. 343). Suspiciousness may be adaptive in certain environments, and determining how much interpersonal trust is appropriate in a given situation may indeed be a 'vexing judgemental dilemma' (Kramer, 1998). Members of minority groups, in particular, may show defensive thinking that is understandable in the broader social context rather than being indicative of mental disorder (see later).

An epidemiological study of a community sample in New Zealand found that 12.6% demonstrated at least some paranoid features (Poulton et al, 2000), and nearly half of American college students report experiences of paranoid thinking (Ellett et al, 2003). Thus, many people manifest mistrust and suspicion from time to time but because these phenomena are transient, modifiable and not significantly disruptive, they are not pathological.

Clinically significant paranoid thinking may therefore best be conceptualised as an overgeneralised form of a common and adaptive psychological process which, in its normal form, has some evolutionary value by facilitating the detection of threats to the self by other people. Conceptual models that emphasise continuity (although not equivalence) with normality may be helpful when attempting to engage people with paranoid personality disorder in treatment.

Other personality disorders

People with other personality disorders may show clinical features that superficially resemble those of paranoid personality disorder.

Schizoid personality disorder

Schizoid personality disorder is characterised by social withdrawal. However, individuals with the disorder are indifferent to other people, not desiring interpersonal contact, rather than being suspicious of them, as in paranoid personality disorder.

Schizotypal personality disorder

This disorder is characterised by a degree of suspiciousness of other people, but also involves distinct oddities of belief and thinking quite different from those seen in paranoid personality disorder.

Avoidant personality disorder

As with paranoid personality disorder, avoidant personality disorder is characterised by a degree of mistrust of other people and consequent social withdrawal. The difference is that the avoidant person is much less ready to see malevolence in other people; their problem is that they lack confidence and believe that they themselves will perform inadequately in social situations.

Narcissistic personality disorder

Narcissistic personality disorder is characterised by an overly inflated sense of entitlement and grandiosity. Generally, there is preoccupation with the need for praise rather than overwhelming suspiciousness of others' intent. Nevertheless, paranoid features redolent of paranoid personality disorder may emerge under stress (Young *et al*, 2003).

Antisocial personality disorder

The key characteristic of antisocial personality disorder is recurrent transgression of others' rights. Individuals with paranoid personality disorder may harm others as part of what they view as revenge or even as a pre-emptive strike. It may be difficult, however, to distinguish the *post hoc* rationalisations of antisocial individuals for their interpersonally harmful behaviours from genuinely paranoid thinking about the malevolent intent of the victims.

Borderline personality disorder

People with borderline personality disorder may develop stress-related paranoid ideation and anger, but, unlike in paranoid personality disorder, these are not enduring features.

Comorbid disorders

Comorbidity of paranoid personality disorder with other personality pathology is common, occurring in more than half of cases (Widiger & Trull, 1998). In forensic populations, antisocial personality disorder is commonly comorbid with paranoid personality disorder (Blackburn & Coid, 1999).

Anxiety disorders

Paranoid personality disorder may initially present with anxiety complaints, but careful mental state examination will reveal the underlying paranoid core features. There is some overlap with anxiety disorders such as social phobia and social anxiety: both may entail social withdrawal and concerns about others' evaluation of the self. The crucial distinction is that in paranoid personality disorder there is a perception of planned harm to self by malevolent others, not merely a preoccupation with negative events in the future or with exposure to public scrutiny. Comorbidity may occur: one study (Reich & Braginsky, 1994) suggests that over half of those with paranoid personality disorder also suffer from panic disorder.

Depression

There is a complex relationship between mood and paranoid thinking. Depressive disorders may present with paranoid symptomatology, often with the underlying theme that the persecution by others is in some way deserved: so-called 'bad-me paranoia' (Chadwick *et al*, 2005). A careful longitudinal history will distinguish the disorders; if clear symptoms and signs of a depressive illness are present, these need to be vigorously treated before a diagnosis of paranoid personality disorder can be made with any confidence.

Delusional disorder

In practice, delusional disorder is generally the most problematic differential diagnosis. By definition, people with paranoid personality disorder do not display persistent psychotic symptoms, whereas delusional disorder is a condition characterised by persistent non-bizarre delusions in the absence of other features of a psychotic illness. This distinction, however, merely begs the question of how to distinguish delusions from the intensely held, idiosyncratic (sometimes called 'overvalued') ideas of a person with paranoid personality disorder. One key distinction is the degree to which reality testing is impaired: in paranoid personality disorder, individuals can at least entertain the possibility that their suspicions are unfounded or that they are overreacting, whereas a diagnosis of delusional disorder is likely warranted when beliefs of persecution are held with incorrigible conviction, resulting in extensive effects on behaviour (Skodol, 2005). To further complicate the issue, delusional disorder may emerge gradually or it may be associated with a precipitating stressful event against a background of a vulnerable paranoid personality, although this is by no means always the case (Blaney, 1999).

In practice, mental health clinicians often disagree about specific cases, and the reliability with which individuals manifesting paranoid behaviour can be differentially classified has not been empirically determined (Haynes, 1986). Genetic studies have similarly been unable to disentangle delusional disorder from paranoid personality disorder (Winokur, 1985), although it now appears that both disorders are probably genetically distinct from schizophrenia (Asarnow *et al*, 2001; Cardno & McGuffin, 2006).

This diagnostic problem can be viewed as part of a wider debate about the boundaries of psychosis, and the resurgent idea that psychotic symptoms are best conceptualised as dimensional phenomena on a continuum with normal experiences (Claridge, 1997; van Os *et al*, 2000; Bentall & Taylor, 2006). In his classic paper, Strauss (1969) suggested four criteria for determining the threshold into clinical psychotic illness:

- the degree of conviction regarding the objective reality of the unusual experience
- the degree to which a cultural or stimulus determination of the experience is absent
- the amount of time spent preoccupied with the experience
- the implausibility of the experience.

Others (Claridge, 1997) have emphasised that the key distinction is not simply the level of symptoms but rather the degree of functional impairment that they cause.

The distinction is challenging and is of more than mere academic interest, having clear clinical implications. Except at times of severe decompensation, people with personality disorders are generally not appropriate candidates for coercive treatment nor, if their behaviour leads to offending, do they generally qualify for consideration of a criminal defence based on lack of criminal responsibility. Those diagnosed with delusional disorder, however, may be candidates for involuntary treatment and may be considered as lacking criminal responsibility should they offend as a result of their disorder (Bronitt & McSherry, 2005).

Although this differential diagnosis will never be easy, the distinction will be assisted by a carefully documented history and chronology of the development of the patient's paranoid thinking, as well as a careful mental state examination.

Other psychotic illnesses

Schizophrenic illnesses must be considered in the differential diagnosis of paranoid personality disorder; the presence of persisting psychotic symptoms and other features of schizophrenia will generally make this differential clear. Other psychotic illnesses that may present with paranoid features include:

- chronic organic psychoses such as those developing in the wake of dementia;
- substance-induced psychoses: be aware, however, that individuals with paranoid personality disorder may well also misuse substances and develop such disorders;
- brief reactive psychoses secondary to acute stressors (Munro, 1999): again, comorbidity may occur and a paranoid personality disorder may confer vulnerability to such brief psychotic episodes (Miller *et al*, 2001), particularly in the context of acute stress such as drastic environmental change (e.g. imprisonment, migration, induction to the military).

Psychological processes

An understanding of paranoid thinking and behaviour in general can assist the clinician in understanding and treating someone with paranoid personality disorder. Although most models have focused on a single specific process, in reality it seems likely that multiple cognitive, behavioural and social processes are usually involved, and these interact and become mutually reinforcing. Thus, the mechanisms discussed below (based on studies involving participants with a variety of paranoid disorders) should not be viewed as exclusive, competing theories but rather as descriptions of various possible alternative pathways to paranoia, the relative importance of each varying between and within individuals over time.

Cognitive biases

People with high levels of paranoid thinking have an externalising personal attributional bias: a tendency to explain negative events in their life by blaming others rather than reflecting on their own potential contribution to circumstances (Bentall *et al*, 2001; Bentall & Taylor, 2006). The normal self-serving bias, whereby negative events are attributed to external circumstances, is exaggerated and distorted (Campbell & Sedikides, 1999), being skewed towards other people and their supposed malevolent intent. There is a corresponding tendency to underuse contextual information when explaining negative outcomes (Gilbert *et al*, 1988).

Bentall & Taylor (2006) suggest that this attributional bias is a psychological defence against underlying low self-esteem, activated when there is perceived threat to the individual's positive view of themselves. Although there is some evidence that self-esteem is generally low in individuals with paranoia in both clinical (Garety & Freeman, 1999) and non-clinical samples (Martin & Penn, 2001; Ellett *et al*, 2003; Combs & Penn, 2004), the relationship between self-esteem, paranoid thinking and behaviour is complex. As mentioned earlier, there is evidence, for example, of subgroups with particularly low self-esteem and low mood who feel the perceived persecution to be justified – 'bad-me paranoia' (Chadwick *et al*, 2005). In such cases it may be that the supposed defence of external attribution of blame is only partially successful in warding off depressive feelings.

Information processing factors

In general, attributions that invoke contextual situational factors require more information and more cognitive resources than external personal attributions. As cognitive load increases, people tend to use external 'paranoid' personal attributions as a kind of default option (Gilbert *et al*, 1988). This may relate to the mooted association between paranoid disorders and brain damage (Munro, 1988). Similarly, perceptual deficits that reduce the availability of relevant social information, most notably in the realm of impaired hearing, have long been associated with increased risk of paranoid thinking (Thewissen *et al*, 2005).

More subtle functional impairments that affect social skills have been linked to paranoia. Deficits in emotional and social perception tasks have been associated with social anxiety and subclinical paranoia (Combs &

Penn, 2004). Paranoid thinking has also been linked to deficits in 'theory of mind': the ability to understand the intentions and mental states of others (Kinderman *et al*, 1998). This may contribute to difficulties in constructing situational (as opposed to personal) attributions for negative social interactions, since failure to understand another's viewpoint may encourage personal attributions. For example, if a colleague passes a person in the street without greeting them, a failure to understand that the colleague may, for example, have been distracted by worry (a situational attribution) may encourage the personal attribution that the colleague is rude.

The hypervigilance of individuals with paranoia appears to be related to an attentional bias whereby they are more likely to both notice and remember (and hence ruminate on) threat-related information. This processing bias that has been demonstrated in both clinical (Garety & Freeman, 1999) and non-clinical (Combs & Penn, 2004) populations.

Interpersonal processes

In 'normal' populations, certain kinds of social situation appear to encourage paranoid thinking. Such situations are likely to severely exacerbate the pathological behaviour and thinking of those with pre-existing paranoid personality traits. A model based on a review of such social effects (Kramer, 1998) proposes that particular social situations are more likely to be appraised in such a way as to lead to 'dysphoric self-consciousness'; this in turn leads to hypervigilance and rumination, and activation of paranoid cognitive biases and behaviours. These may exacerbate the feelings of self-consciousness, and hence feed a vicious cycle (Fig. 4.1). Specific situations that predispose to such cycles include:

- feeling different from the rest of the social group, for example because of gender, ethnicity or level of experience

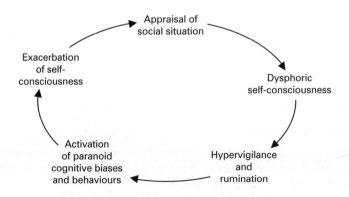

Fig. 4.1 The cycle of dysphoric self-consciousness.

- feeling under the evaluative scrutiny of other people with more power, for example professional seniors
- a sense of uncertainty regarding social status, for example when new to a group.

Similarly, others (Mirowsky & Ross, 1983; Haynes, 1986) have emphasised that paranoid thinking is likely to emerge in situations involving:

- sudden social loss or isolation
- acute disruption of usual social networks
- exposure to environments in which previous social skills may not be useful, for example immigration or imprisonment
- acute sensory deficits
- actual powerlessness and victimisation.

Paranoid personality disorder, by definition, implies enduring features that will be evident even in the absence of such circumstances. However, an understanding of how paranoid thinking can be engendered by such situations not only helps to predict when the features of paranoid personality disorder are likely to become more apparent, but also assists in the differential diagnosis between paranoid personality disorder and normal responses to extraordinary circumstances.

The spiral of escalating paranoia

These various cognitive, behavioural and social processes may become mutually reinforcing, leading to malignant spirals of escalating paranoia and making therapeutic change particularly difficult to effect (Box 4.3). The following self-perpetuating processes are commonly active in those with paranoid personality disorder.

First, it is generally possible to find evidence of malign intent in at least some people some of the time: this is readily taken as confirmatory evidence that the person was 'right all along' to be suspicious. Conversely, apparently benign behaviour in others can be interpreted as a 'front' or as 'trickery'.

Second, it is logically impossible to prove a negative, for example for a spouse to prove that he or she is not having an affair. The very absence of evidence can be interpreted as confirmation of a 'cover up'.

Box 4.3 The self-perpetuating processes of paranoia

- The reality of malign intent in some situations
- The logical impossibility of proving a negative
- Self-fulfilling reciprocal determinism
- The fact that social withdrawal inhibits feedback

Third, people with paranoid personality disorder are generally socially withdrawn, and when they engage in interpersonal encounters they show a tendency to be hypervigilant and suspicious. This may put others off approaching someone with the disorder and may even cause them to be hostile and exclusionary of that person. Such scenarios may confirm the person's suspicions and exacerbate their isolation – a self-fulfilling prophecy termed 'reciprocal determinism' (Haynes, 1986). This dynamic can be seen in querulant persistent complainers, who become increasingly unreasonable in their dealings with organisations and generally elicit progressively more hostile and negative treatment from those in authority (Mullen & Lester, 2006).

Finally, this persistent social withdrawal disrupts social feedback and hence there may be few challenges to the world-view of someone with paranoia: it is difficult to learn from experience that people can be trusted if interpersonal experiences simply never occur.

Hence, paranoid thinking and behaviour can be remarkably resistant to change – a self-sustaining, self-defeating cycle (Kramer, 1998).

The risk of violence

In light of their tendency to view other people's actions as hostile, it would appear obvious that individuals with paranoid personality disorder would be at increased risk of interpersonal violence. Most research data derive from samples with paranoid features that often fall short of a diagnosable paranoid personality disorder and are generally present in combination with other significant risk factors. Therefore, although there is convergent evidence that paranoid traits do indeed increase the risk of violence, it should not be assumed that an individual with paranoid personality disorder is necessarily at high risk of such behaviour.

In cross-sectional studies, paranoid personality features have been associated with histories of both violent (Mojtabai, 2006) and antisocial behaviours in general (Berman et al, 1998), even when antisocial and borderline pathology are statistically controlled for. Similarly, high levels of delinquency in teenagers have been associated with paranoid features such as feeling mistreated, victimised, betrayed and the target of false rumours (Krueger et al, 1994). A large American longitudinal study (Johnson et al, 2000) found that paranoid traits in adolescence predicted violence and criminal behaviour in later adolescence and early adulthood, even after controlling for various possible confounding variables.

In non-clinical populations, a meta-analysis (Bettencourt et al, 2006) concluded that the personality feature of high rumination, which would be expected in paranoid personality disorder, is associated with a tendency to show aggressive behaviour, but only under provoking conditions. This suggests that violence in people with paranoid features generally requires some level of provocation. Note, however, that owing to their various distortions in thinking and perceiving, the threshold for feeling provoked may be abnormally low. Another study (Johnson *et al*, 2000) found that paranoid symptoms were associated with initiating physical fights. There is also ample evidence that specific suspicions about the fidelity of intimate partners, commonly seen as a feature of paranoid personality disorder, are associated with an increased risk of threatening and initiating violence against the partner and others (Mullen, 1995).

Pathways to violence in paranoia

There are various possible explanations for the increased risk of violence in those displaying paranoid thinking. Contemporary models of aggression (Anderson & Bushman, 2002) emphasise the role of biases in cognitive processing, regulation of affect and social information processing. Those with paranoid biases tend to perceive situations to be more provocative than is warranted and to view the world as hostile and threatening; their often fragile self-esteem and their sensitivity to social status may render them hypersensitive to perceived challenges to status as well as to personal safety. Hence, an individual with paranoia may be motivated to engage in both retaliatory and pre-emptive violent strikes on others (Berman *et al*, 1998). They are also likely to be both highly suspicious and unforgiving of perceived attacks, tending to ruminate on the past transgressions of others; such tendencies to bear grudges may also increase their risk of violence. In addition, the 'malignant spiral' discussed earlier, whereby hostility is readily evoked in others by the suspicious, odd behaviour of people with paranoia, may well increase the likelihood that they will encounter actual hostile behaviour from others, which in turn would further increase the likelihood of aggression.

Comorbid disorders are of particular importance when assessing and managing the risk of violence in an individual with paranoia. The combination of a paranoid tendency to see others as threatening with low internal constraints against violence (for example, as part of an antisocial personality structure) is particularly concerning (Blackburn & Coid, 1999). Similar considerations may apply when acute mental illness supervenes in paranoid personality disorder, resulting in lowered inhibitory thresholds for violent behaviour because of psychotic, mood or anxiety symptoms (Kennedy *et al*, 1992; Buchanan *et al*, 1993; Taylor, 1998; Hodgins *et al*, 2003).

As well as violence, paranoid personality features have been associated with other problem behaviours, including stalking (Mullen *et al*, 2000), the uttering of threats (MacDonald, 1963) and abnormal complaining behaviours (Mullen & Lester, 2006).

Treatment of paranoid personality disorder

None of the possible treatments for paranoid personality disorder has been subjected to randomised control trials. Notwithstanding this, the condition should not be viewed as untreatable and there is a degree of consensus with respect to general principles when attempting to safely manage the disorder (Gabbard, 2000; also see Chapter 6, this volume) (Box 4.4).

General principles

Differential diagnosis and comorbid conditions

As discussed above, diagnostic formulation, including consideration of comorbid personality pathology and/or mental illness, is critical in understanding and managing paranoid personality disorder.

Treatment aims

Appropriate long-term treatment goals (Bernstein & Useda, 2007) include helping the patient to:

- recognise and accept their own feelings of vulnerability
- increase their feelings of self-worth
- develop a more trusting view of others
- verbalise their distress, rather than use counterproductive strategies such as shunning or intimidating others.

As with all personality disorders, progress is likely to be slow – some suggest that at least 12 months may be required before determining whether treatment is effective (see Chapter 13, this volume).

Countertransference

Patients with paranoid personality disorder are likely to engender strong countertransference feelings of defensiveness and even aggression in the clinician. Clinicians should avoid reactive counterattacks, as they would probably result in disengagement or even violence. Conversely, they should also beware of minimising the risk of violence because of overoptimism or simple denial, particularly with female patients. They should be open and firm when necessary, and explain why decisions have been made, particularly decisions that may be unwelcome. Resistance should be expected.

Sensitivity to rejection and to authority

Patients with paranoid features are likely to be brought to treatment by others rather than referring themselves. Coercive treatment is generally neither ethically nor legally justified in the absence of comorbid mental illness. It is possible to engage those with paranoid personality disorder in meaningful treatment but a forceful or duplicitous approach is unlikely to bear fruit. The clinician should avoid arousing suspicion: for example, the patient should be informed if contact occurs between different clinicians involved in their care. The source of information contained in the file (whether it is derived from the patient or someone else) should be clearly stated. It is important to help the patient to save face and feel that they have some control over their life and their treatment.

Box 4.4 Treatment of paranoid personality disorder

General principles for the clinician
- Carefully consider differential diagnosis and comorbidity
- Have realistic treatment aims
- Maintain awareness of own feelings
- Take special care regarding the patient's sensitivity to rejection and to authority
- Take care with boundary management
- Monitor the patient's mood symptoms

Psychotherapy
- Generally most useful: the Beck model of cognitive therapy for paranoid personality disorder
- For severe disorder: psychosocial residential treatment with psychotherapy
- With limited evidence base: individual supportive dynamic psychotherapy and schema therapy

Pharmacotherapy
- There is no established drug treatment
- Comorbid conditions should be treated as appropriate

Boundary management

Paranoid individuals may be particularly prone to misunderstanding a clinician's acts of kindness or words of encouragement as a cover for more malevolent intentions. An overly 'warm' therapeutic style is therefore not indicated. Close physical contact, or even overly close seating, should be avoided. An individual with paranoia is likely to require more than the usual amount of body space. In general, group therapy should be avoided (Gabbard, 2000).

Mood symptoms

The clinician should be alert to changes in the patient's mood. For patients who successfully engage in treatment, an understandable sadness (and possibly suicide risk) may emerge as they develop insight into how their paranoid behaviours have isolated them. Antidepressant medication should be considered if there is clinical evidence of an emergent depressive illness.

Psychotherapy

Residential psychosocial treatment with psychotherapy may bring about long-term gains in functioning for individuals with severe personality disorders, including those with paranoid features (Chiesa & Fonagy, 2003). Individual supportive dynamic psychotherapy (Gabbard, 2000) and schema therapy (Young *et al*, 2003) have also been advocated for paranoid personality disorder.

Possibly the most useful for the general psychiatrist, however, is Beck and colleagues' model of cognitive therapy for paranoid personality disorder (Beck *et al*, 2004). The basic tenet is that clinical paranoia can be construed as a systematised and overgeneralised form of an ordinary adaptive psychological process. The core cognitive schema is posited to concern feelings of inadequacy, and so the initial aim of therapy is to enhance the individual's sense of self-efficacy, while openly accepting that they will be mistrusting of clinical intervention, particularly in the early stages. In parallel with this, social skills such as assertion, communication and empathy can also be enhanced. In the longer term, the tendency to attribute blame is challenged and modified, with the aim of terminating the malignant spirals involved. Specific targets might therefore include the beliefs that other people are always malicious and deceptive, or that it is necessary to be constantly on the look-out for threats. The technique of collaborative empiricism, whereby therapist and patient jointly examine the patient's beliefs in the light of objective evidence, may be useful. In this process, the possibility that the patient's suspicions regarding others may contain a kernel of truth should be acknowledged if appropriate (Bernstein & Useda, 2007).

Pharmacotherapy

The role of pharmacotherapy in pure paranoid personality disorder is not well established. If such disorders are viewed as existing on a spectrum with a delusional disorder (Kendler & Gruenberg, 1982) then it might be reasonable to try an antipsychotic medication (Grossman, 2004). However, no such medications are currently formally licensed for this indication.

Obviously, comorbid conditions such as depression and anxiety disorders, or emerging psychotic illnesses, may require appropriate medication.

Conclusion

A certain degree of suspiciousness with respect to the intentions of others is normal, particularly in certain social situations. However, such thinking may be maladaptive and pathological in extent. Paranoid features are found in a variety of contexts: in previously healthy individuals subjected to abnormal stress; in mental illness; and in those with personality disorders, most notably in paranoid personality disorder. Although empirical data regarding paranoid personality disorder are limited, an understanding of underlying psychological processes and adherence to certain management principles can assist psychiatrists in assessing and treating this challenging and disabling condition.

References

American Psychiatric Association (2000) *Diagnostic and Statistical Manual of Mental Disorders (4th edn, text revision) (DSM-IV-TR)*. APA.

Anderson, C. A. & Bushman, B. J. (2002) Human aggression. *Annual Review of Psychology*, **53**, 27–51.

Asarnow, R. F., Nuechterlein, K. H., Fogelson, D., *et al* (2001) Schizophrenia and schizophrenia-spectrum personality disorders in the first-degree relatives of children with schizophrenia: the UCLA Family Study. *Archives of General Psychiatry*, **58**, 581–588.

*Beck, A. T., Freeman, A. & Davis, D. D. (2004) Paranoid personality disorder. In *Cognitive Therapy of Personality Disorders (2nd edn)* (eds A. T. Beck, A. Freeman, D. D. Davis). Guilford Press.

Bentall, R. P., Corcoran, R., Howard, R., *et al* (2001) Persecutory delusions a review and theoretical integration. *Clinical Psychology Review*, **21**, 1143–1192.

*Bentall, R. P. & Taylor, J. L. (2006) Psychological processes and paranoia: implications for forensic behavioural science. *Behavioral Sciences and the Law*, **24**, 277–294.

Berman, M., Fallon, A. E. & Coccaro, E. F. (1998) The relationship between personality psychopathology and aggressive behavior in research volunteers. *Journal of Abnormal Psychology*, **107**, 651–658.

*Bernstein, D. P. & Useda, J. D. (2007) Paranoid personality disorder. In *Personality Disorders: Toward the DSM-V* (eds W. O'Donohue, K. A. Fowler & S. O. Lilienfield). Sage Publications.

Bernstein, D. P., Useda, J. D., Siever, L. J. (1993) Paranoid personality disorder: review of the literature and recommendations for DSM-IV. *Journal of Personality Disorders*, **7**, 53–62.

Bettencourt, B. A., Talley, A., Benjamin, A. J., *et al* (2006) Personality and aggressive behavior under provoking and neutral conditions: a meta-analytic review. *Psychological Bulletin*, **132**, 751–777.

Blackburn, R. & Coid, J. (1999) Empirical clusters of DSM-III personality disorders in violent offenders. *Journal of Personality Disorders*, **13**, 18–34.

Blaney, P. (1999) Paranoid conditions. In *Oxford Textbook of Psychopathology* (eds T. Millon, P. Blaney & R. D. Davis). Oxford University Press.

Bronitt, S. & McSherry, B. (2005) Mental state defences. In *Principles of Criminal Law* (2nd edn) (eds S. Bronitt & B. McSherry). Thomson LBC.

Buchanan, A., Reed, A., Wessely, S., *et al* (1993) Acting on delusions: II. The phenomenological correlates of acting on delusions. *British Journal of Psychiatry*, **163**, 77–81.

Campbell, W. K. & Sedikides, C. (1999) Self-threat magnifies the self-serving bias: a meta-analytic integration. *Review of General Psychology*, **3**, 23–43.

Cardno, A. G. & McGuffin, P. (2006) Genetics and delusional disorder. *Behavioral Sciences and the Law*, **24**, 257–256.

Chadwick, P. D. J., Trower, P., Juusti-Butler, T. M., *et al* (2005) Phenomenological evidence for two types of paranoia. *Psychopathology*, **38**, 327–333.

Chiesa, M. & Fonagy, P. (2003) Psychosocial treatment for severe personality disorder: 36-month follow-up. *British Journal of Psychiatry*, **183**, 356–162.

Claridge, G. (1997) Final remarks and future directions. In *Schizotypy: Implications for Illness and Health* (ed. G. Claridge). Oxford University Press.

Combs, D. R. & Penn, D. L. (2004) The role of subclinical paranoia on social perception and behavior. *Schizophrenia Research*, **69**, 93–104.

Ellett, L., Lopes, B. & Chadwick, P. (2003) Paranoia in a nonclinical population of college students. *Journal of Nervous and Mental Disease*, **191**, 425–430.

Gabbard, G. O. (2000) Cluster A personality disorders. In *Psychodynamic Psychiatry in Clinical Practice* (ed. G. O. Gabbard). American Psychiatric Press.

Garety, P. A. & Freeman, D. (1999) Cognitive approaches to delusions: a critical review of theories and evidence. *British Journal of Clinical Psychology*, **38**, 113–154.

Gilbert, D. T., Pelham, B. W., Krull, D. S. (1988) On cognitive busyness: when person perceivers meet persons perceived. *Journal of Personality and Social Psychology*, **54**, 733–740.

Grossman, R. (2004) Pharmacotherapy of personality disorders. In *Handbook of Personality Disorders* (ed. J. J. Magnavita). John Wiley & Sons.

Haynes, S. N. (1986) A behavioral model of paranoid behaviors. *Behavior Therapy*, **17**, 266–287.

Hodgins, S., Hiscoke, U. L. & Freese, R. (2003) The antecedents of aggressive behavior among men with schizophrenia: a prospective investigation of patients in community treatment. *Behavioral Sciences and the Law*, **21**, 523–546.

Johnson, J. G., Cohen, P., Smailes, E., *et al* (2000) Adolescent personality disorders associated with violence and criminal behavior during adolescence and early adulthood. *American Journal of Forensic Psychiatry*, **157**, 1406–1412.

Kendler, K. S. & Gruenberg, A. M. (1982) Genetic relationship between paranoid personality disorder and the 'schizophrenic spectrum'. *American Journal of Psychiatry*, **139**, 1185–1186.

Kennedy, H. G., Kemp, L. I. & Dyer, D. E. (1992) Fear and anger in delusional (paranoid) disorder: the association with violence. *British Journal of Psychiatry*, **160**, 488–492.

Kinderman, P., Dunbar, R. I. & Bentall, R. P. (1998) Theory-of-mind deficits and causal attributions. *British Journal of Psychology*, **89**, 191–204.

*Kramer, R. M. (1998) Paranoid cognition in social systems: thinking and acting in the shadow of doubt. *Personality and Social Psychology Review*, **2**, 251–275.

Krueger, R. F., Schmutte, P. S., Caspi, A., *et al* (1994) Personality traits are linked to crime among men and women: evidence from a birth cohort. *Journal of Abnormal Psychology*, **103**, 328–338.

MacDonald, J. M. (1963) The threat to kill. *American Journal of Psychiatry*, **120**, 125–130.

Martin, J. A. & Penn, D. L. (2001) Brief report: social cognition and subclinical paranoid ideation. *British Journal of Clinical Psychology*, **40**, 261–265.

Miller, M. B., Useda, J. D., Trull, T. J., *et al* (2001) Paranoid, schizoid and schizotypal personality disorders. In *The Comprehensive Handbook of Psychopathology (3rd edn)* (eds H. E. Adams & P. B. Sutker). New Plenum.

Mirowsky, J. & Ross, C. E. (1983) Paranoia and the structure of powerlessness. *American Sociological Review*, **48**, 228–239.

Mojtabai, R. (2006) Psychotic-like experiences and interpersonal violence in the general population. *Social Psychiatry and Psychiatric Epidemiology*, **41**, 183–190.

Mullen, P. (1995) Jealousy and violence. *Hong Kong Journal of Psychiatry*, **5**, 18–24.

*Mullen, P. E. & Lester, G. (2006) Vexatious litigants and unusually persistent complainants and petitioners: from querulous paranoia to querulous behaviour. *Behavioral Sciences and the Law*, **24**, 333–349.

Mullen, P., Pathe, M. & Purcell, R. (2000) *Stalkers and their Victims*. Cambridge University Press.

Munro, A. (1988) Delusional (paranoid) disorders: etiologic and taxonomic considerations. I. The possible significance of organic brain factors in etiology of delusional disorders. *Canadian Journal of Psychiatry*, **33**, 171–174.

Munro, A. (1999) Reactive and cycloid psychoses: the acute and transient psychotic disorders. In *Delusional Disorders: Paranoia and Related Illnesses* (ed. A. Munro). Cambridge University Press.

Poulton, R., Caspi, A., Moffitt, T. E., *et al* (2000) Children's self-reported psychotic symptoms and adult schizophreniform disorder. *Archives of General Psychiatry*, **57**, 1053–1058.

Reich, J. & Braginsky, Y. (1994) Paranoid personality traits in a panic disorder population: a pilot study. *Comprehensive Psychiatry*, **35**, 260–264.

Skodol, A. E. (2005) Manifestations, clinical diagnosis, and comorbidity. In *The American Psychiatric Publishing Textbook of Personality Disorders* (eds J. M. Oldham, A. E. Skodol & D. S. Bender). American Psychiatric Publishing.

*Strauss, J. S. (1969) Hallucinations and delusions as points on continua function. *Archives of General Psychiatry*, **21**, 581–586.

Taylor, P. J. (1998) When symptoms of psychosis drive serious violence. *Social Psychiatry and Psychiatric Epidemiology*, **33**, S47–S54.

Thewissen, V., Myin-Germeys, I., Bentall, R. P., *et al* (2005) Hearing impairment and psychosis revisited. *Schizophrenia Research*, **76**, 99–103.

Torgersen, S. (2005) Epidemiology. In *The American Psychiatric Publishing Textbook of Personality Disorders* (eds J. M. Oldham, A. E. Skodol & D. S. Bender). American Psychiatric Publishing.

*van Os J., Hanssen, M., Bijl, R. V., et al (2000) Strauss (1969) revisited: a psychosis continuum in the normal population? *Schizophrenia Research*, **45**, 11–20.

Widiger, T. A. & Frances, A. J. (2002) Toward a dimensional model for the personality disorders. In *Personality Disorders and the Five-Factor Model of Personality (2nd edn)* (eds P. T. Costa & T. A. Widiger). American Psychological Association.

Widiger, T. A. & Trull, T. J. (1998) Performance characteristics of the DSM-III–R personality disorder criteria sets. In *DSM-IV Sourcebook* (eds T. A. Widiger, A. J. Frances, H. A. Pincus, *et al*). American Psychological Association.

Winokur, G. (1985) Familial psychopathology in delusional disorder. *Comprehensive Psychiatry*, **26**, 241–8.

Young, J., Klosko, J. & Weishaar, M. (2003) *Schema Therapy: A Practitioner's Guide*. Guilford Press.

*Publications of particular interest for further reading.

CHAPTER 5

Personality disorder in older people: how common is it and what can be done?

Aparna Mordekar and Sean A. Spence

Summary There has been little systematic study of personality disorders in older people (65 years of age and above). However, with an ageing population worldwide we should expect to find increasing numbers of people with Axis II disorders surviving into old age. With this in mind, we undertook a qualitative review of the literature concerning personality changes and disorders in older people, their prevalence and possible amelioration.

Although one's core personality is thought to remain stable over the adult years, modest variation may arise in terms of its expression with advancing age. For instance, an increase in obsessive–compulsive traits is common among older people and may reflect not so much a change in intrinsic personality as an adaptation of the person to failing powers or altered relationships and environments (Engels *et al*, 2003). The neurological substrate of reduced adaptability has also been variously investigated in the context of cerebrovascular pathology (Stone *et al*, 2004) and falling levels of central neurotransmitters (e.g. dopamine; Volkow *et al*, 1998).

Personality disorder (Box 5.1) is a controversial concept, but the diagnosis remains pertinent in older people, provided that a suitable account of long-standing dysfunction can be established that pre-dates presentation. In simple terms, personality disorder may be construed as a long-standing pattern of maladaptive interpersonal behaviour (Kroessler, 1990). So, although it might be considered very late for the condition to present in old age (perhaps marking the culmination of many unhappy events for the individual), there might at least be the advantage of a considerable longitudinal history and pattern of behaviour for the examiner to investigate at the time of assessment.

Diagnosing personality disorders in older people is confounded by factors that are less likely to be present in younger age groups (Box 5.2).

Box 5.1 Diagnostic categories of personality disorder

DSM-IV (American Psychiatric Association, 1994)

Cluster A: 'eccentric'

- Paranoid
- Schizoid
- Schizotypal

Cluster B: 'flamboyant'

- Antisocial
- Borderline
- Histrionic
- Narcissistic

Cluster C: 'anxious'

- Avoidant
- Dependent
- Obsessive–compulsive

ICD-10 (World Health Organization, 1992)

- Paranoid
- Schizoid
- Dissocial
- Emotionally unstable
- Histrionic
- Anankastic
- Anxious
- Dependent

Prevalence

There are relatively few prevalence data concerning personality disorders in older people, yet ICD-10 asserts that such disorders are stable and enduring over time (World Health Organization, 1992: p. 200). Hence, by inference, personality disorder 'should' be seen among this stratum of the population. However, as age advances, certain 'problem' behaviours associated with personality disorder (e.g. impulsivity, aggression, promiscuity, fighting and law-breaking) might be expected to decline in frequency, while comorbid psychiatric disorders might enhance the expression of other dysfunctional traits: there is, for instance, a predominance of social withdrawal and major depressive and dysthymic disorders among older people (Devanand, 2002).

Box 5.2 Barriers to diagnosis

- Lack of co-informant
- Co-informant with little knowledge of patient's early life
- Unreliable patient and/or co-informant
- Cognitive impairment of patient and/or co-informant
- Co-informant's characteristics (e.g. shame, minimisation, embarrassment, guilt) that affect their account
- Severe physical illness in patient
- Axis I and Axis II similarities, e.g. paranoid personality disorder v. paraphrenia; dissocial personality v. frontotemporal dementia

The prevalence of personality disorder among older people in the community has been estimated to be about 10% (Abrams & Horowitz, 1996). Among older in-patients, personality disorder has been described in 6% of those with organic mental disorders and 24% of those with major depressive disorder (Kunik *et al*, 1994). Cluster C personality disorders (mainly the anxious and dependent types) were the most common. Patients with early-onset depression are more likely to exhibit personality dysfunction, mainly avoidant, dependent and 'not otherwise specified' (Kunik *et al*, 1994; Abrams & Horowitz, 1996). There is also some evidence that among older patients with major depressive disorder, personality disorder is associated with a recurrent pattern of (depressive) illness (Kunik *et al*, 1994). A study of 76 older people with dysthymia found 31% (24) to have personality disorder. Of these, 17% (4) had obsessive–compulsive personality disorder, 12% (3) had avoidant personality disorder and 5% (1) had borderline personality disorder (Devanand *et al*, 2000).

As alluded to above, there is thought to be a reduction with age in certain dissocial behaviours and a possible decline in cluster B personality disorders. If true, such a decrease might be attributable to:

- a reduction in dramatic behaviour intrinsic to ageing
- age-related neurobiological changes that affect the manifestation of dissocial conduct
- increasing physical incapacity, reducing the ability to 'act out'
- population attrition through death by suicide or other behaviours connected with personality disorder (e.g. recklessness)
- omission from studies of older people with antisocial personality disorder who are in prison or forensic psychiatric hospitals (Fazel *et al*, 2001)
- a cohort effect, whereby older age groups derive from cohorts who had lower (pre-existing) levels of personality disorder than their younger comparators.

It is also possible that the natural history of the disorder is one of gradual improvement. Certainly, there is an anecdotal belief that certain personality disorders, for example borderline personality disorder, may 'burn out' with age. Indeed, the outcome of the latter is generally better than may be routinely acknowledged (Stone, 1993). Two-thirds are clinically well at follow-up, although they may retain mild residual symptoms (Stone *et al*, 1987). One study found that only a quarter of people with an initial diagnosis of borderline personality disorder retained this full diagnosis at long-term follow-up (Zanarini *et al*, 2003). As the individual ages, it seems that impulsivity resolves first; next to improve is interpersonal functioning, and affective symptoms are the last to reduce or disappear.

Personality disorder among older prisoners in England and Wales has been studied by Fazel *et al* (2001). The prevalence was 34% (in total), with avoidant and antisocial categories contributing most (8.3% each), followed by anankastic (7.9%), schizoid (6.4%) and paranoid (3.4%).

Personality disorder as a risk factor for abuse

If someone has a difficult personality, does this place them at increased risk of abuse as they become older and perhaps infirm? Of the potential risk factors for elder abuse identified by the House of Commons Health Committee (2004), social isolation and a poor relationship with a carer might reflect personality difficulties; others, however, relate more to the perpetrator than the victim, for example dependence of the abuser on the person they abuse and a history of mental health problems, personality disorder, or drug and alcohol problems in the abuser. Although the public perception might be that older people are at greater risk of abuse in residential and nursing care, over two-thirds of elder abuse happens in the victims' own homes (Fig. 5.1).

Older people with anxious and dependent personality disorders are particularly prone to abuse (Kurrle *et al*, 1991), as are those undergoing organic personality change (Hansberry *et al*, 2005). This may be because of their disinhibition, inability to communicate and/or lack of decisional capacity.

Comorbidity associated with personality disorder

Personality disorder is often associated with an Axis I psychiatric disorder, and this may compound problems for the potential patient and their carer(s). The link between depression and personality disorder seems well established (Devanand, 2002). Also, many patients with late-onset schizophrenia have never married, live alone and may have exhibited abnormal premorbid personality traits (Fuchs, 1999).

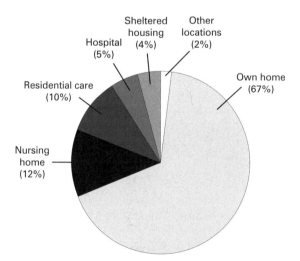

Fig. 5.1 Place of residence of people subjected to elder abuse in the UK (House of Commons Health Committee, 2004).

Affective disorder

Consistent data suggest a strong relationship between personality disorder and depression (Box 5.3). In one study (Kunik *et al*, 1994), the rate of personality disorder with comorbid major depression was 24%. In older people with personality disorder, there is a high rate (73%) of adult-onset rather than late-onset (geriatric) depression (45%) (Camus *et al*, 1997).

In a sample of older patients with dysthymic disorder, only a minority had a comorbid personality disorder, mainly the obsessive–compulsive or avoidant subtypes (Devanand *et al*, 2000).

Anxiety disorder

Anxiety is a frequent concomitant of depression. Individuals with cluster C personality disorders seem more prone to developing anxiety disorder, phobias and acute stress disorder. A study of personality disorder in 347 patients with anxiety disorder reported that the most common subtypes were avoidant (13%), obsessive–compulsive (11%) and dependent (8%) (Sanderson *et al*, 1994).

Somatisation disorder

Somatoform disorders are common in older adults and are complicated by the frequency of concurrent physical illness. A community cross-sectional study found that patients who presented with somatisation were more likely to be depressed (Bogner *et al*, 2009). Improvement in hypochondriacal complaints with treatment, yet persistence of less intense hypochondriacal concerns after remission, suggests that these features may represent an admixture of state and trait phenomena in elderly people with depression (Kramer-Ginsburg *et al*, 1989).

Substance misuse

Certain personality disorders, especially those in clusters B and C, are more likely to involve problem alcohol use. In a study by Speer & Bates (1992), it was found that older people are more likely to have the 'triple diagnosis' of personality disorder, alcohol dependence and depression.

Diogenes syndrome

Some people consider Diogenes syndrome to be an end stage of personality disorder. It refers to extreme self-neglect, unaccompanied by a medical or psychiatric condition sufficient to account for the condition. It can be seen as the response of someone with a particular personality type to old age and loneliness. It might also be a reaction to stress in older people with certain personality characteristics, such as the schizotypal or anankastic (Rosenthal *et al*, 1999).

Box 5.3   Personality disorder and depression: a case example

A 69-year-old widow was referred for depressive symptoms following social stressors (a son had emigrated). She had shown little response to antidepressants prescribed by her general practitioner. It transpired that she had withheld information regarding contact with psychiatric services in early adult life for recurrent self-harm (lacerations to her wrists). Placing her recent stressors in the context of her longer-term problems helped her to adjust (she had experienced separations before and survived). Her antidepressant medication was adjusted and she received follow-up with the community mental health team. Her depression responded well and she lived independently in her own home.

Dementia

Of course, personality changes occur in organic disorders even if they are not classified as personality disorder. Changes such as apathy and dysphoria have been described in Alzheimer's disease (Landes *et al*, 2005). Frontotemporal dementia is characterised by personality changes such as lack of insight, apathy and disinhibition. Not all individuals experience such change, but in those that do, three patterns have been reported: change at the onset of dementia; ongoing change with disease progression; and change into disturbed behaviour (Petry *et al*, 1989). Carers often describe personality changes such as becoming 'out of touch', reliant on others, childish, irritable, unreasonable, unhappy, cold and cruel (Wattis, 1998). Some of these features may be attributable to organic changes, whereas others are a reaction to dementia. It is also possible that the dementing process 'releases' underlying behavioural propensities that the individual may have been better able to control when well.

Management of personality disorder

The literature on the management of personality disorder in older people is very sparse: the basic principles are listed in Box 5.4. However, as

---

Box 5.4   Principles of treating personality disorder in older people

- Form a therapeutic alliance
- Treat any comorbid Axis I disorder
- Adopt a consistent approach
- Use supportive cognitive psychotherapy
- Establish good links with other professionals
- Involve significant others where possible

---

mentioned earlier, personality disorder is commonly accompanied by an Axis I disorder, and judicious treatment of the latter may ameliorate certain aspects of the personality disturbance.

Role of medication in treatment

Medications are often used to treat the functional illnesses comorbid with personality disorders. The mainstays of pharmacological treatment of depressive disorders are obviously the antidepressants. However, because of the frailty and physiological changes that occur with age, they are often started at low doses and increased slowly. The most commonly used antidepressants are the selective serotonin reuptake inhibitors (SSRIs), owing to their safer side-effect profile and less frequent interactions with other medications. Kunik *et al* (1994) reported that older in-patients both with and without personality disorder who had major depression benefitted equally from treatment, primarily antidepressant medication or electroconvulsive therapy (ECT) (research on the clinically important topic of ECT for depression in older in-patients with personality disorder is sparse). Conversely, Thompson *et al* (1987) found that concomitant personality disorder in older patients with major depression decreased the likelihood of response to psychotherapy.

Low-dose antipsychotic drugs are mainly used to control agitation and psychotic symptoms (Bouman & Pinner, 2002). Their appropriate use in older people has become an area of increasing debate: typical antipsychotics are generally more likely to induce extrapyramidal side-effects, but there are concerns over the safety of the atypicals in this age group (Herrmann & Lanctot, 2006). The use of minimal effective doses seems vital here (as elsewhere in medicine).

Role of psychotherapy in treatment

Some expressions of troublesome personality traits will resolve with treatment of an associated or underlying functional disorder. However, when a patient has persistent or residual symptoms of personality disorder, a consistent approach from an experienced therapist may be of benefit.

As with younger patients with personality disorder, forming a therapeutic alliance can be difficult. Supportive, dynamic and cognitive approaches may be applicable, depending on the presenting complaint. It is important to have a consistent approach, with firm boundaries and good communication between the professionals involved. It is also important to involve the carers and to modify (if appropriate and possible) their reactions to untoward behaviour (Davison, 2002).

Research suggests that the current generation of older adults are inclined to believe that talking therapy can help most people with depression and that they prefer psychological therapies to medication (Rokke & Scogin,

1995). So, although older people may be initially less inclined to discuss their psychological problems, they appear not to be resistant to the idea of psychological intervention.

Nevertheless, the theoretical study and clinical use of psychotherapies with older people have been slow to develop, mainly because of ageism, negative stereotypes about the treatability of older people and a perceived lack of psychotherapeutic theories for later life (Hepple, 2004). The predominance of organic or biological models of old age may have biased the field towards 'brain-based' rather than 'psyche-based' explanations for illnesses in old age.

Cognitive–behavioural therapy

There is some evidence to suggest that adapted cognitive–behavioural therapy (CBT) is effective in addressing negative thoughts, identifying the dysfunctional cycles that can arise and intervening in unhelpful thinking patterns of older people (Thompson *et al*, 1987). Barrowclough *et al* (2001) demonstrated the effectiveness of CBT *v.* supportive counselling for anxiety symptoms.

Evans (2007) has suggested how CBT might be modified to accommodate the degree of cognitive change and sensory and physical impairment encountered among older people.

Cognitive analytic therapy

In old age, people often face great challenges related to disability and loss – their social roles diminish and vanish, partners and friends die. These can precipitate lowered self-esteem and depression. Again, antecedent cluster C personality traits might constitute predisposing factors. Cognitive analytic therapy (CAT) can offer a coherent way of linking past and present, and may be well suited to work in later life because of its emphasis on the interpersonal and the need to find shared meaning and understanding in therapy across generational and cultural boundaries (Hepple, 2004). Cognitive analytic therapy has been applied to late-life problems of patients with narcissism, borderline personality traits and post-traumatic syndromes (Hepple & Sutton, 2004).

For a more extensive discussion of CAT, see Chapter 18, this volume.

Psychodynamic therapy

Psychodynamic therapy is at least as effective as CBT in treating depression in older people (Thompson *et al*, 1987), but the patient's age can affect the nature of the transference and countertransference. In most cases, one might anticipate that the patient will be older – perhaps by a great deal – than the therapist, and this may be worth considering at the outset, during patient allocation and supervision.

Dialectical behaviour therapy

Older people with personality disorder who become depressed have been shown to be less responsive to depression-specific therapies (Robins, 2003). In such cases, it appears that dialectical behaviour therapy may show promise (Lynch, 2000). An adaptation of behavioural therapy, dialectical behaviour therapy aims to promote change in emotion 'dysregulation' (Robins, 2003). Lynch found that it reduced interpersonal stress, hopelessness, and avoidant, detached and emotional coping strategies, and also reduced dependency on, and desire to please, others.

Supportive psychotherapy

Supportive psychotherapy may be helpful for individuals with personality disorders who manifest low self-esteem and low self-confidence; it may also assist them in problem-solving and reducing the risk of future relapses or deterioration (Bloch, 2006). Psychodynamically oriented supportive therapy may help people to strengthen their 'ego function' and promote a better adaptation to reality (Rockland, 2003). Personality changes often occur in dementia, and supportive psychotherapy may help affected patients and also provide some support for their carers (Junaid & Hegde, 2007).

Family therapy

Family therapy may help the families of people with dementia accompanied by personality change; it may be especially useful when counselling relatives before the diagnosis is revealed (Qualls, 2000). It can also inform awareness of family dynamics that are affecting the patient (Hepple, 2004).

Nidotherapy

There is growing evidence that nidotherapy may help to achieve a better fit, within the community, for younger people with personality disorders. It comprises a systematic adjustment of the environment to suit the needs of the individual (see Chapter 20, this volume). The principles of nidotherapy might be applied to an older population to facilitate better coping skills and social functioning by manipulating their physical and social environment. In my opinion, the most obvious way of doing this is to offer patients access to residential care.

Conclusion

The literature concerning personality disorder among older people is currently quite sparse. This might be because personality disorders themselves have been rather contentious and, traditionally, old age psychiatry services have tended to focus on dementia and the major Axis I disorders. However, it is likely that a greater number of patients with persistent Axis II disorders will survive into old age. Now would be a good time for psychiatric researchers to investigate the complex needs and issues associated with ageing in this group of people.

References

Abrams, R. C. & Horowitz, S. V. (1996) Personality disorders after age 50: a meta-analysis. *Journal of Personality Disorder*, **10**, 271–281.

American Psychiatric Association (1994) *Diagnostic and Statistical Manual of Mental Disorders (4th edn) (DSM-IV)*. APA.

Barrowclough, C., King, P., Colville, J., *et al* (2001) A randomised trial of effectiveness of cognitive–behavioural therapy and supportive counselling for anxiety symptoms in older adults. *Journal of Consulting and Clinical Psychology*, **69**, 756–762.

Bloch, S. (2006) Supportive psychotherapy. In *An Introduction to the Psychotherapies* (4th edn) (ed. S. Bloch), pp. 215–236. Oxford University Press.

Bogner, H. R., Shah, P. & de Vries, H. F. (2009) A cross-sectional study of somatic symptoms and the identification of depression among elderly primary care patients. *Journal of Clinical Psychiatry*, **11**, 285–291.

Bouman, W. P. & Pinner, G. (2002) Use of atypical antipsychotic drugs in old age psychiatry. *Advances in Psychiatric Treatment*, **8**, 49–58.

Camus, V., de Mendonca Lima, C. A., Gaillard, M., *et al* (1997) Are personality disorders more frequent in early onset geriatric depression? *Journal of Affective Disorder*, **46**, 297–302.

Davison, S. E. (2002) Principles of managing patients with personality disorder. *Advances in Psychiatric Treatment*, **8**, 1–9.

Devanand, D. P. (2002) Comorbid psychiatric disorders in late life. *Biological Psychiatry*, **52**, 236–242.

Devanand, D. P., Turret, N., Moody, B. J., *et al* (2000) Personality disorders in elderly patients with dysthymic disorder. *American Journal of Geriatric Psychiatry*, **8**, 188–195.

Engels, G. I., Duijsens, I. J., Haringsma, R., *et al* (2003) Personality disorders in the elderly compared to four younger age groups: a cross-sectional study of community residents and mental health patients. *Journal of Personality Disorder*, **17**, 447–459.

Evans, C. (2007) Cognitive behavioural therapy with older people. *Advances in Psychiatric Treatment*, **13**, 111–118.

Fazel, S., Hope, T., O'Donnell, I., *et al* (2001) Hidden psychiatric morbidity in elderly prisoners. *British Journal of Psychiatry*, **179**, 535–539.

Fuchs, T. (1999) Patterns of relation and premorbid personality in late paraphrenia and depression. *Psychopathology*, **32**, 70–80.

Hansberry, M. R., Chen, E. & Gorbien, M. J. (2005) Dementia and elder abuse. *Clinics in Geriatric Medicine*, **21**, 315–332.

Hepple, J. (2004) Psychotherapies with older people: an overview. *Advances in Psychiatric Treatment*, **10**, 371–377.

Hepple, J. & Sutton, L. (eds) (2004) *Cognitive Analytic Therapy in Later Life: A New Perspective on Old Age*. Brunner-Routledge.

Herrmann, N. & Lanctot, K. L. (2006) Atypical antipsychotics for neuropsychiatric symptoms of dementia: malignant or maligned? *Drug Safety*, **29**, 833–843.

House of Commons Health Committee (2004) *Elder Abuse: Second Report of Session 2003–04. Volume 1: Report, together with Formal Minutes*. TSO (The Stationery Office) (http://www.publications.parliament.uk/pa/cm200304/cmselect/cmhealth/111/11101.htm).

Junaid, O. & Hegde, S. (2007) Supportive psychotherapy in dementia. *Advances in Psychiatric Treatment*, **13**, 17–23.

Kramer-Ginsberg, E., Greenwald, B. S., Aisen, P. S., *et al* (1989) Hypochondriasis in the elderly depressed. *Journal of the American Geriatric Society*, **37**, 507–510.

Kroessler, D. (1990) Personality disorder in the elderly. *Hospital and Community Psychiatry*, **41**, 1325–1329.

Kunik, M. E., Mulsant, B. H., Rifai, A. H., *et al* (1994) Diagnostic rate of comorbid personality disorder in elderly psychiatric inpatients. *American Journal of Psychiatry*, **151**, 603–605.

Kurrle, S. E., Sadler, P. M. & Cameron, I. D. (1991) Elder abuse: an Australian case series. *Medical Journal of Australia*, **155**, 150–153.

Landes, A. M., Sperry, S. D. & Strauss, M. E. (2005) Prevalence of apathy, dysphoria and depression in relation to dementia severity in Alzheimer's disease. *Journal of Neuropsychiatry and Clinical Neurosciences*, **17**, 342–349.

Lynch, T. R. (2000) Treatment of elderly depression with personality disorder comorbidity using dialectical behaviour therapy. *Cognitive and Behavioural Practice*, **7**, 468–477.

Petry, S., Cummins, J. L., Hill, M. A., *et al* (1989) Personality alterations in dementia of Alzheimers type: three year follow up study. *Journal of Geriatric Psychiatry and Neurology*, **2**, 203–207.

Qualls, S. H. (2000) Therapy with ageing families: rationale, opportunities and challenges. *Aging & Mental Health*, **4**, 191–199.

Robins, C. (2003) Dialectical behavior therapy for borderline personality disorder. *Psychiatric Annals*, **32**, 608–616.

Rockland, L. H. (2003) *Supportive Therapy: A Psychodynamic Approach*. Basic Books.

Rokke, P. D. & Scogin, F. (1995) Depression treatment preferences in younger and older adults. *Journal of Clinical Geropsychology*, **1**, 243–257.

Rosenthal, M., Stelian, J., Wagner, J., *et al* (1999) Diogenes syndrome and hoarding in the elderly: case reports. *Israel Journal of Psychiatry and Related Sciences*, **36**, 29–34.

Sanderson, W., Wetzler, S., Beck, A., *et al* (1994) Prevalence of personality disorders among patients with anxiety disorders. *Psychiatry Research*, **51**, 167–174.

Speer, D. C. & Bates, K. (1992) Comorbid mental and substance disorders among older psychiatric patients. *Journal of the American Geriatric Society*, **40**, 886–890.

Stone, M. H. (1993) Long-term outcome in personality disorders. *British Journal of Psychiatry*, **162**, 299–313.

Stone, M. H., Hurt, S. W. & Stone, D. K. (1987) The PI–500: Long term follow-up of borderline in-patients meeting DSM-III criteria. I: Global outcome. *Journal of Personality Disorders*, **1**, 291–298.

Stone, J., Townend, E., Kwan, J., *et al* (2004) Personality change after stroke: some preliminary observations. *Journal of Neurology, Neurosurgery and Psychiatry*, **75**, 1708–1713.

Thompson, L., Gallagher, D. & Breckenridge, J. S. (1987) Comparative effectiveness of psychotherapies for depressed elders. *Journal of Consultant and Clinical Psychology*, **55**, 385–390.

Volkow, N. D., Gur, R. C., Wang, G., *et al* (1998) Association between decline in brain dopamine activity with age and cognitive and motor impairment in healthy individuals. *American Journal of Psychiatry*, **155**, 344–349.

Wattis, J. (1998) Personality disorder and alcohol dependence. In *Seminars in Old Age Psychiatry* (eds R. Butler & B. Pitt), pp. 163–179. Gaskell.

World Health Organization (1992) *The ICD-10 Classification of Mental and Behavioural Disorders: Clinical Descriptions and Diagnostic Guidelines*. WHO.

Zanarini, M. C., Frankenburg, F. R., Hennen, J., *et al* (2003) The longitudinal course of borderline psychopathology: 6-year prospective follow-up of the phenomenology of borderline personality disorder. *American Journal of Psychiatry*, **160**, 274–283.

CHAPTER 6

Management of common personality disorders in the acute setting

Leonard Fagin

Summary General principles of management of patients with personality disorders admitted in crisis are discussed. The role of the acute ward in the overall plan of care, the clinical thresholds to consider in deciding whether admission is appropriate and the main elements of the in-patient care plan are outlined. The management of patients with borderline personality disorder, who constitute the majority of such admissions, is discussed in detail, and that of patients with paranoid, antisocial and hysterical and histrionic personality disorders, who require admissions less frequently, is also assessed.

The management and treatment of personality disorders has caused considerable controversy among psychiatrists in the UK. In Chapter 11, Gwen Adshead outlines the main issues relating to the status of personality disorders as nosological entities and their treatability. Guidance from the National Institute for Mental Health in England helpfully raised many issues relating to this often-excluded group, which prevalence studies suggest constitutes 10–13% of the population (National Institute for Mental Health in England, 2003), and guidelines now exist for the treatment of cluster B disorders (Kendall *et al*, 2009; National Collaborating Centre for Mental Health, 2009). However, these reports and guidelines offer little advice about the role of the acute in-patient setting in the lifetime experiences of people with personality disorders.

The use of acute psychiatric wards in the treatment of personality disorders has been viewed as at the very least, unhelpful, and at worst, harmful. In a review of the literature on the usefulness of hospital admission for suicidal patients with borderline personality disorder, Paris (2004) concluded that there is no evidence to suggest that admission to this setting has any effect in reducing risks, has unproven benefits in terms of safety and is, in many cases, counterproductive in terms of self-harming and suicidal behaviour. Other reviews have endorsed this general conclusion.

For example Krawitz & Batcheler (2006) went so far was to say that 'A strong consensus exists that overly defensive treatment measures can actually increase the long term risk in working with adults with borderline personality disorder'.

However, several studies show more positive outcomes of hospital admission in the treatment of borderline personality disorder (e.g. Bateman & Fonagy, 1999, 2001; Chiesa et al, 2002; Vaslamatzis et al, 2004; McGowan, 2008). These have been primarily concerned with units that provide a more specialised intervention than the non-specialist and diagnostically heterogeneous environment of an acute psychiatric ward.

While the debate on specialist services for personality disorder continues, most clinicians in adult psychiatry have to face the fact that, like it or not, they may have to manage people with personality disorders in acute settings at some time, either because of crises that lead to emergency admission, or because Axis II personality disorders complicate other presentations, such as depression or schizophrenia, and require complex handling if the basic issues are to be appropriately tackled (Norton & Hinshelwood, 1996; Mulder, 2002). Hayward et al (2006) conducted a number of assessments of a group of psychiatric in-patients in a London ward and found that 54% of them met the DSM-IV criteria for personality disorder. Among in-patients with drug, alcohol and eating disorders, Moran (2002, 2005) estimated that the prevalence of personality disorders was frequently above 50% and often in excess of 70%.

My aim in this chapter is not to suggest that all personality disorders are always treatable in acute in-patient settings. Rather, I look at the resources available in those environments that can respond to the extremes of personality difficulties, both for patients admitted with this sole diagnosis in a state of crisis and for those in whom personality disorder is an added dimension of another psychiatric diagnosis. My approach is to look at the possibility of acute clinical management strategies in certain subtypes of personality disorder and, if favourable circumstances allow, to extend beyond this, incorporating a longer-term outlook. This model of care has shown promising results (Chiesa et al, 2002). Although I agree that acute in-patient units are generally unsuitable for long-term work with people with personality disorders, I concur with Norton & Hinshelwood (1996) when they state that 'an admission, whilst problematic, can be conceived as an opportunity'. In all of these presentations, the question for staff is whether the patient can embark on meaningful change in their distorted behavioural and emotional patterns in an appropriate therapeutic environment. For this to take place, staff will have to enlarge their skills base (see Chapter 12, this volume). They may also be supported and supervised by local specialist teams dedicated to the assessment, management and treatment of personality disorder (National Institute for Mental Health in England, 2003). Considerations of the views of service users (Haigh, 2002, 2006; Castillo, 2003) have highlighted stigma, lack of information, and concerns about lack of knowledge and care within professional systems.

> **Box 6.1** Principles in the treatment of personality disorders
>
> Staff should devote effort to achieving adherence to the treatment that:
> - is well structured
> - has a clear focus
> - has a theoretical basis that both staff and patient understand
> - is relatively long term
> - is well integrated with other services available to the patient, using the care programme approach as a main means of networking, communicating and reviewing plans between different elements of the service
> - involves a clear treatment alliance between staff and patient
>
> (After Bateman & Tyrer, 2002)

Management principles

Bateman & Tyrer (2002) and Davison (2002) have identified the guiding principles of effective therapy for people with personality disorders, and aspects of these can be taken into account when we envisage the role of the acute ward in the management of care (Box 6.1).

Nicholson & Carradice (2002) helpfully outline three levels of working with patients with personality disorders in the acute psychiatric setting.

The first of these is direct work, i.e. assessment and formulation of goals. This involves working with the individual (or the group), finding out as much as possible about the person's history, the circumstances that led to their admission and the involvement of the community care team.

The second level is indirect work, i.e. formal and informal liaison with staff. The clinician uses ward rounds and other contacts with ward staff, carers and community teams as opportunities to share views and feelings and discuss management issues.

The third level is strategic work. Through multidisciplinary supervision and training, and organisational support, hospitals can contribute to therapeutic aims and becomes less reactive to risk.

One of the controversial points in this area is the clinical thresholds that need to be set as indicators for in-patient admission (Bateman & Tyrer, 2002), particularly taking into account the possible deleterious effect on the patient or others of such an intervention (Box 6.2). Translated to an in-patient service, the main elements of psychiatric interventions are listed in Box 6.3.

Part of the problem created by patients with Axis II disorders is that they are, on the whole, very unpopular with staff, and therefore do not contribute to the creation of a therapeutic alliance. When a patient's role switches from that of victim to that of perpetrator, equally extreme responses can be provoked in staff, from being a 'kind defender' to a 'cruel attacker' (Norton & Dolan, 1995).

83

Box 6.2   Indicators for in-patient admission of people with personality disorders

- Crisis intervention, particularly to reduce risk of suicide or violence to others
- Comorbid psychiatric disorder such as depression or brief psychotic episode
- Chaotic behaviour endangering the patient and the treatment alliance
- Need to stabilise existing medication regimes
- Review of the diagnosis and the treatment plan
- Full risk assessment

It is essential that the in-patient unit has the capacity, in terms of skills, staffing and clinical pressures, to manage the admission

---

Not everybody can work with patients with personality disorders. Duggan (2002) has identified key competencies that help staff work effectively with these individuals. They include emotional resilience, clarity about personal and interpersonal boundaries, and ability to tolerate the intense emotional impact that these patients can have on them. Added to these is effective and regular supervision, both at individual and team level.

Box 6.3   Key elements of psychiatric intervention in an acute setting

- Informality
- Careful assessments by experienced staff, focusing on present crisis and need for containment
- Involvement of significant others, carers, relatives and other agencies in the assessment
- Early care plan, with specified goals agreed and communicated to all staff and the patient, paying special attention to perceived or real inconsistencies.
- Anticipation of crises, especially about impulsive discharge, self-harm, drug use, sexual promiscuity or aggression, and establishment of an agreed multi-disciplinary response
- A focus on immediate needs, mostly of a practical nature
- Clear boundaries regarding intolerable behaviour, including aggression, suicidal gestures, use of illicit substances or alcohol and absconding
- Effective use of in-patient groups
- Treatment of psychiatric symptoms with medication when necessary
- Staff support groups and supervision looking at countertransference reactions, particularly for junior staff, who may become overinvolved
- Early discharge arrangements when crisis has been overcome
- Readiness to discharge if goals are not met
- Referral to community or specialist services on discharge, with close and careful handover through the care programme approach
- Short duration of admission
- Consideration of comorbidity of a personality disorder if treatment for an Axis I disorder does not meet with the predictable response

---

The different characteristics of personality configurations make it impossible to state formulaic approaches to problems. Therefore, it may be prudent first to visit currently defined diagnostic categories and then, with the help of descriptive clinical pictures, to try to see whether the in-patient acute environment can contribute to their management. I here take on board the point made by a number of commentators critical of these nosological entities, but accept that for the moment they are the best we have (Coid, 2003) and, following most researchers, I have relied on the DSM-IV classification (American Psychiatric Association, 1994).

Common personality disorders in acute practice

In the rest of this chapter, I will confine myself to making a few clinical suggestions on the most common of the personality disorders likely to present in acute settings: borderline and paranoid personality disorders. I do not broach the subject of how personality issues can be dealt with when they complicate an Axis I diagnosis, although I believe that many of the points are equally valid in these circumstances. I will also address some specific issues arising in patients with other, less common personality disorders, such as schizoid, antisocial, and hysterical and histrionic types. I have not included, for brevity's sake, those with obsessive–compulsive, avoidant and dependent personality disorders, as they are very rarely admitted to hospital, but I have discussed them in an earlier version of this chapter (Fagin, 2004).

Borderline personality disorder

This group, consisting predominantly of female patients, are likely to be admitted in a crisis, usually with suicidal or self-harming intent. Borderline personality disorder has a number of recognised features:

- impulsive and sometimes manipulative self-destructive behaviour, pathological attachments tinged with dread of abandonment
- unstable self-image
- affective lability
- transient circumscribed psychotic-like or magical thinking
- overwhelming feelings of anger and feelings of entitlement.

These features make patients with the disorder most likely to present after-hours to a busy, and possibly overwhelmed, on-call junior doctor. The fears of what may happen if patients are not contained inevitably lead to admission. The patients' histories typically reveal parental rejection and abandonment, as well as sexual abuse at an early stage of development, with recent incidents of assault or neglect as triggering factors.

Patients with borderline personality disorder provoke the most extreme countertransferential feelings in staff, who will report that they feel abused and deceived (see Chapter 12, this volume). The difficulties posed by these patients when they are suicidal are particularly troublesome (Matsberger, 1999), especially if they make accusations against staff suggesting that they do not care enough, are insensitive, have lost hope or secretly wish them to die. In a culture of risk management and serious incident investigations, this may be difficult to bear. It can cause staff to feel that they have more responsibility for keeping these suicidal individuals alive than do the patients themselves, a condition which Hendin (1981) described as coercive bondage. The catch-22 is that analysis of completed suicides by patients with borderline personality disorder has shown that perceived rejection by caregivers has often been the precipitating cause (Kullgren, 1988).

These negative features should be put into context. Studies of the natural course of this illness are rare, but analyses of data on patients in contact with psychiatric services report generally good outcomes over prolonged periods of observation (Stone, 1990; Zanarini *et al*, 2010). Guidelines for services and treatment can be found in the National Institute for Health and Clinical Excellence's guideline CG78 (National Collaborating Centre for Mental Health, 2009). Difficulties arise when specialist interventions are not easily available in all districts.

The role of the acute in-patient setting

Reported clinical experience indicates that there is a role for the in-patient unit where patients are often taken in an emergency, if a graded and well-informed response can be agreed between staff and patient. The approach, however, requires good team functioning and clarity of purpose, as without these, caring for people with borderline personality disorder is likely to expose any team problems. Good leadership is also required, and in particular a good understanding of purpose between the senior nurse and the consultant psychiatrist (Piccinino, 1990). The aim is to restore to the patient a sense of responsibility and reliance on their previous good internal resources (Wester, 1991). Admissions should be brief (Nehls, 1994*a,b*), mostly to deal with the emergent problems that have precipitated the crisis. Patterns of impulsive responses and wild fluctuations in attitudes and attachments to and from staff should be witnessed and discussed. Once the emotional crisis subsides, these can be worked through in focused individual and group therapy, with an emphasis on problem-solving. A major source of argument is over the nature of response to suicidal and self-harming behaviour. Clear understanding of the meaning of that behaviour and the aims of staff response can help patients in a number of ways, for example by enabling them to:

- improve their interpersonal skills during conflicts
- increase their internal regulation of unwanted emotions
- develop skills to tolerate emotional distress until change occurs
- learn self-management (Gallop, 1992).

A difficult balance needs to be arrived at between ensuring that the patients are safe by observation, and the avoidance of collusion with their feelings of helplessness and their abdication of responsibility for their behaviour (Sederer & Thornbeck, 1986). These patients are likely to cause major rifts in the team, splitting it between those who believe the patient to be manipulative and in need of firm, controlling interventions, and those who become overprotective and tolerant beyond reasonable limits (Kaplan, 1986; O'Brien, 1998). The importance of staff discussions and support groups in these circumstances cannot be overstressed. Staff have to be prepared for regular re-admissions, and it is helpful to keep a historical perspective, looking at changes over time, as this can give hope when they feel despondent about possible eventual change when all they see are repeated similar presentations.

Discharge planning

In all of this, staff need to remember that, on discharge, these patients are likely also to be a concern for community clinicians, and that effective communication and sharing of ideas should be established between in-patient and community teams. Likewise, family members are likely to be enmeshed and entangled in the presentation and management of the in-patient admission, and sometimes contribute to splitting or undermining of coherent staff approaches. In both these scenarios, the care programme approach (CPA) meeting, where clear boundaries, expectations and responsibilities as well as contingency planning are discussed, can become a very useful tool.

As noted above, a major hurdle to be overcome in the care of patients with borderline personality disorder is the sense of hopelessness they provoke by repeated acting out, incessant demands, crossing of boundaries and weak therapeutic alliances. This leads many patients to sabotage well-prepared care plans and to present only in states of major upheaval. In this situation, the in-patient ward represents the only constancy, a safe place able to contain and hold, even if this creates an ambiguous and sometimes intolerable attachment. This contrasts with the usual experience of most people with borderline personality disorder, who have tenuous parental relationships that often end in their being abandoned to their own devices. They are in fact 'soothed' and supported by the notion that this safety net is available. Slowly, over time, many are able to take in and appreciate this approach, and to some extent take over the 'soothing' role without being precipitated into a crisis.

Another point to bear in mind is that these patients form a very heterogeneous group, and that set and inflexible responses will not always be appropriate. Sometimes patients just need to be emotionally contained, at other times supported. On occasions where risk-taking behaviour is predominant, boundaries will need to be firmly clarified and adhered to

(Rouse, 1994). Staff will have to intuit when patients are ready to benefit from some degree of confrontational and interpretative techniques. Before these can be attempted, patients need to perceive that their internal feelings are empathically validated, particularly if recent events open up old wounds relating to early childhood traumas.

Management principles

Box 6.4 summarises several of the principles of technique suggested by Gabbard (2000) that broadly apply to most patients with borderline personality disorder. These principles are enlarged in Table 6.1.

I have already indicated the difficulties that patients with borderline personality disorder pose for staff in in-patient environments. A not uncommon scenario is where patients perceive themselves to be 'special' and different from others, and therefore requiring extra attention. Or they may form a clique with other like-minded individuals, and purposefully disrupt the therapeutic milieu by sabotaging collaborative activities, undermining staff or disparaging their work in the unit. Others simply display passive resistance and go into monumental sulks. Overall, the treatment plan should aim to avoid regression and support the contention that patients can eventually restore their adaptive functions and control chaotic, self-destructive urges. Medication is used only to help people take back control over their feelings. The structure of the hospital day implies the rediscovery of order and a predictable pattern of interactive opportunities with individual staff and groups. The focus is on understanding the precipitants of the crisis, the pattern of responses and how these link up with previous traumatic experiences.

When the furore has died down, patients may be able to look at alternative ways of responding, accept the consequences of their actions, and validate remaining ego strengths and abilities. When setting limits, staff will need to be able to say 'No' without malice, explaining that this

---

Box 6.4 Principles of management of borderline personality disorder patients in in-patient units

- Maintain flexibility
- Establish conditions to make the patient safe
- Tolerate intense anger, aggression and hate
- Promote reflection
- Set necessary boundaries
- Establish and maintain the therapeutic alliance
- Avoid splitting between psychotherapy and pharmacotherapy (Table 6.1)
- Avoid or understand splitting between different members of staff, either in hospital or in the community
- Monitor countertransference feelings

Table 6.1 Principles of management – an elaboration

Principle	Actions
Maintain flexibility	Take into account the patient's ego strength, psychological mindedness, level of intellect and emotional state when deciding whether to use interpretive or supportive techniques. Be prepared to make mistakes and to use a trial-and-error approach. Be aware of a potential lack of responsiveness in staff, which may be a defence against the extreme feelings that these patients engender. Patients are likely to respond very negatively to stereotypical or rigid stances, so staff need to be spontaneous as far as possible, yet keep professional boundaries (not an easy task).
Establish conditions that keep the patient, family, staff and therapeutic relationship safe	Agree with patient and staff risk levels that would determine the need for admission or discharge, in terms of suicidal, aggressive or inappropriate behaviour, use of drugs and alcohol, and crossing of professional boundaries, and discuss alternative management strategies if hospital admission is terminated.
Tolerate intense anger, aggression and hate	Remember that most patients are trying to re-establish their relationship with the rejecting parent by creating a sado-masochistic attachment to staff. Attempts to avoid such projections, either by defensive countermeasures, trying to prove that the staff are in fact good, or by angry retorts and rejections are likely to lead to disengagement.
Promote reflection	'What triggered that extreme reaction?' 'How do you think I felt when you attacked me in that way?' 'What do you think are the consequences of cutting your wrists?'
Establish and maintain the therapeutic alliance	Regularly revisit the aims and goals of the therapeutic contract, especially when either the patient or staff have lost their way.
Avoid splitting between psychotherapy and pharmacotherapy	Patients' responses to prescribed medication must form part of the therapeutic interactions and be discussed openly if medication is resisted, sabotaged or misused. Patients may need reminding that the aims of medication are modest: to alleviate the most distressing symptoms and allow time and opportunity to reflect and share feelings.
Avoid or understand splitting between members of staff, either in hospital or in the community	Recognise that patients may display completely different attitudes, both loving and attacking, within short periods, which can be quite perplexing to staff. Patients are projecting these aspects of themselves onto others, as a way of trying to control these fragmented parts of themselves.
Monitor counter-transference feelings	Enable staff to share embarrassing or difficult feelings prompted by their involvement with these patients

is in the interests of the patient and not, as patients may often construe it, a sadistic means of control. If there are attempts at self-harm such as wrist slashing, staff may need to convey calmly that, although patients are responsible for their behaviour, the staff will be there to do reparative minor surgery if necessary.

Medication

Polypharmacy is not uncommon in people with borderline personality disorder admitted to hospital (Lieb *et al*, 2004), despite the fact that NICE guidelines recommend that 'drug treatment should not be used specifically for borderline personality disorder or for the individual symptoms or behaviour associated with the disorder (for example, repeated self-harm, marked emotional instability, risk-taking behaviour and transient psychotic symptoms)' (National Collaborating Centre for Mental Health, 2009: p. 10).

In a Cochrane review of 27 randomised trials, Lieb *et al* (2010) suggest that the NICE guidelines be reassessed in the light of their findings that specific symptoms in borderline personality disorder benefit from a pharmacological as well as psychotherapeutic approach. Although they found no evidence to support the use of selective serotonin reuptake inhibitors (SSRIs) for affect dysregulation (emotional instability) or impulsive behaviour, they do advise that SSRIs be used if there is a comorbid major depressive episode. Mood stabilisers such as topiramate, valproate semisodium and lamotrigine show beneficial outcomes for patients with affect dysregulation, as do aripiprazole, olanzapine and haloperidol. There is also evidence of positive results with omega-3 fatty acids and, to a lesser extent, flupentixol decanoate. Aripiprazole, but not olanzapine, has shown beneficial effects in controlling impulsivity. However, these two antipsychotics have been used to good effect in patients with cognitive or perceptual symptoms such as suspiciousness and depersonalisation. The rationale suggested is to treat the three different elements of disturbance in borderline personality disorder with medication (Box 6.5) only when other measures appear insufficient to ensure patient safety.

Although the benefits of medication in borderline personality disorder remain modest, a number of studies have reported improvements when

---

Box 6.5   Medication strategies in borderline personality disorder

- Use medication only when other strategies do not ensure patient safety
- The effect of psychotropic medication is modest: explain this to the patient and family
- Use SSRIs only when there is a comorbid depressive disorder
- Use the rationale of focusing on mood disturbances, behavioural problems or cognitive functioning
- Symptoms of affect dysregulation may benefit from mood stabilisers such as topiramate, valproate semisodium and lamotrigine and from the antipsychotics aripiprazole, olanzapine and haloperidol; there is also evidence of positive results with omega-3 fatty acids and, to a lesser extent, flupentixol decanoate
- Impulsivity may be controlled with aripiprazole but not olanzapine
- Cognitive or perceptual symptoms may respond to aripiprazole or olanzapine

(Adapted from Lieb *et al*, 2010)

medication is used for comorbid psychiatric disorders in combination with other therapeutic approaches, including cognitive–behavioural and dialectical behaviour therapies. However, such psychological techniques will be more likely used after the patient has been discharged from in-patient care (American Psychiatric Association, 2002).

Paranoid personality disorder

In paranoid personality disorders (Chapter 4, this volume), the key features are ego-syntonic, so the 'patient' sees no problem with their viewpoint. It is common for such individuals to be brought to the attention of psychiatric services by relatives, friends or work colleagues, who lose patience with their constant suspiciousness and accusations. Hyperawareness of 'what may lie beneath the surface' and rigidity of response can make people with this disorder intolerable to those around them, and they require considerable expenditure of energy and time when they become patients (Gabbard, 2000).

A common reason for admission of individuals with paranoid person-alities is that their suspicions have incited them to attack someone, often a close relative or work colleague. Initial assessment is likely to involve a differential diagnosis of paranoid schizophrenia, but once this alternative has been discarded, the challenge is to see how admission, even if brief, can be used as a platform for further psychiatric or psychological interven-tions. More often than not, such admissions simply confirm the patient's suspicions about services, resulting in a wasted opportunity. Their response will greatly depend on the ability of staff to contain the patient's paranoid projections without counterattacking or responding in a defensive manner. Staff will need to withstand the onslaught of accusations and demeaning remarks. Any success in this regard has the possible corollary of establish-ing a bridge of contact that can be crossed at some time in the future. One way of handling this is to acknowledge the efforts patients have to expend to keep those around them at a safe emotional distance. This approach may eventually allow the patients to acknowledge their own fears and weakness-es, something that they desperately defend themselves against. This shift, which will happen in the patients' own time and in an enabling therapeutic framework, will permit patients to contemplate an alternative view to their previously rigid and stereotypical perception of the world around them.

The propensity to violence that brought the paranoid patient to hospital will remain during the admission and requires strategies to address it (Table 6.2).

Antisocial personality disorder

Admission to a general psychiatric unit is inadvisable for people with antisocial personality disorder, because of the likelihood that they will

Table 6.2 Strategies to prevent risk of violence in paranoid personalities

Strategy	Actions
Help patients save face	Staff must be particularly aware of patients' low self-esteem and their need to keep this hidden from themselves as well as the outside world
Avoid arousing further suspicion	Staff should explain clearly each decision that they make and should avoid ingratiating friendliness
Be prepared to be openly firm when necessary	This may involve straight-talking; when decisions have to be made that could be perceived as persecutory, staff should clearly explain how they have come about and in whose interests they would be
Help patients to feel they are in control	Staff must openly acknowledge why patients have construed the world around them as they have and must respect their need for autonomy
Encourage verbalisation rather than physical acting out	Staff should sense and support patients' experience of anger and discuss with them the consequences of violence
Give plenty of breathing space	Avoid close sitting arrangements and physical contact
Tune in to own countertransference denial of violence	Be aware of your own aggressive and provocative feelings and remember that women are as likely as men to assault staff (Tardiff *et al*, 1997)

Adapted from Gabbard (2000).

disrupt the treatment of others by flouting agreed rules and boundaries and undermining therapeutic activities and the ability of staff. Some patients charm staff into thinking that they are benefiting from their care, whereas they are going through the motions without any real change; some convince staff that they are victims of circumstances or only 'bad' when they use drugs or alcohol. These individuals may take advantage of the kindness of staff or their need to be helpful, prompting them to play down the patient's ruthlessness, even in the light of previous negative experience.

Needless to say, they arouse extreme negative responses in staff. To some degree this depends on the setting: countertransference in a hospital is different from that in a correctional institution. Antisocial personalities tend to elicit in staff very polarised feelings: from the desire to punish and seek retribution to the illusion that they can defeat evil by their kindness and endeavour; from outrage to admiration, hopelessness to fear (Lion, 1999). Added to this are the dangers of being deceived, as these patients regularly lie and distort facts, thereby disabling any semblance of a trusting therapeutic alliance.

Patients admitted in crisis, should be assessed rapidly and the decision taken either not to treat but take risk-management measures or, if there is scope for intervention, to refer to the relevant service as soon as

---

Box 6.6 Predictors of response to therapeutic approach in antisocial personality disorder

Predictors of positive response

- Presence of anxiety
- Axis I diagnosis of depression
- Axis I diagnosis of psychosis other than depression or organic condition

Predictors of negative response

- History of arrest for a felony
- History of repeated lying, use of aliases, conning
- Unresolved legal situation on admission
- History of conviction for a felony
- Hospitalisation as an alternative to imprisonment
- History of violence to others
- Diagnosis on Axis I of organic brain impairment

(After Gabbard & Coyne, 1987)

---

possible. While this is happening it is important that strict boundaries and conditions are set regarding aggression, sexual acting out, theft and drug importation, with consequences if these are transgressed. Staff's countertransference feelings of disbelief, rationalisation and collusion must be carefully monitored. Trepidation about the possibility of an assault may lead to loosening of agreed boundaries for fear of provoking a reaction. Any breaking of rules needs to be confronted immediately, so that patients are aware of the consequences of their actions, and they should be encouraged to think and talk before taking impulsive action. Unfortunately this is not always feasible.

Gabbard & Coyne (1987) have produced a list of predictors (Box 6.6), that can be used in in-patient units to assess potential treatability, and they advise not to be led by 'gut feeling responses'.

Lion's (1999) advice for dealing with antisocial personality disorder is summarised in Box 6.7

Hysterical and histrionic personality disorders

Hysterical and histrionic conditions are not properly distinguished in DSM-IV. Hysterical conversion disorder is subsumed under conversion or somatoform disorder and is not related to hysterical personality disorder.

Gabbard (2000) describes both hysterical personality disorder and histrionic personality disorder. He attributes to them shared behavioural characteristics, such as a tendency to labile and shallow emotionality, attention-seeking, disturbed sexual functioning, dependency and helplessness, and self-dramatisation. However, he differentiates hysterical personality disorder as being healthier, as histrionic personality is more

---

Box 6.7 Dealing with patients with antisocial personality disorder

- Remain sceptical, particularly during assessments
- Do not deny or normalise dangerousness: a charismatic patient can lure staff into a forgiving or permissive response to unacceptable behaviour
- Be aware of polarities in feeling: a patient's assertiveness or even violence can arouse secret awe and admiration one moment, but disgust and punishment the next
- Be aware of the risk of sexual seduction by patients
- Ensure that less experienced staff are supervised by a more experienced clinician

(After Lion, 1999)

---

florid in every way, less subtle and more impulsive, functioning at a much more primitive level. This differentiation is often reflected in individuals' respective success or failure to maintain relationships and work commitments, and in differences of degree of erotic transference wishes.

Although traditionally seen as disorders affecting mostly women, hysterical and histrionic personality disorders have also been extensively documented in men. These have fallen into two broad subtypes: the hyper-masculine Don Juan, unable to commit himself to any relationship, and the passive effeminate man (homosexual or heterosexual), usually impotent. In both genders, the cognitive style is impressionistic, unable to elaborate detail about the people or world around them, indicating a defensive emotional detachment (*la belle indifférence*), although, paradoxically, individuals may present with shallow emotionality.

Women with histrionic personality disorders tend to have a history of maternal rejection, which draws them to their fathers for dependency needs. They become 'Daddy's little girl' and repress their own sexual maturation and identity.

Women with hysterical personality disorder have usually had more satisfying early relationships with their mother, but develop intense rivalry and compete for their father's attention. They are more likely to have a history of actual incest. In adulthood, they appear to be unaware of their attempts at seductiveness. As a result, their own sexuality and their experiences of intimacy are disturbed and unsatisfactory, as is their choice of partners. It is usually a relationship crisis, leading to dramatic acts of impulsive self-harm, that results in admission to an acute hospital setting via the emergency department.

The story is similar for men. In men with histrionic personalities, maternal (and paternal) unavailability may lead them to emulate their mothers, adopting a passive, effeminate role, or their fathers, mimicking hypermasculine cultural stereotypes of masculinity. In those with hysterical personalities, feelings of sexual inadequacy keep men attached to their mothers, again either adopting effeminate or celibate lifestyles, or overcompensating by shallow efforts at becoming tough 'real men'.

Both men and women with these disorders pose difficulties in in-patient settings, as they often engage in rivalrous relationships with other patients and erotic transferences to staff. They usually see themselves as special, tend to take over groups, where they need to be at the centre of all discussions, and take on other people's problems as part of their own, in a self-referential manner. If thwarted in their attempts, they are likely to become increasingly dramatic, and sometimes engage in risk-taking behaviour in order to attract attention. This often provokes negative countertransference feelings in staff, who try to ignore their demands, which only reinforces the cycle.

Although long-term work with these patients is the province of the out-patient clinic or psychotherapy department, two principles of management can be applied in the in-patient unit that might help patients take on longer-term work.

First, the initial assessment should be used as an opportunity to challenge the patient's cognitive style. These individuals will assume that doctors and nurses intuitively know what is happening with them. Although history-taking can be a frustrating experience for these patients, it allows them to describe, perhaps for the first time, their internal world, feelings and expectations.

Second, erotic transference must be effectively managed. Eroticised feelings towards staff can sometimes be very insistent and pervasive, and in an in-patient unit, nursing staff are particularly vulnerable to overt or covert advances. Many careers have been blighted because of inappropriate crossing of sexual boundaries, which can also be devastating to patients.

The management of transference involves a close examination of countertransference feelings. There are large hurdles to overcome if this is to be dealt with appropriately, as there seems to be no tradition in the UK of openly discussing sexualised feelings, which are often ignored or denied in patients and staff (Gabbard, 2000). Nurses in particular have no vehicle for expressing their concern and no support system to rely on, and any suggested breaking of boundaries is immediately responded to in a punitive manner, with suspension or dismissal. Sometimes staff are so frightened of these consequences that they respond to a patient's advances with aggression or aloofness, which the patient reads as evidence that sexual desires are dangerous or dirty.

Another common response by staff is to tell the patient that their feelings are not real, when to the patient they are extraordinarily real. A more appropriate response is to communicate to the patient that sexual or loving feelings do occur but cannot be reciprocated. This acknowledges the reality of the feelings, but places them within a therapeutic process that can help staff to understand some of the patient's inner thoughts and feelings, even if at times it is embarrassing or painful for the patient not to have their desires fulfilled.

95

Conclusion

People with borderline personality disorders present particular challenges to staff in in-patient units, and the management of problems presented by these patients needs to be in the therapeutic armamentarium of the general psychiatrists and multidisciplinary staff who work in such units. Although I do not advocate that the in-patient unit is the place of choice for the treatment of personality disorders, I do suggest that the experience on the unit of positive management of the crisis that leads to admission can, in the long-term, help patients by reducing their morbidity and acting out behaviours. I also believe that in-patient units offer a setting in which evaluation of risk and adequate assessments that might determine treatability can take place, leading to possible referrals to appropriate therapeutic units or services.

References

American Psychiatric Association (1994) *Diagnostic and Statistical Manual of Mental Disorders (4th edn) (DSM–IV)*. APA.

American Psychiatric Association (2002) *Practice Guidelines for the Treatment of Psychiatric Disorders*. APA.

Bateman, A. & Fonagy, P. (1999) The effectiveness of partial hospitalisation in the treatment of borderline personality disorder: a randomised controlled trial. *American Journal of Psychiatry*, **156**, 1563–1569.

Bateman, A. & Fonagy, P. (2001) Treatment of borderline personality disorder with psychoanalytically oriented partial hospitalization: an 18-month follow-up. *American Journal of Psychiatry*, **158**, 36–42.

Bateman, A. W. & Tyrer, P. (2002) *Effective Management of Personality Disorder*. Department of Health (http://www.dh.gov.uk/prod_consum_dh/groups/dh_digitalassets/@dh/@en/documents/digitalasset/dh_4130843.pdf).

Castillo, H. (2003) *Personality Disorder: Temperament or Trauma?* Jessica Kingsley.

Chiesa, M., Fonagy, P., Holmes, J., et al (2002) Health service utilisation costs by personality disorder following specialist and non-specialist treatment: a comparative study. *Journal of Personality Disorders*, **16**, 160–173.

Coid, J. (2003) Epidemiology, public health and the problem of personality disorder. *British Journal of Psychiatry*, **182** (suppl. 44), s3–s10.

Davison, S. E. (2002) Principles of managing patients with personality disorder. *Advances in Psychiatric Treatment*, **8**, 1–9.

Duggan, M. (2002) *Developing Services for people with Personality Disorder: The Training Needs of Staff and Services*. National Institue for Mental Health in England.

Fagin, L. (2004) Management of personality disorders in acute in-patient settings. Part 2: Less-common personality disorders. *Advances in Psychiatric Treatment*, **10**, 100–106.

Gabbard, G. O. (2000) *Psychodynamic Psychiatry in Clinical Practice*. American Psychiatric Press.

Gabbard, G. O. & Coyne, L. (1987) Predictors of response of antisocial patients to hospital treatment. *Hospital and Community Psychiatry*, **38**, 1181–1185.

Gallop, R. (1992) Self-destructive and impulsive behaviour in the patient with a borderline personality disorder: rethinking hospital treatment and management. *Archives of Psychiatric Nursing*, **6**, 178–182.

Haigh, R. (2002) *Services for People with Personality Disorder: The Thoughts of Service Users*. Department of Health (http://www.dh.gov.uk/assetRoot/04/13/08/44/04130844.pdf).

Haigh, R. (2006) People's experiences of having a diagnosis of personality disorder. In *Personality Disorder and Community Mental Health Teams: A Practitioner's Guide* (eds M. J. Sampson, P. A. McCubbin & P. Tyrer), pp. 161–177. John Wiley & Sons.

Hayward, M., Slade, M. & Moran, P. A. (2006) Personality disorders and unmet needs among psychiatric inpatients. *Psychiatric Services*, **57**, 538–543.

Hendin, H. (1981) Psychotherapy and suicide. *American Journal of Psychotherapy*, **35**, 469–480.

Kaplan, C. A. (1986) The challenge of working with patients diagnosed as having a borderline personality disorder. *Nursing Clinics of North America*, **21**, 429–438.

Kendall, T., Pilling, S., Tyrer, P., *et al* (2009) Borderline and antisocial personality disorders: summary of NICE guidance. *BMJ*, **338**, b93.

Krawitz, R. & Batcheler, M. (2006) Borderline personality disorder: a pilot survey about clinician views on defensive practice. *Australasian Psychiatry*, **14**, 320–322.

Kullgren, G. (1988) Factors associated with completed suicide in borderline personality disorder. *Journal of Nervous and Mental Diseases*, **176**, 40–44.

Lieb, K., Zanarini, M. C., Schmahl, C., *et al* (2004) Borderline personality disorder. *Lancet*, **364**, 453–461.

Lieb, K., Völlm, B., Rücker, G., *et al* (2010) Pharmacotherapy for borderline personality disorder: Cochrane systematic review of randomised trials. *British Journal of Psychiatry*, **196**, 4–12.

Lion, J. R. (1999) Countertransference in the treatment of the antisocial patient. In *Countertransference Issues in Psychiatric Treatment* (ed. G. O. Gabbard), pp. 73–84. American Psychiatric Press.

Matsberger, J. (1999) Countertransference in the treatment of the suicidal borderline patient. In *Countertransference Issues in Psychiatric Treatment* (ed. G. O. Gabbard), pp. 27–43. American Psychiatric Press.

McGowan, J. (2008) Working with personality disorders in an acute psychiatric ward. In *Cognitive Behaviour Therapy for Acute Inpatient Mental Health Units: Working with Clients, Staff and the Milieu* (eds I. Clarke & H. Wilson), pp. 92–111. Routledge.

Moran, P. (2002) *The Epidemiology of Personality Disorder*. Department of Health (http://www.dh.gov.uk/assetRoot/04/13/08/45/04130845.pdf).

Moran, P. (2005) Developments in the epidemiological study of personality disorders. *Psychiatry*, **4** (3), 4–7.

Mulder, R. T. (2002) Personality disorder and treatment outcome in major depression: a review. *American Journal of Psychiatry*, **159**, 408–411.

National Collaborating Centre for Mental Health (2009) *Borderline Personality Disorder: Treatment and Management (NICE Clinical Guideline 78)*. National Institute for Health and Clinical Excellence.

National Institute for Mental Health in England (2003) *Personality Disorder: No Longer a Diagnosis of Exclusion. Policy Implementation Guidance for the Development of Services for People with Personality Disorder*. Department of Health.

Nehls, N. (1994a) Brief hospital treatment plans: innovations in practice and research. *Issues in Mental Health Nursing*, **15**, 1–11.

Nehls, N. (1994b) Brief hospital treatment plans for persons with borderline personality disorder: perspectives of in-patient psychiatric nurses and community mental health centre clinicians. *Archives of Psychiatric Nursing*, **8**, 303–311.

Nicholson, J. M. & Carradice, A. (2002) Clinical psychology provision for inpatient settings: a challenge in team working? *Clinical Psychology*, **18**, 25–30.

Norton, K. & Dolan, B. (1995) Acting out and the institutional response. *Journal of Forensic Psychiatry*, **6**, 317–332.

Norton, K. & Hinshelwood, R. D. (1996) Severe personality disorder: treatment issues and selection for in-patient psychotherapy. *British Journal of Psychiatry*, **168**, 723–731.

O'Brien, L. (1998) Inpatient nursing care of patients with borderline personality disorder: a review of the literature. *Australian and New Zealand Journal of Mental Health Nursing*, **7**, 172–183.

Paris, J. (2004) Is hospitalization useful for suicidal patients with borderline personality disorder? *Journal of Personality Disorders*, **18**, 240–247.

Piccinino, S. (1990) The nursing care challenge: borderline patients. *Journal of Psychosocial Nursing*, **28**, 22–27.

Rouse, J. D. (1994) Borderline and other dramatic personality disorders in the psychiatric emergency service. *Psychiatric Annals*, **24**, 598–602.

Sederer, L. & Thornbeck, J. (1986) First do no harm: short term inpatient psychotherapy of the borderline patient. *Hospital and Community Psychiatry*, **37**, 692–697.

Stone, M. H. (1990) *The Fate of Borderline Patients*. Guilford Press.

Tardiff, K., Marzuk, P. M., Leon, A. C., *et al* (1997) Violence by patients admitted to a private psychiatric hospital. *American Journal of Psychiatry*, **154**, 88–93.

Vaslamatzis, G., Coccossis, M., Zervis, C., *et al* (2004) A psychoanalytically oriented combined treatment approach for severely disturbed borderline patients: the Athens Project. *Bulletin of the Menninger Clinic*, **68**, 337–349.

Wester, J. M. (1991) Rethinking inpatient treatment of borderline patients. *Perspectives in Psychiatric Care*, **27**, 17–20.

Zanarini, M., Frances, R., Frankenburg, D., *et al* (2010) Time to attainment of recovery from borderline personality disorder and stability of recovery: a 10 year follow up study. *American Journal of Psychiatry*, **167**, 663–667.

CHAPTER 7

Personality disorder in women

Jaydip Sarkar and Rebecca Lawday

Summary   This chapter explores differences in the way in which personality disorders manifest in the two genders and considers possible biopsychosocial reasons underlying such differences. It looks at common clinical presentations in women with personality disorders and attempts to provide an understanding of these. It concludes by highlighting the need for gender-specific services and approaches, and for workforce development and support to meet the needs of this group.

Numerous studies have shown an association between personality disorder and gender (Box 7.1), but explanations for this take various standpoints. For example, researchers have suggested:

- gender bias in the diagnostic criteria for certain personality disorders
- differences in rates of personality disorders in the two genders
- differing behavioural manifestation of traits across gender lines
- differences in trait distribution across the two genders
- clinician bias in diagnosing certain personality disorders.

Let us consider each of these in turn. First, there is indeed evidence that gender bias within the American Psychiatric Association's DSM

Box 7.1   Gender differences in personality disorders

- Women have higher rates of histrionic, borderline and dependent personality disorders
- Men have higher rates of antisocial, narcissistic, schizoid and obsessive–compulsive personality disorders
- Men have higher rates of DSM cluster A disorders, but rates for clusters B and C are the same for the two genders
- There is diagnostic as well as clinician bias in the international criteria for antisocial personality disorder in men and histrionic personality disorder for women
- Gender differences are seen in major traits, e.g. impulsivity manifests as impulsive aggression and interpersonal exploitation in antisocial but in self-destructive acts and mood instability in borderline personality disorder

---

diagnostic criteria leads to disproportionately high rates of histrionic personality disorder among women, although the five-factor model of personality (openness, conscientiousness, extraversion, agreeableness and neuroticism) is less prone to this (Samuel & Widiger, 2009). Stereotypically feminine traits have been caricatured in the DSM diagnosis. Some have made feminist claims that healthy women can earn the diagnosis of histrionic personality disorder because of the gender-biased criteria constructed by a task-force comprised largely of men (Kaplan, 1983). Although this is an extreme position, there is evidence that the criteria of antisocial personality disorder are heavily loaded in favour of characteristics associated with being male (Paris, 2004).

Second, genuine and significant gender differences (beyond any biases) have been found in the rates of narcissistic personality disorder (Paris, 2004) and antisocial personality disorder (Samuels et al, 2002), which are higher among men, and borderline (Paris, 2004) and histrionic personality disorder (Samuel & Widiger, 2009), which are higher among women. Large-scale community studies (Torgersen et al, 2001; Samuels et al, 2002) have also found differences in how the DSM clusters of personality disorder diagnoses (cluster A, B or C) are distributed in the two genders. Cluster A disorders are more common in men, owing to high rates of schizoid personality disorder. Clusters B and C are equitable for the genders, because of high rates of antisocial personality disorder in men and borderline personality disorder in women (for cluster B), and dependent personality disorder for women and obsessive–compulsive personality disorder for men (for cluster C).

Third, there is evidence that the same trait can manifest itself differently. Not only does, impulsivity as a trait, for example, manifest as impulsive violence/aggression and interpersonal exploitation in antisocial personality disorder, but in self-destructive acts and mood instability in borderline personality disorder (Paris, 2004). It may also manifest itself as aggression towards others in antisocial men but as sudden mood swings and self-destructive acts in antisocial women. These differences do not reflect diagnostic bias and have been consistently confirmed in epidemiological studies (Schwartz et al, 1990; Torgersen et al, 2001).

Fourth, Looper & Paris (2000) suggest that similar underlying psycho-pathology on a trait level can lead to different behavioural presentations in males and females. Their hypothesis was developed for cluster B disorders (antisocial personality disorder, narcissistic personality disorder, borderline personality disorder, histrionic personality disorder). In these, impulsivity is a common feature but it is present in different degrees of severity and its interactions with other personality dimensions, gender and culture all influence its expression.

Fifth, even experienced clinicians tend to make certain diagnoses in a gender-biased manner, from the same clinical information diagnosing histrionic personality disorder for women but antisocial personality disorder for men (Morey *et al*, 2002). It is thought that the pull of global impressions that rely heavily on a few central features of a disorder outweighs carefully considered diagnostic criteria (Ford & Widiger, 1989; Kim & Ahn, 2002).

Clinical presentations and underlying factors

In clinical experience, features of personality disorder in clinical samples of women tend to be classified as mainly emotionally unstable (borderline), histrionic and dependent. However, in our experience a combination of features is more commonly seen in clinical practice. We illustrate this section with a number of fictitious case vignettes showing how women with different characteristics of personality disorder might present on psychiatric evaluation. All of these styles of coping, interacting and behaving can be understood as reactions to complex trauma interacting with already established personality traits and attachment styles.

Personality

It has been suggested that personality is a complex, multilayered capacity that evolves out of the interplay between heritable temperaments and early-life experiences of care and safety (Caspi *et al*, 2002). As with all human behaviour, personality is shaped by the interaction of genes and environment. The resultant matrix of multiple capacities and experiences is then established into a life-script which directs the individual's perception of self and others, and expectations of the future (McAdams & Pals, 2006). Within such a framework, personality disorders represent the characteristic adaptations that an infant/child born with certain temperamental features makes in response to early-life challenges – positive and negative – posed by carers. These adaptations represent the infant's attempts to ensure survival (McAdams & Pals, 2006). Characteristic adaptations relate largely to the capacity for managing emotions and interpersonal relationships (because of the prolonged period of dependency), and provide frameworks of learning and behaviour later in life (Sarkar & Adshead, 2006). Traumatic childhood conditions due to abusive and neglectful parenting generate characteristic modes of thinking, feeling, perceiving, relating and behaving that, although appropriate in the context of survival, can become the only available template for managing emotions and interpersonal relationships in future, even when relationships are not abusive, settings not traumatic and survival not at stake. These adaptations, so helpful to a child, in an adult are labelled personality disorder.

Temperamental predispositions (dispositional traits)

Vulnerability models of personality development emphasise the genetic predisposition that we have to particular personality traits. Studies of normal personality have consistently revealed that 40–60% of the variability in personality traits appears to be heritable (Loehlin & Nichols, 1976; Loehlin & Gough, 1990). A similar picture appears to have emerged in the personality disorder literature (Livesley *et al*, 1993, 1998), which describes heritability effects in emotional dysregulation (47%), dissocial behaviour (50%), inhibitedness (48%) and compulsivity (38%).

Evolutionary psychology provides the best understanding of the gender-specific trajectories that occur in women with personality disorders. It holds that psychological attributes that confer on their bearers significant benefits in terms of survival and reproduction have become ingrained in the genes and transmitted as evolved modules of problem-solving relating to these challenges (Tooby & Cosmides, 1992). Women are typically physically less powerful than men. So in struggles for survival, it is suggested that evolution has conferred on females the protection of apparently genetically encoded high levels of fear, which discourages them from engaging in life-threatening physical combat with males (McLean & Anderson, 2009). As a result, girls and women react differently to stressful challenges of life than do boys and men.

It has also been suggested that girls have a biologically rooted temperamental vulnerability owing to the possession of a trait of negative affectivity, which is characterised by psychological instability and proneness to anxiety, anger and sadness (Rothbart & Bates, 2006). In addition, they are less able to control negative affect (Muris *et al*, 2007). This makes it more likely that girls will experience internalising symptoms (symptoms that lead to negative perceptions and ruminations, dysphoria and anxiety) and a tendency to internalise negative and destructive impulses (Lonigan & Phillips, 2001). These may well be reasons why women target their bodies, the container of their negative emotions: what Erikson (1968) calls 'inner space'. As the body is the container of negativity, much of female psychopathology is experienced and manifested through an 'embodiment of emotions'. Women with personality disorders display high rates of self-harm, eating disorders, somatisation disorders, and conversion and dissociative disorders. These disorders are often chronic, with episodes of acute exacerbation during periods of heightened reactivity to environmental stressors.

Salient life stressors and characteristic adaptations

Biological predispositions of this nature create a breeding ground for typical manifestations of psychopathology in the face of life stressors such as abusive or neglectful parental care. One particular stressor, childhood sexual abuse, is strongly associated with later personality disorder (Weiler & Widom, 1996). Girls experience far greater levels of childhood sexual abuse than boys, but they are less likely than boys to develop serious and enduring mental illnesses (schizophrenia and bipolar affective disorder) as a result (Spataro *et al*, 2004). We believe that trauma-informed theories proffer explanations of women's tendency to concentrate their distress on their bodies. For women whose experiences include boundary violations such as childhood sexual abuse, their sense of identity may reside in their bodies. The domain of control, of communication, of affection and of self is located in the physical. Psychic or emotional stress is easier to conceive and control when it is physical.

Other periods of high stress are: the onset of female fecundity with menarche; the onset of adolescence, which 'gives a second chance for reassurance of gender identity' (Welldon, 1991), greater gender socialisation and separation; pregnancy and its consequent instinctual maternal tasks; and finally menopause or any condition that ends the capacity to bear children. These times on the biological clock, with their associated socially meaningful tasks, interact with the individual's 'inner space', so that onset or exacerbation of psychological disorders is observed in vulnerable individuals during these periods (McLean & Anderson, 2009). Examples include eating disorders, substance misuse, self-harm, offending behaviours, sexual perversions and abuse of dependent children (Welldon, 1991; Pedersen, 2004; McLean & Anderson, 2009). The post-natal period has been described as particularly overwhelming. For women who had hoped that a baby might 'fill an emptiness', as is often described by those with borderline personality disorder, it can also be a time of great disappointment (Pines, 2010).

Interpersonal strategies and attachment styles

Developmental trauma can create a disordered template for later relationships. As Herman writes (1992), 'Repeated trauma in adult life erodes the structure of the personality already formed, but repeated trauma in childhood forms and deforms the personality'. Experience of multiple and potentially life-threatening trauma (most trauma involving childhood abuse and neglect is of this kind) leads to a bimodal distribution of physiological changes and symptoms: autonomic hyperarousal and intrusive re-experiencing alternate with hypoarousal and avoidance (van der Kolk, 1994). This affects the nature and quality of emotional attachments, so that the individual is typically excessively anxious (or clingy), avoidant (distant) or disorganised (fluctuating between the two) in how they relate to the presence of others (Fonagy et al, 1991).

Numerous studies have identified factors that protect against the damaging influence of psychological trauma. These include higher IQ, a supportive family network and sociodemographic factors that reduce the risk of poverty and social disadvantage. However, the most influential may well be healthy early childhood attachment experiences and a sub-sequent 'secure' adult attachment style. The early attachment relationship between an infant and their primary caregiver has been demonstrated to be relatively fixed in later infanthood (Ainsworth et al, 1978) related to overall functioning in relationships at age 6 (Main et al, 1985), and to be linked to later adult relational styles (Hazan & Shaver, 1987). In terms of intergenerational findings, mothers' working models of attachment have also been linked to their infants' security of attachment (Main *et al*, 1985).

John Bowlby (1969), inspired by Konrad Lorenz's 1950s studies of imprinting in baby geese, believed that the human baby is equipped with a set of built-in behaviours that helps keep the parent nearby (feeding alone is not the basis of attachment). The inner representation of this parent–child bond becomes an important part of personality. It serves as an internal working model of the availability, support and interaction of attachment figures, and becomes the basis for future close relationships in infancy, childhood, adolescence and adult life. From close observations of 1- and 2-year-old children, Bowlby's student Mary Ainsworth proposed specific styles of attachment: secure attachment and two types of insecure attachment, 'avoidant and resistant' and 'ambivalent' (Ainsworth *et al*, 1978). Insecure attachment occurs when the parent/primary carer consistently fails to respond sensitively to the infant. Ainsworth's three-fold taxonomy of attachment styles has been translated into terms of adult romantic relationships as follows (Hazan & Shaver, 1987).

Secure adults find it relatively easy to get close to others and are comfortable depending on others and having others depend on them. They do not often worry about being abandoned or about someone getting too close to them. Avoidant (also described as 'dismissive') adults are uncomfortable being close to others: they find it difficult to trust others completely or to allow themselves to depend on others. They are nervous when anyone gets too close, and partners often want them to be more intimate than they feel comfortable being. Anxious/ambivalent (also described as 'preoccupied') adults find that others are reluctant to get as close as they would like. They often worry that their partner does not really love them or want to stay with them. They want to merge completely with the other person, and this desire sometimes scares people away.

Insecure styles disrupt the ability to communicate in relationships, to think about one's own and other people's thinking (to mentalise; Fonagy *et al*, 1991; Bateman & Fonagy, 2004) and to regulate affect. Insecure styles of relating can have an impact on a mother's attachment with her own child.

Relationships in which women are violent are likely to repeat or remind them of their early attachment experiences: as caregivers, they are now in the position of power; as mothers, they may see in their children reminders of the stresses and failures of their maternal attachment. Attachment models therefore emphasise the drive for relationships and the importance of emotional safety and security in all humans.

A model of social interaction

Personality disorder in women can be explained in terms of the nature (evolutionary purpose) and the nurture (attachment style) aspects of social interaction. Inability to establish healthy and appropriate 'social distances' from others can result in pathologies of overinvolvement (moving towards others), underinvolvement or hostility (moving away from others) and inconsistent involvement (alternately moving towards and away from others).

Moving towards others

From an evolutionary perspective, it might be said that women require relationships, partly for care and comfort, but in large part to meet their need for safety and provisioning. This is related to the findings introduced above that women tend to be less aggressive and dominant, with higher levels of innate fear and anxiety (McLean & Anderson, 2009), but it might also be a reflection of the culturally sanctioned tendency in most societies for women rather than men to have the role of caretaker.

In some, this natural desire for relationships can become pathological. Clinginess and overdependence are the hallmark of dependent personality disorder and, to some extent, histrionic personality disorder (which are more common in women), whereas avoidance and dismissiveness feature strongly in antisocial and narcissistic personality disorders (which are more common in men). People with dependent personality disorder rely on others even for mundane everyday decisions in their lives and subjugate their autonomy and agency to the will of another. Those with histrionic personality disorder use their bodies, through sexual seductiveness, physical appearance and rapidly changing shallow emotionality, to engage in relationships, which tend to be stormy (American Psychiatric Association, 2000). But the key pathology in both these disorders remains an inability to be on their own because of excessive fear being alone/lonely (Box 7.2).

Possessiveness and dependency

As noted above, in species terms, females need relationships, even if they are with abusive males, to fulfil their evolutionary purpose of procreation. Females pay a far greater price in evolutionary struggles, by bearing children, nursing them and caring for them to near adulthood. Contributions by males are generally much lower and they have a choice in deciding how much. A child produced by a casual encounter involves, at minimum, a 9-month investment by the mother, but only a small amount of semen from the father. Thus, for men, casual sex is the best way to maximise evolutionary survival of their genes, whereas for women, supportive male relationships are necessary to maximise the chances of survival of their offspring into adulthood, and thus the survival of her genes. This might explain why female jealousy is typically centred on relationships ('Do you love her'?), whereas male jealousy is focused on sex ('Did you sleep with him?'). It also explains the ubiquitous female–female jealousy and envy that characterises competition for males, much as inter-male violence tends to characterise competition for suitable women (Tooby & Cosmides, 1992).

105

Box 7.2 Case vignette 1: Ruth

Ruth has an extensive history of victimisation and boundary violations both within and outside of her family. When her mother put her forward as a child model for a clothing catalogue neither expected that she would be exposed to and used in pornography. Although she was, her mother did not prevent it for fear of losing the status that Ruth's local fame ensured. In the absence of boundaried parenting, Ruth came to rely on others, usually older men, to define who she was, how she was and whether or not she was worthy of love and attention. Now she presented less as someone who required attention, being normally fairly quiet in nature, but she clearly craved affirmation and both consciously and unconsciously she found seductive ways of ensuring she achieved the affirmation she craved.

Ruth described herself as being 'all things to all people'. She became a mother early because her older partner had wanted more children. She sought the 'unconditional love' promised by romantic notions of motherhood and described being bitterly disappointed when her child was not just invalidating of Ruth's needs, but herself needy. Her relationship with her child appeared to become the template by which she entered all relationships – wholly and with high expectations but with angry reactions when these came at a cost or compromise to herself.

Ruth became prone to extreme outbursts of anger when she considered that she had been rejected, especially when this was also coupled with shame. An example she gave was a fight she initiated when she made a futile attempt to entice the father of her child back into her life by being naked when he came to pick up their daughter for a weekend. She struggled with jealousy and assumed that if someone else was in favour with a friend or family member then there was no room for her. Ruth was absolutely committed to psychotherapeutic treatment but often became angry with her therapist when asked to change in any way. The therapist's role became to model and provide examples of consistent and boundaried relationships.

Pregnancy brings about the need for additional resources and safety for the offspring. Males invest in their own genes (own children), but not those of other males. It is possible to know, from their behaviour or appearance, when certain animals are ovulating, this is not the case for women. Consequently, evolutionary strategies involve many male-specific possessive behaviours that have the potential to take the form of psychopathological states. These can assume ritualistic proportions and involve hypersensitivity to the prospect of other males gaining sexual access to their female partners, leading to pathological jealousy, delusions of infidelity (or mate-guarding) and treating women as property, either as slaves or by laws and customs that strictly control sexual partners in certain societies. The evolutionary underpinning of these phenomena is discussed by Wilson & Daly (1992) in a aptly titled chapter 'The man who mistook his wife for a chattel'.

The greater a woman's dependence on a man for protection and provision, the higher the likelihood of domestic abuse and violence, often a complicating feature of dependent personality disorder, where patients volunteer to do unpleasant things for others (American Psychiatric Association, 2000). Many women with this condition reach a state of learned helplessness (Seligman, 1971) such that they accept their condition as 'normal' or 'usual'. Such pathological levels of fear, anxiety and self-blame underlie submission in most sadomasochistic relationships, masochistic (or self-defeating) personality disorder (contained in DSM-III; American Psychiatric Association, 1980), and sexual and other forms of bondage. The combination of exploitative and submissive partners in relationships is commonly encountered in secure women's wards.

Battered women and domestic violence

A pathological extension of this condition is battered woman syndrome. This is not yet a recognised psychiatric diagnosis in international classificatory systems, yet it is recognised in law, on the basis of expert psychiatric testimony, as a defence against the crime of murder for women who kill their partners (Rix, 2001). Battered person syndrome describes any person who, because of constant and severe domestic violence, usually involving physical abuse by a partner, becomes severely depressed and/or is unable to take any independent action that would allow them to escape the abuse. The condition explains why abused people may not seek assistance from others, fight their abuser, or leave the abusive situation, being often led to believe that the abuse is their fault. Such individuals may refuse to press charges against their abuser, or refuse all offers of help, perhaps even becoming aggressive or abusive to those who offer it.

Moving against others

Women with antisocial or narcissistic personality disorders are often dismissive of the needs of others and tend to drive people away through deception and violence (in antisocial personality disorder) or an extreme preoccupation with themselves (in narcissistic personality disorder). Childhood risk factors for development of antisocial and narcissistic personality disorders include poverty-related maltreatment, physical discipline by the mother, and reduced affection and maternal care in infancy (McLoyd, 1990). Evolutionary psychiatry suggests that such treatment of her offspring is the female's competitive response to resource shortages, particularly as they affect her subsequent reproductive success. Thus, poverty can create a self-perpetuating cycle of these personality disorders (Campbell *et al*, 2001).

Women are seven times more likely than men to be sexually or physically abused (Peugh & Belenko, 1999). A woman has two avenues for obtaining necessary resources for survival and procreation: through attachment to a provisioning male, as discussed above, or through her own independent means. One potential 'side-effect' of the former is further abuse, relationship difficulties, coercion and addiction, factors highly relevant to female crime (Home Office, 2007) (Box 7.3).

Box 7.3   Case vignette 2: Victoria

Victoria has been living in secure hospitals since she was first admitted 15 years ago after making threats to kill her daughter. Her background was one of extreme neglect and of problems in foster care. She experienced multiple episodes of abuse and was described as 'uncontrollable' by early adolescence. She became involved in drug use and criminality and was known to burn herself regularly with cigarettes and had tried to set fire to herself. When she was 17 she gave birth to a premature baby girl and social services assumed parental responsibility because of Victoria's history. The baby remained in neo-natal care and Victoria was permitted to visit to encourage bonding. She recalls now being very scared of the implications of having a baby and fearful of her own emotions, feeling out of control, especially when experiencing an intense desire to kill the baby.

The anxiety and anger she experienced in the post-natal period were quickly projected onto institutions that served to protect the child from her. When Victoria and her boyfriend (the baby's father) were refused access to the neo-natal ward because they were drunk, they fought each other and the boyfriend ran off. Left alone outside the hospital, Victoria set a fire that was reckless and life-threatening. Incarcerated for this arson, she began making threats to find and kill her child.

Since her admission, Victoria's emotional experience has continued to fluctuate dramatically, and she has become reliant on the structure of the hospital's procedures and staff to contain her distress. She talks now of fearing leaving hospital, saying that she knows no other way, has not had a chance to build a life in the community and does not feel confident in her basic skills to cope. In more reflective moments she says that by committing to moving on from hospital she risks people not attending to her needs, being alone, losing control and harming others, and in committing to rehabilitation she thinks it unfair that she should be asked to take responsibility for the failings of others in her past.

Crime and violence

Their lower threshold for fear generally inhibits crime in females (Bartlett, 2009), and they carry out significantly fewer crimes than males (International Criminal Police Organisation, 1994). The need to provide for themselves in poverty-stricken and violent environments (Farrington & Painter, 2004) are key factors in the disproportionately higher levels of property damage/ arson and drug-related offences, rather than crimes of physical violence, committed by women (Chesney-Lind, 1997; Campbell *et al*, 2001; Bartlett, 2009). If women do carry out violent crimes, these are more likely to involve low-risk strategies: simple and aggravated assaults rather than intentional grievous bodily harm, murder (Kruttschnitt, 1993) and weapons offences (Steffensmeier, 1993; Miller, 1998).

Perversions of care and attachments

In a book entitled *Perversion: The Erotic Form of Hatred*, Stoller (1975) refers to a fantasy of revenge that is hidden in an act or behaviour whereby the abused becomes triumphant. Some of the low-risk strategies referred to in the previous section involve the targeting of intimate others, particularly the individual's partner or children. There is a violent perversion of care that can end in serious harm to the victim. In adult sexual relationships, this can involve the killing of the partner, although in cases where women kill in such situations there are conflicting findings on whether the homicide is precipitated by a history of victimisation of the woman by the man – indeed, substance misuse by the woman is a common contributing factor (Jurik & Winn, 1990; Weizmann-Henelius *et al*, 2003). Children can become the victims of physical and emotional abuse when an adult (usually the mother) caring for them fabricates symptoms of medical illnesses in the children, for psychological and material gains. This rare form of abuse was originally called Munchausen syndrome by proxy but has more recently become known as fabricated or induced illness (Adshead & Bluglass, 2005). In the murder of a child by a parent, mothers are disproportionately more likely to have committed the act (Liem & Koenraadt, 2008).

Perversion of attachment relationships appears to stem from a combination of antisocial traits and narcissism. The latter characteristically involves a sense of entitlement and the expectation of automatic compliance with expectations in relationships in which other people serve as an element of the individual's extended self (World Health Organization, 1992; American Psychiatric Association, 2000).

It has been suggested that in women with personality disorders, there is often a perversion of key human instincts. Examples given include moral perversion (crime and delinquency), social perversion (prostitution), maternal perversion (fabricated or induced illness; Box 7.4) and nutritional perversion (eating disorders) (Welldon, 1991). Where such perversions are kept secret, there is a sense of control and power in deception by presenting a façade to society (whose expectations of women does not allow for disclosure).

Alternately moving towards and away from others

Borderline personality disorder captures the difficulty people have in determining the right socioemotional distance from others. Those with the disorder vacillate between tendencies to get too close to others and to withdraw from them or ward them off. Intensely strong emotional memories of early life experiences leave them frightened at the possibility of being abused in a relationship. This leads to withdrawal from or aggression towards the object of their attachment. When close to another, they may make many attempts to avoid real or imagined abandonment and rejection (American Psychiatric Association, 2000). Conversely, there may be attempts to provoke rejection in order to test the strength of the socioemotional bonds, so as to be 'in control' of potential disappointments.

There is now substantial evidence of neurobiological dysregulation in key brain areas with regard to affective instability and impulsivity. Adequate serotonin (5-HT) activity in key prefrontal areas, i.e. the orbitofrontal and

Box 7.4   Case Vignette 3: Stacey

In Stacey's early years, she was regularly presented by her mother to the health visitor or general practitioner with differing health concerns. She had some early experiences of both stress and neglect in the home, which she does not recall, but she knows that she was an anxious child. Although she described her mother as both frightening and smothering, she did not feel able to distance herself from her, refusing school and social activities with other children. When Stacey was 8 years old her mother was admitted to hospital under the Mental Health Act. Stacey's father was known but absent, and she was brought up by family members, who described her as 'fragile'. When stressed (normally by being alone and/or being forced to integrate with other children), Stacey developed a tendency to express this physically, looking for concrete physical evidence that her needs were being met by those caring for her. She did not appear to be aware of the impact of stress psychically, but was aware of the need to be heard and not ignored or neglected.

She continued to be presented to health professionals throughout her childhood with regular injuries, apparently both self-inflicted and caused by fights with cousins. Stacey recalled these trips to hospital as being validating, but the residual anger she held at her mother's removal by health professionals was projected onto those offering her physical interventions. The more she protested at the lack of care she experienced from the NHS, the less help she received. When she received a diagnosis of somatisation disorder at the age of 20 she lost this opportunity for validation.

Stacey maintained her interest in the physical and decided to become a nurse. She performed well in the theoretical aspects of her training, but when faced with the need to care for others on placement this appeared to trigger a stress response and associated anger. To protect herself from the uncertainty and loneliness she feared, she did not express her anger outwardly. Instead she internalised it, her body again taking over control of self and of expression – this is when Stacey began to secretly cut herself.

anterior cingulate cortex, is known to regulate impulsivity. Not only are there substantial differences in serotonergic transmission between men and women with borderline personality disorder (New *et al*, 2003; Soloff *et al*, 2003); there is also decrease in the volumes of key prefrontal cortices that regulate impulsivity (Lieb *et al*, 2004). In addition, there is volume reduction in the amygdala and hippocampus, two key limbic areas involved in storage of memories (Bohus *et al*, 2004), the experience of fear, and the operationalisation and rationalisation of experience.

Self-harm and violence

Impulsivity and affective instability result in alterations in perceptions of self and others that are associated with considerable aggression towards self and others, both physical and/or psychological. Trait-like features such as affective instability and impulsivity interact with states of acute life crises to manifest pathological behaviours such as self-mutilation, suicidality and micropsychotic episodes of mood-congruent delusions and hallucinations (Bohus *et al*, 2004). Violence by people with borderline personality disorder tends to be impulsive and either unplanned or without any sophisticated planning. In contrast, violence in antisocial or narcissistic personality disorder is often instrumental and premeditated, frequently characterised by exploitation and lack of empathy. In borderline personality disorder, the violence is often directed against the self, as fear of the other prevents its discharge outwards. In the analytic literature, this tendency has been referred to as 'retroflexed homicide' or homicide turned against oneself (Menninger, 1933). The instability in the direction of discharge of affects and urges is set in sharp relief in instances of joint homicide–suicide. After committing a homicide, often of an intimate partner or child, the perpetrator turns the violence on him- or herself, taking (or attempting to take) their own life (Liem & Koenraadt, 2008).

Attachment relationships provide a degree of calm, joy and sense of safety mediated by the endogenous opiate system, and this might explain the reduced numbers of opioid receptors found in the brains of individuals who have experienced high levels of stress in childhood (van der Kolk, 1994). It might also partly underlie the need of some people for significant levels of stress in adulthood, through aggression or self-harm, to achieve an effective experience of the release of endogenous opiates (Box 7.5). This process may become addictive, as may be the case for sports fanatics, particularly when individuals have few alternative means of self-soothing.

Box 7.5   Case vignette 4: India

India presented to forensic psychiatric services because she feared her own capacity to kill. India had a confused concept of death, her mother dying when she was aged 6. She and her younger sister were looked after by their grandmother and their father, but India's father was required to go away to work. India was 14 when her grandmother became ill. India began to become preoccupied with death and assumed that she was responsible for the safety of herself, her grandmother and her now 10-year-old sister.

She started to become involved in internet forums focused on death and was introduced to sadomasochistic imagery and self-harm via such sites. India found that she could control the frightening thoughts and violent death imagery she was experiencing by cutting herself. She also found relief in the care she received (and obviously craved) as a result. Her thoughts became increasingly intrusive and unwanted.

When her grandmother died, India reported that she wondered whether her obsession with death had somehow caused both her mother's and her grandmother's deaths. From this time, India's compulsive safety-seeking behaviours increased, including presenting herself to the police and hospital, requesting that she be detained for the safety of others.

Dissociation and identity disturbance

Dissociation and identity disturbance are related in large part to 'disconnection' in the normal integration of various aspects of mental processes, such as impulses, memories and identities (World Health Organization, 1992). These disturbances are the consequence of multi-levelled brain dysfunctions. The amygdala is involved in the storage of implicit bodily (somatosensory) sensations (or 'gut feelings') that provoke emotionality, whereas the hippocampus stores explicit memories, including those with emotional memories. This suggests a two-fold disturbance in the regulation of affects and impulses in dissociation and identity disturbance.

First, there is enhanced emotionality of an undifferentiated and poorly nuanced nature (amygdalar dysfunction), associated with poor verbal memories of experiences (hippocampal damage) that cause the emotional outburst. Second, abnormalities in serotonin transmission in key prefrontal regulatory areas (the orbitofrontal and anterior cingulate cortex) allow impulses and affects generated to be manifested behaviourally without the ability to contain or make meaning of them.

Clinically, there appears to be a bimodal response to salient stressors (van der Kolk, 1994). Frenzied and agitated states with increased tendency to engage in fight or flight behaviours are interspersed with dissociation or disconnection from the environment, with sudden reduction in levels of arousal, affect and identity. Although there is seemingly purposeful engagement in goal-directed behaviours during these periods, the individual later has limited capacity to provide a proper account of their mental state or behaviour at the time (Box 7.6). In fact, along with alteration of memories and affect, individuals experience altered identities and tend to act and relate differently during these periods. In extreme cases, they assume different identities with little or no memories of other identities, a condition called dissociative identity disorder.

Treatment planning

Given the wealth of differences in biology, sociological influences, psychological experience and presentation between women and men, we support the argument for women-only mental health services for personality disorder, with gender-specific individual and systemic approaches to treatment.

An understanding of women's needs in psychotherapeutic approaches should be linked to the issue of disempowerment:

'The term *gender* refers to the economic, social, political and cultural attributes and opportunities, associated with being male and female. In most societies, men and women differ in the activities they undertake, in access to and control of resources, and in participation in decision-making. And in most societies, women as a group have less access than men to resources, opportunities and decision-making' (Desprez-Bouanchaud *et al*, 1987: pp. 20–21).

Box 7.6 Case vignette 5: Avril

Avril presented to hospital emergency departments and to the police for a year or more with increased problematic alcohol use and suicidal gestures. Eventually she was admitted after speaking to a crisis team, reporting simple visual hallucinations and use of benzodiazepines. Avril had managed to maintain a level of stability and occupational competence in the preceding few years, having secured a job in a factory. However, before this she had spent some years working in the sex industry, mostly performing sexual acts for men in bars and clubs. She reported an early introduction to prostitution, having been involved in an age-inappropriate relationship with a bar-owner when she was 14. She learned to use both alcohol and dissociative strategies (cutting off) to cope with sexual encounters. She left this line of work when she lost a pregnancy. She continued to use dissociative strategies and alcohol to avoid intrusive symptoms such as flashbacks and nightmares. At work, Avril now kept herself to herself – relying on her rote memory to get the work done while remaining detached. Outside of work she drank – without a drink she would dissociate to varying degrees: from a general numb presentation, disconnection from conversations and looking 'spaced-out', to using breath control and self-strangulation to induce unconsciousness and occasionally splitting off with brief psychotic experiences. She had few friends and trusted only a couple of people.

In treatment settings it is difficult not to replicate such experiences, given the lack of control patients often have over decision-making in their care and the tendency of stretched services to reject patients who 'test' the system. The issue of treatment readiness and responsivity has historically meant that patients with complex presentations that include personality disorder have been excluded from services (National Institute for Mental Health in England, 2003). If attention is not paid to the need for careful management of change, the building of therapeutic relationships and the establishment of safety, the likelihood of therapeutic success is limited.

The model of care designed and refined for the women's secure service in which we work is based on a review of approaches to personality disorder and dominated by the staged approach described by many writers in the field but using the language of John Livesley (2003) and Marsha Linehan (1993). Livesley writes, 'evidence suggests that the non-specific component makes the greatest contribution to change; an approach based on generic mechanisms promises to provide the most effective way to manage and treat core pathology' (Livesley, 2003: p. 115). The approach, although set down with individual therapy in mind, has been used to structure an overarching systemic treatment model within our setting (Lawday, 2009). The model can be described as integrative eclecticism, in that we understand that when attempting to provide treatment for women with complex presentations such as personality disorder, intervention styles and approaches across professional divides, across individuals and across time will vary to some extent. We suggest that the focus remains on the natural stages of treatment, with (wherever possible) approaches working in harmony with a recognition of theses stages or phases of change. In institutions, procedures for the management of decisions, discussion of approaches and interactions, and shared understanding of treatment should reflect the complexity of the patient group.

We recommend that therapists undertaking individual therapy with women who have personality disorders ensure they have appropriate and adequate supervision and that they reflect on the stages of treatment, handling sensitively the temptation to embark on highly exploratory treatments too early. The pace and movement of therapy will be dictated by the patient. This can happen in an open exchange of views about the help needed at each stage of treatment, and/or it may happen through more complicated, non-verbal ways of relating and through periods of disengagement.

The language of change is important, and the therapist should consider it and share it with the patient. In our service, we talk about early-stage 'change management', which is important for patients from other institutions who will lose established relationships in the transition to our service, as well as for patients who are having their first experience of an in-patient healthcare setting. The next stages dictate the approaches used and opportunities provided across professional groups and in the given setting. These stages are described as 'safety and containment', 'control and regulation', 'exploration and change' and 'integration and synthesis' (see Livesley, 2003).

Conclusion

Given the complexity of experience, of relating and of environmental and social pressures that face women with a diagnosis of personality disorder, even an integrated model of treatment is optimistic. However, real change has been observed in women who present with problems that they want help to change. The pessimism and possibility for hopelessness that can exist in the interplay between doctor, therapist and client can be self-fulfilling, especially where systems are set up to encourage failure (by excluding women, especially women with personality disorders). Assessment and treatment protocols should allow for an understanding and acceptance of the complexity of these disorders, while offering a relatively straightforward approach to their management.

Key concepts to consider in assessment and formulation for a woman who presents with personality disorder include: social construction of gender (her own experience); disposition and traits; salient life stressors (especially those in which her gender played a pivotal role); interpersonal style (attachment style and strategies to manage traumatic re-experiencing); behavioural expressions; and her current environment and support systems. Treatment should then, where possible, be clear, consistent, staged and collaborative, with a sense of empowerment at its heart.

References

Adshead, G. & Bluglass, K. (2005) Attachment representations in mothers with abnormal illness behaviour by proxy. *British Journal of Psychiatry*, **187**, 328–333.

Ainsworth, M. D. S., Blehar, M. C., Waters, E., *et al* (1978) *Patterns of Attachment: A Psychological Study of the Strange Situation*. Lawrence Erlbaum.

American Psychiatric Association (1980) *Diagnostic and Statistical Manual of Mental Disorder (3rd edn) (DSM-III)*. American Psychiatric Association.

American Psychiatric Association (2000) *Diagnostic and Statistical Manual of Mental Disorder (4th edn, Text Revision) (DSM-IV-TR)*. American Psychiatric Association.

Bartlett, A. (2009) Gender, crime and violence. In *Forensic Mental Health: Concepts, Systems and Practice* (eds A. Bartlett & G. McGauley). Oxford University Press.

Bateman, A. & Fonagy, P. (2004) *Psychotherapy for Borderline Personality Disorder: A Practical Guide*. Oxford University Press

Bohus, M., Schmahl, C. & Lieb, K. (2004) New developments in the neurobiology of borderline personality disorder. *Current Psychiatry Reports*, **6**, 43–50.

Bowlby, J. (1969) *Attachment and Loss, Vol. 1: Attachment*. Hogarth Press.

Campbell, A., Muncer, S. & Bibel, D. (2001) Women and crime: an evolutionary approach. *Aggression & Violent Behaviour*, **6**, 481–497.

Caspi, A., McClay, J., Moffitt, T., *et al* (2002) Role of genotype in the cycle of violence in maltreated children. *Science*, **297**, 851–854.

Chesney-Lind, M. (1997) *The Female Offender: Girls, Women and Crime*. Sage Publications.

Desprez-Bouanchaud, A., Doolaege, J. & Ruprecht, L. (1987) *Guidelines on Gender-Neutral Language*. UNESCO.

Erikson, E. (1968) *Identity: Youth and Crisis*. Norton.

Farrington, D. & Painter, K. (2004) *Gender Differences in Risk Factors for Offending* (RDS Research Findings 196). Home Office.

Fonagy, P., Steele, M. & Steele, H. (1991) Maternal representations of attachment during pregnancy predict the organisation of infant–mother attachment at one year of age. *Child Development*, **62**, 891–905.

Ford, M. & Widiger, T. (1989) Sex bias in the diagnosis of histrionic and antisocial personality disorders. *Journal of Consulting and Clinical Psychology*, **57**, 301–305.

Hazan, C. & Shaver, P. (1987) Romantic love conceptualized as an attachment process. *Journal of Personality and Social Psychology*, **52**, 511–524.

Herman, J. (1992) *Trauma and Recovery*. Basic Books.

Home Office (2007) *The Corston Report: A Review of Women with Particular Vulnerabilities in the Criminal Justice System*. Home Office.

International Criminal Police Organisation (1994) *International Crime Statistics 1994*. ICPO Interpol General Secretariat.

Jurik, N. & Winn, R. (1990) Gender and homicide: a comparison of men and women who kill. *Violence and Victims*, **5**, 227–242.

Kaplan, M. (1983) A woman's view of DSM-III. *American Psychologist*, **38**, 786–792.

Kim, N. & Ahn, W. (2002) Clinical psychologists' theory-based representations of mental disorders predict their diagnostic reasoning and memory. *Journal of Experimental Psychology*, **131**, 451–476.

Kruttschnitt, C. (1993) Violence by and against women: a comparative and cross-national analysis. *Violence and Victims*, **8**, 253–270.

Lawday, R. (2009) Self harm in women's secure services: reflections and strategies for treatment design. In *Managing Self Harm: Psychological Perspectives* (ed. A. Motz). Routledge.

Lieb, K., Zanarini, M., Schmahl, C., *et al* (2004) Borderline personality disorder. *Lancet*, **364**, 453–461.

Liem, M. & Koenraadt, F. (2008) Filicide: a comparative study of maternal versus paternal child homicide. *Criminal Behaviour and Mental Health*, **18**, 166–176.

Linehan, M. M. (1993) *Cognitive Behavioural Treatment of Borderline Personality Disorder*. Guilford Press.

Livesley, W. J. (2003) *Practical Management of Personality Disorder*. Guilford Press

Livesley, W. J., Jang, K. L., Jackson, D. N., *et al* (1993) Genetic and environmental contributions to dimensions of personality disorder. *American Journal of Psychiatry*, **55**, 941–948.

Livesley, W. J., Jang, K. L. & Vernon, P. A. (1998) The phenotypic and genetic architecture of traits delineating personality disorder. *Archives of General Psychiatry*, **55**, 941–948.

Loehlin, J. C. & Gough, H. G. (1990) Genetic and environmental variation on the California Psychological Inventory vector scales. *Journal of Personality Assessment*, **54**, 463–468.

Loehlin, J. C. & Nichols, R. C. (1976) *Heredity, Environment, and Personality: A Study of 850 Sets of Twins*. University of Texas Press.

Lonigan, C. & Phillips, B. (2001) Temperamental influences on the development of anxiety disorders. In *The Developmental Psychopathology of Anxiety* (eds M. Vasey & R. Dadds). Oxford University Press.

Looper, K. & Paris, J. (2000) What are the dimensions underlying cluster B personality disorders? *Comprehensive Psychiatry*, **41**, 432–437.

Main, M., Kaplan, N. & Cassidy, J. (1985) Security in infancy, childhood and adulthood: a move to the level of representation. *Monographs of the Society for Research in Child Development*, **50**, 66–104.

McAdams, D. & Pals, J. (2006) A new Big Five: fundamental principles for an integrative science of personality. *American Psychologist*, **61**, 204–217.

McLean, C. & Anderson, E. (2009) Brave men and timid women? A review of the gender differences in fear and anxiety. *Clinical Psychology Review*, **29**, 496–505.

McLoyd, V. C. (1990) The impact of economic hardship on black families and children: psychological distress, parenting, and socioemotional development. *Child Development*, **61**, 311–346.

Menninger, K. (1933) Psychoanalytic aspects of suicide. *International Journal of Psychoanalysis*, **14**, 376–390.

Miller, J. (1998) Up it up: gender and the accomplishment of street robbery. *Criminology*, **36**, 37–65.

Morey, L., Warner, M. & Boggs, C. (2002) Gender bias in the personality disorders criteria: an investigation of five bias indicators. *Journal of Psychopathology and Behavioural Assessment*, **24**, 55–65.

Muris, P., Meesters, C. & Blijlevens, P. (2007) Self-reported reactive and regulative temperament in early adolescence: relations to internalizing and externalizing problem behaviour and 'Big Three' personality factors. *Journal of Adolescence*, **30**, 1035–1049.

National Institute for Mental Health in England (2003) *Personality Disorder: No Longer a Diagnosis of Exclusion*. Department of Health.

New, A., Hazlett, E., Buchsbaum, M., *et al* (2003) M-CPP PET and impulsive aggression in borderline personality disorder. *Biological Psychiatry*, **53**, 104S.

Paris, J. (2004) Gender differences in personality traits and disorders. *Current Psychiatry Reports*, **6**, 71–74.

Pedersen, C. (2004) Biological aspects of social bonding and the roots of human violence. *Annals of New York Academy of Sciences*, **1036**, 106–127.

Peugh, J. & Belenko, S. (1999) Substance-involved women inmates: challenges to providing effective treatment. *Prison Journal*, **79**, 23–44.

Pines, D. (2010) *A Woman's Unconscious Use of Her Body: A Psychoanalytical Perspective*. Routledge.

Rix, K. (2001) Battered woman syndrome and the defence of provocation. *Journal of Forensic Psychiatry*, **12**, 131–149.

Rothbart, M. & Bates, J. (2006) Temperament. In *Handbook of Child Psychology: Vol 3 Social, Emotional and Personality Development* (eds N. Eisenberg, W. Damon & R. M. Lerner). John Wiley & Sons.

Samuel, D. & Widiger, T. (2009) Comparative gender biases in models of personality disorder. *Personality and Mental Health*, **3**, 12–25.

Samuels, J., Eaton, W. W., Bienvenu, O. J., *et al* (2002) Prevalence and correlates of personality disorders in a community sample. *British Journal of Psychiatry*, **180**, 536–542.

Sarkar J & Adshead G. (2006) Personality disorders as disorganisation of attachment and affect regulation. *Advances in Psychiatric Treatment*, **12**, 297–305.

Schwartz, M., Blazer, D., George, L., *et al* (1990) Estimating the prevalence of borderline personality disorder in the community. *Journal of Personality Disorders*, **4**, 257–272.

Seligman, M. E. P. (1971) Phobias and preparedness. *Behaviour Therapy*, **2**, 307–320.

Soloff, P., Kelly, T., Strotmeyer, S., *et al* (2003) Impulsivity, gender and response to fenfluramine challenge in borderline personality disorder. *Psychiatry Research*, **119**, 11–24.

Spataro, J., Mullen, P. E., Burgess, P. M., *et al* (2004) Impact of child sexual abuse on mental health: prospective study in males and females. *British Journal of Psychiatry*, **184**, 416–421.

Steffensmeier, D. (1993) National trends in female arrests 1960–1990: assessment and recommendations for research. *Journal of Quantitative Criminology*, **9**, 411–441.

Stoller, R. J. (1975) *Perversion: The Erotic Form of Hatred*. Random House.

Torgersen, S., Kringlen, E. & Cramer, V. (2001) The prevalence of personality disorders in a community sample. *Archives of General Psychiatry*, **58**, 590–596.

Tooby, J. & Cosmides, L. (1992) The psychological foundations of culture. In *The Adapted Mind* (eds J. Barkow, L. Cosmides & J. Tooby). Oxford University Press.

van der Kolk, B. (1994) The body keeps the score: memory and the evolving psychobiology of post traumatic stress. *Harvard Review of Psychiatry*, **1**, 253–265.

Weiler, B. & Widom, C. (1996) Psychopathy and violent behaviour in abused and neglected young adults. *Criminal Behaviour and Mental Health*, **6**, 253–271.

Weizmann-Henelius, G., Viemero, V. & Eronen, M. (2003) The violent female perpetrator and her victim. *Forensic Science International*, **133**, 197–203.

Welldon, E. V. (1991) Psychology and psychopathology in women: a psychoanalytic perspective. *British Journal of Psychiatry*, **158** (suppl. 10), 85–92.

Wilson, M. & Daly, M. (1992) The man who mistook his wife for a chattel. In *The Adapted Mind* (eds J. H. Barkow, L. Cosmides & J. Tooby). Oxford University Press.

World Health Organization (1992) *The ICD-10 Classification of Mental and Behavioural Disorders: Clinical Descriptions and Diagnostic Guidelines*. World Health Organization.

CHAPTER 8

Personality disorder in adolescence

Gwen Adshead, Paul Brodrick, Jackie Preston and Mayura Deshpande

Summary There is considerable debate about the diagnosis of personality disorder in adolescence. It is argued that, because personality is still developing in the teenage years, it is impossible to state with certainty that a young person's personality is disordered. Alternatively, some researchers and clinicians argue that it is possible to diagnose emerging personality disorder on the basis of trait theories of personality. We review the evidence for both sides of the debate.

Disorder of personality in adolescence is a complex concept. On the one hand, it may be hard to distinguish personality pathology from normal developmental impermanence and instability. A developmental perspective demands that we keep an open mind about pathology trajectories, and balance resilience against vulnerability factors (Werner 1993). On the other hand, a small subgroup of young people do seem to present with emerging psychopathology that resembles adult personality disorder, where early diagnosis is likely to lead to early interventions and thus improve prognosis. The challenge lies in getting the formulation right. An inaccurate diagnosis of personality disorder in a young person may focus attention away from interventions that improve the caregiving environment at home, or stigmatise a young person in ways which ultimately do more to increase their problems. In this chapter, we will explore these issues in some detail, basing our views on our work in a residential secure unit for young people.

Difficulties in diagnosing personality disorder in adolescents

A key debate about the diagnosis of personality disorder in adolescents is between those who argue that personality is not fully formed until early adulthood, and those who argue that some personality traits are present and stable from early childhood.

Continuity and traits

Theories of personality development and continuity from childhood to adulthood are summarised by Caspi *et al* (2005). Certain clusters of adult traits, such as neuroticism, extraversion, conscientiousness, agreeableness and openness (the so-called 'Big Five' personality traits; Ehrler *et al*, 1999), have been identified in pre-school children. Their presence in childhood predicts later behaviours (Shiner, 2005), suggesting continuity of certain traits. Other studies have described the longitudinal relationship between childhood personality traits and behaviour and adult personality traits (John *et al*, 1994; Caspi *et al*, 2003, 2005; Shiner & Caspi, 2003).

A chief criticism of trait-based personality theory for adolescence is that it seems reductive and does not account for how personalities change over time. Prospective studies of the Big Five traits in children tend to use outcome data based on adult reports, which may reflect adult personality and mood, rather than the childhood trait (Lewis, 2001; Kroes *et al*, 2005).

Change and development

Personality change from adolescence to adulthood is robustly reported in a variety of lifespan and longitudinal studies (Vaillant, 1983; Soldz & Vaillant, 1999; Sroufe *et al*, 2005). There is also evidence that personality traits and diagnoses can change considerably in childhood and early adolescence (10–15 years of age), but that there is less change and more stability in later adolescence (16–21 years) (Klimstra *et al*, 2009).

In adolescence, it may be more helpful to think of the personality as a complex organisation of various psychological functions, differentiated into hierarchical levels. It may be that change in adolescence takes place at a different level of personality function, especially at the levels of character adaptations or beliefs and values and cognitions (McAdams & Olsen, 2010; Box 8.1). The narrative level of the personality is the level of meaning and subjective experience of identity, what McAdams (2008) has called the 'storied self'. Such narratives begin to emerge in late adolescence and are crucially related to the development of a 'moral' identity that makes ethical choices in social groups (Tappan, 1989). The development of these moral narrative identities may be relevant to the issue of rule-breaking and conformity in adolescence.

Attachment, abuse and disordered formation of the personality

Studies of development based on attachment theory have proved relevant to understanding how the caregiving environment can produce problematic behaviours in vulnerable children: behaviours that are the basis of the diagnosis of emerging personality disorder. The caregiving environment provided by parents and other adults acts as a growth medium in which the growing child's forebrain will develop through a process of arborisation, dendritisation and neuronal pruning. If the milieu is hostile, frightening

---

Box 8.1 Levels of personality functioning and interventions

Disorders may occur at any level: people with personality disorder typically have high levels of negative traits, limited sense of agency, and impoverished self-narratives characterised by passivity, hostility and a sense of threat.

Level 1

The person as an actor: traits, dispositions, temperament (limited interventional options: medications for symptomatic relief)

Level 2

The person as an agent: motivations, intentionality, individual characteristics (effective interventions address cognition, values, beliefs, goals, e.g. cognitive–behavioural therapy, dialectical behaviour therapy)

Level 3

The person as an author: the storied, reflective self (effective interventions address the social and self-reflexive self: group therapies, therapeutic communities, mentalisation-based therapy, cognitive analytic therapy)

(McAdams & Olsen, 2010)

---

or absent through neglect, these neuronal processes are affected (Rice & Barone, 2000; Schore, 2001).

There is a body of evidence linking insecure attachment patterns to various forms of personality pathology (for a review see Sarkar & Adshead, 2006). An important longitudinal study is the Minnesota project by Sroufe *et al* (2005), which has followed up a high-risk group of children into early adulthood. These authors have focused on childhood as a time of developmental complexity, arguing that successful psychological maturity is associated with high degrees of differentiation and complexity in terms of representations of 'self' and 'other'. In their sample, insecure attachment is strongly associated with the later development of personality pathology in adolescence. This confirmed earlier studies which found that dismissing attachment traits in adolescence are associated with elevated risk of developing traits of narcissistic and antisocial disorders, conduct disorder and substance misuse problems (Rosenstein & Horowitz, 1996). In contrast, preoccupied adolescents were more likely to have traits of histrionic, borderline and schizotypal personality disorder.

Childhood and adolescent experience of trauma is also relevant to personality pathology, especially experiences that induce high levels of fear or shame, or both (Lee *et al*, 2001). Evidence comes from the adolescent community surveys of Johnson *et al* (1999), who have followed up a large cohort of children in the community into their early 20s. The strength of this research is that it starts from a study of the 'normal', i.e. not those selected because of perceived behavioural difficulties. This research group has shown clearly that childhood maltreatment, including neglect, substantially increases the risk of developing a personality disorder in adolescence (Johnson *et al*, 2008). They found no difference between genders in terms of the range of maltreatment or the types of personality disorder that develop.

Neurobiology, genes and the development of the personality

There are neurological reasons why diagnosis of personality disorder in children and adolescents may be complex. The brain continues to develop throughout adolescence in terms of myelination and formation of synaptic networks (Rice & Barone, 2000). This implies that the neural bases for many psychoregulatory systems will still be in development. Such systems will not be fully functional or yet fully 'calibrated' to the individual's needs or environment, and may be expressed as immature psychological defences such as denial or somatisation (Heilbrunn, 1979; Northoff *et al*, 2007). The development of the frontal lobe in adolescence may continue to be influenced by the nature of attachment relationships, which may be subject to change as parents get older or grandparents die (Sunderland, 2006).

Magnetic resonance imaging studies have found that when the brains of adolescents are compared with the brains of young adults there are significant maturational changes in the frontal, temporal and occipital lobes (Sowell *et al*, 1999). Areas of the brain responsible for response inhibition, emotion regulation, planning and organisation are continuing to develop, hence the increased impulsivity so often seen in adolescence. It has been suggested that adolescents are motivated to take part in novel adult experiences, but lack the contextual knowledge to guide their decision-making, seeming to be more impulsive (Chambers *et al*, 2003). Adolescent neural networks are also responding to exposure to high levels of sex hormones, with attendant effects on mood regulation. In contrast to pre-school children (where similar struggles with mood and impulse regulation are the norm), language, spatial awareness and sensory functions are largely mature by adolescence (Blakemore & Choudhury, 2006).

Yet another problematic aspect of personality disorder diagnosis in childhood and adolescence is revealed by research into gene–environment interactions, which indicate that the caregiving environment influences the expression of genetic neuropharmacological vulnerability. For example, studies in boys have found evidence of an interaction between genetic vulnerability and adverse environments. A hostile caregiving environment makes antisocial behaviour much more likely in boys with variations in allele length for serotonergic proteins than in those without this mutation (Livesley *et al*, 1993; Caspi *et al*, 2002; Kim-Cohen *et al*, 2006).

Finally, given the prevalence of substance misuse among some adolescents, it is vital to consider the relevance of this in relation to psychopathology and diagnosis. Adolescents are motivated to use psychoactive substances that reduce anxiety, increase confidence and allow for attachment to peer groups. The immediate effects of drug and alcohol use on behaviour and social function are well documented, and are a major area of clinical and social work practice. However, the full and long-term extent of the effects of psychoactive substances on forming and developing neural networks, especially in the prefrontal cortex, is not yet known. It is possible that ethanol, in particular, is neurotoxic to processes such as synaptogenesis and dendritisation, and that it makes the adolescent brain increasingly vulnerable to environmental challenges that in turn may increase the likelihood of adult psychiatric disturbance (Olney *et al*, 2000).

Emerging personality disorder and child and adolescent mental health services

The factors discussed in the previous section have two main implications for child and adolescent mental health services (CAMHS). First, if young people's brains are changing, then any psychopathology is also likely to be changing. Therapeutic formulations and diagnoses need to be flexible and responsive to change. Axis I and Axis II disorders commonly co-occur. In adolescence, this 'transaction' between Axis I and Axis II disorders is likely to be more pronounced, such that each makes the other more likely to develop, and both suggest a vulnerable psychological self-regulating system (Shiner, 2009).

The other issue is that the parents' state of mind or beliefs about how they provide care and how the child elicits care are key influences on the child's development and behaviour (Lewis, 2001). Children's behaviour is affected not so much by what parents do, as what they believe about their children and their relationship with those children. There is evidence that suggests it is the mother's 'mindedness' about her child that affects the way in which the child develops an emotional language and theory of mind that are part of their personality structure (Meins, 1997). Support for the parents is therefore an important aspect of helping young people with emerging personality pathology. In addition, parents of children with conduct or hyperactivity problems are likely to have significant personality pathology themselves (Wolff & Acton, 1968; Lahey *et al*, 1988; Nigg & Hinshaw, 1997; Kuperman *et al*, 1999). The most die-hard genetic reductionist must accept that if personality problems are largely genetic, then both the genes and the environment come from the parents. If a child has, for example, callous and unempathic traits, then at least one of the parents probably does too, with potentially dire effects on the caregiving milieu in which the child grows up.

Current thinking about personality disorder favours a dimensional approach to understanding the pathology, i.e. personality disorders are extreme dimensions of normal traits, which can vary in severity (Tyrer & Johnson, 1996). If the traits of extraversion, conscientiousness, agreeableness, openness to experience and neuroticism are referred to

Table 8.1 Positive and negative personality traits: Big Five *v.* Bad Five

Big Five	Bad Five
Found dimensionally in the general community	*Found dimensionally mainly in populations with diagnosed personality disorders and associated with significant harm*
1 Extraversion: outgoing personality, sociability	1 Avoidance of others and mistrust
2 Conscientiousness: seeing things through	2 Impulsivity and attentional problems
3 Agreeableness: likeability, prosocial stance	3 Antisocial attitudes: contempt for social relations, especially for need and vulnerability
4 Openness to experience	4 Rigidity of thought and lack of curiosity
5 Neuroticism: anxiety and tendency to hyperarousal when stressed	5 Emotional dysregulation: unpredictable, unmodulated affects when stressed

Source: Shiner, 2009.

as the Big Five, then it is possible to conceive of a set of 'Bad Five' traits (Table 8.1). These would include: avoidance of others and mistrust; impulsiveness and attentional problems; antisocial attitudes and contempt for others; rigidity of thinking and lack of curiosity about anything; and emotional dysregulation, resulting in unmodulated and negative affect in response to unpredictable stimuli (Shiner, 2009).

Shiner (2009) describes how these traits may be manifest in childhood and adolescence in terms of DSM-IV clusters (Table 8.2). Cluster A involves avoidance, rigidity and variations in reality testing (what Shiner calls the 'peculiar factor'). Cluster C involves avoidance and internalised emotional dysregulation, characterised by preoccupying anxieties. Cluster B (which, as in adult services, tends to draw most attention) combines antisocial attitudes and contempt for others, impulsivity and emotional dysregulation.

Table 8.2 Personality disorder clusters (DSM-IV) and personality traits

Cluster	Personality disorder	Cluster traits
Cluster A	Paranoid Schizoid Schizotypal	Avoidance, rigidity, impairment of reality testing
Cluster B	Antisocial Borderline Histrionic Narcissistic	Antisocial attitudes, impulsivity, emotional dysregulation
Cluster C	Avoidant Dependent Obsessive–compulsive	Avoidance, preoccupied anxiety

Source: American Psychiatric Association, 1994.

The self-destructive and antisocial aspects of personality disorder are of greatest concern, because they have the potential to cause most distress in adults around the young people, and are therefore most likely to generate referral to CAMHS and/or forensic services. However, children and adolescents are also vulnerable to developing other types of personality dysfunction. Young people with Cluster A and C disorders also need interventions, since any Axis II disorder increases the chance of developing an Axis I disorder (Crawford *et al*, 2008). In addition, any personality disorder in adolescence increases the risk of violent acting out, with potentially disastrous consequences for the young person (Johnson *et al*, 2000).

Prevalence of personality disorder in children and adolescents

Despite scepticism about whether personality disorder can really exist in children, there are studies which indicate that personality disorder diagnoses in adolescents have validity and stability over time (Brent *et al*, 1990; Bernstein *et al*, 1993; Levy *et al*, 1999).

The personality disorders that present to adolescent services appear to resemble those that present to adult services. As always, prevalence rates are affected by selection bias in relation to services selected for study and the recruitment of participants. For example, the Bernstein *et al* (1993) study of personality disorder in a community-based sample of children and adolescents found a prevalence of 31%: the most common was obsessive–compulsive personality disorder. Only 17% of the cohort had a severe disorder, most commonly narcissistic personality disorder. By contrast, Levy *et al* (1999) found that 61% of an adolescent in-patient sample had a Cluster B personality disorder, mainly borderline personality disorder. There were very few patients with Cluster C diagnoses. Neither study screened for antisocial personality disorder.

Kasen *et al* (1999) completed a prospective longitudinal study of personality pathology in children aged 9–13 years over three follow-up points in a 10-year period. Their prevalence data indicate that about 15% of adolescents had a Cluster B personality disorder before young adulthood. Prevalence rates were comparable across genders. The prevalence of personality disorder at the start of the study was 9.6% for Cluster A, 16.7% for Cluster B, and 8.2% for Cluster C. However, the prevalence of the disorders changed over time: for example, at the start of the study, 7.6% of boys and 9.4% of girls had a Cluster B diagnosis, but 9 years later, the prevalence was 22.4% of boys and 11.9% of girls. The prevalence had increased in both genders, but considerably more among the boys.

Most studies of personality disorder in in-patient settings focus on Cluster B disorders: borderline or antisocial psychopathology. We have reviewed some of the data on antisocial personality symptoms here, but emphasise that other personality psychopathology may be emergent in adolescence, yet ignored because it does not cause social disruption.

Emerging antisocial personality traits and related disorders

Conduct disorder in children and later antisocial personality disorder and psychopathy are interrelated but are distinct clinical concepts. There has been considerable interest in the relationship of early childhood behavioural problems and later antisociality since the early studies of Robins (1966) showed that a small subgroup of children with conduct disorder show persistently antisocial behaviour in adulthood. The diagnosis of antisocial personality disorder requires evidence of childhood history of rule-breaking and irresponsibility.

Frick and colleagues (Frick *et al*, 1994; Salekin & Frick, 2005) demonstrated that children with severe behavioural disturbance can sometimes show callous–unemotional traits, and that these traits are different from traits in the behavioural definitions for conduct disorder. Frick (1998) suggested that the coexistence of attention-deficit hyperactivity disorder, childhood-onset conduct disorder and callous–unemotional traits is highly correlated with the construct of psychopathy. However, there are no empirical data supporting the progression of these factors into adult psychopathy, which is characterised by affective deficits, multiple forms of criminality and increased risk of severe violence (Frick, 2002).

Farrington (2005*a,b*) reports a prospective study of 400 boys up to adulthood using the Hare Psychopathy Checklist Screening Version (PCL-SV). His group found that high PCL-SV scores at age 48 years were predicted by childhood environmental (rather than personality) factors between ages 8 and 10, including physical neglect, poor parental supervision, a disrupted family, large family size, a convicted parent, and a mother with depression. Such studies confirm that childhood adversity is a good predictor of later antisociality and is as important as any genetic influence.

Delinquency in young women is often overlooked. In a meta-analytic review, Fontaine *et al* (2009) examined 46 empirical studies that examined the developmental trajectories of antisocial behaviour in females. They found similar trajectories to the adolescent male research, with the addition of a further category, adolescent delayed onset, where females had apparently not shown antisocial behaviour until later in adolescence. The emergence of antisocial behaviour at this time was considered to be associated with a decrease in familial and school control over the young women, an association with delinquent peer groups and hormonal changes due to puberty. Caspi *et al* (1993) suggest that there may be specific biological risk factors for delinquency in women (e.g. early menarche).

Offending and personality disorder in adolescents

The peak age for minor offending is 17–18 and so it is not unusual to find an adolescent male who has committed an offence. However, there is a subgroup of adolescent offenders who commit the majority of offences. These can be divided into:

- those who behave antisocially only during adolescence (and effectively 'grow out' of their antisocial behaviour);
- those that persist in acting antisocially as they get older.

Research into offending trajectories indicates that only 5–10% of adolescents who show antisocial characteristics follow the trajectory into adulthood. They are referred to as the early-onset life course group (Moffitt & Caspi, 2001; Laub & Sampson, 2003). This group are clinically distinct and have a poorer prognosis than the adolescence-limited group, who engage in antisocial behaviour for only a limited period during adolescence. The latter are believed to show antisocial behaviour as a part of gaining independence, seeking status and becoming free of parental supervision.

The evidence indicates that the early-onset group have experienced severe family adversity and a coercive parenting style (Moffitt & Caspi, 2001). This group are thought to be exposed to severe environmental adversity over a prolonged period of time. A follow-up study of males who had been aggressively antisocial in childhood, but had shown little delinquency in adolescence, reported that at age 26 they tended to be socially isolated and to have adjustment and mood problems and financial difficulties, rather than severe antisocial behaviour *per se* (Moffitt *et al*, 2002).

Vizard *et al* (2004) propose the existence of severe personality disorder in children and adolescents, on the basis of studies of the characteristics of young people who have committed sexual assaults or other serious crimes. They hypothesise that callous and unemotional personality traits arise as a consequence of a combination of genetic, perinatal and early developmental difficulties which become progressively more disabling as the individual matures. The authors outline a multifactorial pathway for the development of severe personality disorder involving early attachment difficulties, poor peer relationships, and early and serious child abuse, which manifest as aggression and sexualised behaviours in childhood. They emphasise the therapeutic importance of early detection.

Assessment of personality in childhood and adolescence

Given that the diagnostic process is complex in adolescents, it is not clear whether assessment tools that are based on adult assessment of personality disorder will be either valid or reliable. Nor is it clear whether there is value in assessment tools that are standardised on clinical populations.

In children, both temperament and behaviour can be assessed using a variety of tools, although these are rarely used outside research protocols. Most research studies of emerging personality pathology have utilised assessment tools based on those for adults (Shiner *et al*, 2003). There is uncertainty about the use of such tools in ordinary clinical services.

However, some specialist services for adolescents do use personality assessment tools (Box 8.2). These include the NEO Personality Inventory – Revised (NEO-PI-R; Costa & McCrae, 1992), which assesses Big Five traits in adolescents (De Clercq & De Fruyt, 2003; Allik *et al*, 2004), and the Millon Adolescent Clinical Inventory (MACI; Millon *et al*, 2006). The MACI is a self-report measure based on the Millon Clinical Multiaxial Inventory. Constructs have been validated against DSM-IV diagnostic criteria and address three different types of reported difficulties: personality traits, expressed concerns and behaviours.

Measures of attachment may be helpful in terms of making sense of personality pathology and suggesting interventions in family dynamics. A variety of measures of both attachment and personality disorder in adolescents are described by Westen *et al* (2006).

Forensic CAMHS and some youth offender services use youth versions of risk assessment instruments, such as the Hare Psychopathy Checklist – Youth Version (PCL-YV; Forth, 2005) and the Structured Assessment of Violence Risk in Youth (SAVRY; Borum *et al*, 2005). There are ethical concerns about their routine use because they can be used in stigmatising ways that reduce young people's access to general adolescent services.

Management of adolescent personality disorder

Work with children and adolescents differs from that with adults, in that services take a more systemic approach. An especially significant difference from adult services is the statutory involvement of the education system, and the need to work with family members who are still involved in

---

Box 8.2 Some personality disorder assessment tools used in adolescence

- Hare Psychopathy Checklist – Youth Version: young people's version of standard measure of psychopathy (Forth, 2005)
- Millon Adolescent Clinical Inventory: developed to be used in teenagers (Millon *et al*, 2006)
- Minnesota Multiphasic Personality Inventory – Adolescence (MMPI-A): an empirically based measure of adolescent psychopathology (Butcher *et al*, 2006)
- NEO Personality Inventory – Revised: a general measure of Big Five personality traits (Costa & McCrae, 1992)

the young person's social network. However, the treatment of a young person with an emerging personality disorder should follow the principles of CAMHS generally. In particular, it is important to screen for Axis I disorders such as depression or psychotic disorders, especially in children and adolescents with emerging borderline personality disorder, where depression is likely to be a comorbid condition.

Specific interventions for personality disorder in adolescents are similar in principle to those for adults, although few have been subjected to the same level of empirical evaluation. The National Institute for Health and Clinical Excellence (NICE) guidelines for borderline personality disorder noted that there has been only one published randomised controlled trial of interventions for adolescents with personality disorder, which may be because clinicians are reluctant to diagnose young people with the disorder (National Collaborating Centre for Mental Health, 2009a). Similarly, there is no mention of any evidence relating to the treatment of comorbid personality disorders in young people with depression or eating disorders, even though these are common comorbidities in adulthood. Such a lack of evidence makes treatment complex, especially since the transition between adolescence and adulthood may be a critical period for intervention.

Dialectical behaviour therapy

Dialectical behaviour therapy (DBT) has been adapted for a wide range of clinical populations, including adolescents. Programmes offering DBT to adolescents have been adapted in a number of ways, but no one version has been shown to be superior.

There is preliminary evidence to support an adapted version of DBT with adolescents who meet criteria for borderline personality disorder (Rathus & Miller, 2002). Adolescent DBT (DBT-A) differs from adult DBT in that it is designed to be delivered over fewer sessions (24 sessions over 12 weeks, compared with typically weekly sessions over 12 months for adults), includes parents in the therapy programme, places a greater emphasis on the family and focuses on teaching a smaller number of skills. The language used is adapted to be more appropriate for an adolescent.

Involvement of the family or carers in skills training is common to many of these adaptations. Teaching other family members can enable them to act as skills coaches to generalise skills in the young person's everyday environment. Although individuals are encouraged to work towards changing their own environment during DBT, it is recognised that adolescents may not always have the autonomy to effect this.

Rathus & Miller (2002) found that adolescents engaging in DBT were admitted to hospital less often, had higher rates of treatment completion and reduced suicidal ideation and symptoms of borderline personality disorder compared with those who received treatment as usual. There was a significant reduction in behavioural incidents when DBT was used on an adolescent in-patient unit, when compared with a unit run on psycho-dynamically oriented principles (Katz *et al*, 2004). James *et al* (2011) offered DBT to a community sample of adolescents in the 'looked after' system (i.e., in the care of a Local Authority). The authors found a significant reduction in self-reported depression scores (Beck Depression Inventory), hopelessness (Beck Hopelessness Scale) and episodes of self-harm.

Dialectical behaviour therapy has also been shown to have some positive effects in female juvenile rehabilitation settings (Trupin *et al*, 2002). This study highlighted both the impact of DBT on the young people and changes in the staff's reactions to them. Staff who had completed in-depth training in DBT showed a reduction in punitive interventions.

STEPPS

Another programme for improving emotion regulation is Systems Training for Emotional Predictability and Problem Solving (STEPPS; Blum *et al*, 2009). This has been used with adolescents to good effect (Schuppert *et al*, 2009). Compared with treatment as usual, adolescents who completed the STEPPS programme reported feeling a greater sense of control over their mood swings. The STEPPS programme, like DBT-A, involves training not just the young person, but also family, friends and professionals, with a shared understanding of the skills so that the network of people closest to the young person learn to reinforce and support the newly acquired skills.

Treatments for conduct disorder

A variety of interventions for conduct disorder have been evaluated both in the USA and the UK (Breston & Eyber, 1998; National Collaborating Centre for Mental Health, 2009*b*). These include parent training, cognitive problem-solving training with young people, programmes that combine work with parents and children, family therapy and treatment in foster care. All these interventions have been shown to be effective for selected groups. Family therapy and treatment in foster care have both been found to reduce behaviour problems and offending. There is a large evidence base for group-based training programmes for parents, probably due to an effect on parental negativity towards their child.

Multisystemic therapy

Multisystemic therapy is used with children and adolescents at risk of antisocial behaviours. It has been subject to a number of treatment trials, and shown to be effective with selected groups of young people and their families. It is a family- and community-based treatment programme, with the aim of improving communication, parenting skills, prosocial peer relationships, school performance and social networks. The outcome is to keep young people in their family homes rather than incarcerated in prison settings or hospitals (Henggeler *et al*, 1992; Littell, 2005). Families have

129

reported increased family cohesion, and young people have fewer arrests and self-reported offences.

Are psychological therapies effective?

It is possible to provide adolescents with psychological interventions that improve problematic behaviours. However, it is not clear whether these interventions effect change in underlying personality structures. Given the role of insecure attachment in the development of disordered personalities, it seems important to provide a secure base for therapy, and to promote curiosity and learning of new cognitions and appraisals, both of self and others. Young people with different attachment styles may present with different symptom profiles and behavioural challenges.

Conclusions and questions

It seems clear that for a small number of adolescents, a diagnosis of personality disorder can be confidently made. There is significant health morbidity among affected adolescents. Just as for adults, young people who have a personality disorder have high rates of early mortality, especially those with borderline or antisocial personality disorders (Kjelsberg & Dahl, 1998; Pajer, 1998). Therefore, these disorders are deserving of more time and attention from researchers, clinicians and policy makers.

However, the diagnosis of personality disorder is a double-edged sword (Box 8.3). Although early identification and treatment are likely to

---

Box 8.3 Pros and cons of personality disorder diagnosis

Pros

- Early diagnosis means early intervention
- Improved diagnosis means improved treatment planning and implementation
- The personality disorder diagnosis reflects a developmental account of the young person and their experience
- Personality disorder is a real disability: we may contribute to stigma and myths if we do not name it when we need to
- There are effective treatments for personality disorder

Cons

- Tendency of personality disorder diagnoses to 'stick' and not be revised as the young person changes
- People with personality disorder diagnoses are often refused access to services
- The diagnosis is a stigmatising label, and puts the young person at risk of rejection by services and ignorant professionals
- The diagnosis does not reflect the trauma histories in young people
- It is pointless to make a diagnosis if there is no treatment service

---

ameliorate a lifetime of potential suffering for the individual and society, a personality disorder diagnosis is a stigmatising label that can follow a young person for a considerable time and, paradoxically, block their access to treatment and services (Castillo, 2000). An alternative lexicon has sprung up in recent decades, with clinicians appearing to prefer to use diagnoses that emphasise trauma rather than challenging behaviours, such as the widespread use of the term 'complex post-traumatic stress disorder' instead of emerging borderline personality disorder, particularly when there is a history of prolonged trauma as an antecedent. Similarly, young people with significant antisocial traits continue to be labelled as having conduct disorder or mixed disorder of conduct and emotions or even reactive attachment disorder, rather than antisocial personality disorder.

This approach illustrates the continuing reluctance of clinicians to diagnose personality disorder in young people whose personalities are still developing. Clearly, it is unprofessional to use diagnoses in thoughtless and unhelpful ways, and it is valuable to promote recovery and coping skills in all mental disorders, including personality disorder. The difficulty with not using the personality disorder diagnosis is that this may obscure clinical need, often in relation to the most difficult symptoms such as hostility and rage attacks. It may also allow professionals to avoid looking at their own negative reactions to difficult young people, especially those who have been cruel or hostile to others.

Whichever diagnostic descriptors are used, clinicians are likely to meet young people with symptoms and signs of antisocial or borderline personality disorder. Therefore there must be more debate and consensus on which descriptive diagnoses are most useful. A move from purely categorical to more dimensional diagnostic systems would help to partly overcome this. Adolescents with these syndromes must not be denied interventions and treatments merely because of the fears of labelling and perpetuation of stigma.

There are a number of research questions to pursue. The principal of these regard the prevention of antisocial personality disorder in adolescence and the identification of high-risk cases (Harrington & Bailey, 2004). We also do not know why girls subjected to trauma are more likely to develop borderline personality disorder, whereas boys are likely to develop conduct disorder and eventually antisocial personality disorder. Nor can we identify which young people will present with which disorder, at which point in their lives and why. Related to this are ethical questions about identifying children and adolescents as being at 'high risk' or antisocial, especially on the basis of their genes.

Research in the area of personality disorder in the young is bound to focus on aetiology and pathogenesis. In recent years, gene–environment interactions have received increasing attention as efforts are made to unravel the complex interplay between the two. However, future research must focus on bridging the gap between gene and environment, since a purely genetic or purely environmental view is unlikely to provide the answer. Since it is also unlikely that we will be able to alter genetic profiles any time soon, we may be under an extra duty to intervene in children's adverse environments.

On this basis, services should be designed to intervene early and to address the adolescent's environment – the home, school and neighbourhood. Therapeutic interventions for children and adolescents must focus on helping to increase their resilience as much as on treating the disorder, and on the development of a prosocial identity. The emphasis must shift to the preventive, in the form of interventions for parents and caregivers. Environmental adversity in childhood increases the risk of the development of a whole range of problems (Axis I and Axis II disorders) in childhood and adolescence that may persist into adulthood. These disorders are costly, not only for the young people and their families but for all of us.

References

Allik, J., Laidra, K., Realo, A., *et al* (2004) Personality development for 12–18 years of age: changes in mean levels of and structures of traits. *European Journal of Personality*, **18**, 445–462.

American Psychiatric Association (1994) *Diagnostic and Statistical Manual of Mental Disorders (4th edn) (DSM-IV)*. APA.

Bernstein, D., Cohen, P., Velez, N., *et al* (1993) Prevalence and stability of the DSM-III-R personality disorders in a community survey of adolescents. *American Journal of Psychiatry*, **150**, 1237–1242.

Blakemore, S. J. & Choudhury, S. (2006) Development of the adolescent brain: implications for executive function and social cognition. *Journal of Child Psychology and Psychiatry*, **47**, 296–312.

Blum, N. S., Bartels, N. E., St John, D., *et al* (2009) *Systems Training for Emotional Predictability and Problem Solving (STEPPS – UK Version): Group Treatment Program for Borderline Personality Disorder*. Level One Publishing (http://www.steppsforbpd.com).

Borum, R., Bartel, P. & Forth, A. (2005) Structured assessment of Violence Risk in Youth (SAVRY). In *Mental Health Screening and Assessment in Juvenile Justice* (eds T. Grisso, G. Vincent & D. Seagrave), pp. 311–323. Guilford Press.

Brent, D., Zelenak, J., Bukstein, O., *et al* (1990) Reliability and validity of structured interviews for personality disorder in adolescence. *Journal of the American Academy of Child & Adolescent Psychiatry*, **29**, 349–354.

Breston, E. & Eyber, S. (1998) Effective psychosocial treatment of conduct disordered children: 29 years, 82 studies and 5,272 kids. *Journal of Clinical Child Psychiatry*, **27**, 180–189.

Butcher, J., Williams, C. L., Graham, J. R., *et al* (2006) *Minnesota Multiphasic Personality Inventory – Adolescence*. Pearson Education.

Caspi, A., Lynan, D., Moffitt, T., *et al* (1993) Unravelling girls' delinquency: biological, dispositional and contextual contributions to adolescent misbehaviour. *Developmental Psychology*, **29**, 19–30.

Caspi, A., McClay, J., Moffitt, T., *et al* (2002) The role of the genotype in the cycle of violence in maltreated children. *Science*, **297**, 851–854.

Caspi, A., Harrington, H., Milne, B., *et al* (2003) Children's behavioural styles at age 3 are linked to their adult personality traits at age 26. *Journal of Personality*, **71**, 495–514.

Caspi, A., Roberts, B. & Shiner, R. (2005) Personality development: stability and change. *Annual Review of Psychology*, **56**, 453–484.

Castillo, H. (2000) *Personality Disorder: Temperament or Trauma?* Jessica Kingsley.

Chambers, R. A., Taylor, R. P. & Potenza, M. N. (2003) Developmental neurocircuitry of motivation in adolescence: a critical period of addiction vulnerability. *American Journal of Psychiatry*, **160**, 1041–1052.

Costa, P. & McCrae, R. (1992) *Revised NEO Personality Inventory (NEO-PI-R) and the NEO Five-Factor Inventory Professional Manual.* Psychological Assessment Resources.

Crawford, T., Cohen, P., First, M., *et al* (2008) Comorbid Axis I and Axis II disorders in early adolescence. *Archives of General Psychiatry*, **65**, 641–648.

De Clercq, B. & De Fruyt, F. (2003) Personality disorder symptoms in adolescence: a five factor model perspective. *Journal of Personality Disorders*, **17**, 269–292.

Ehrler, D., Evans, J. G. & McGhee, R. L. (1999) Extending Big-Five theory into childhood: a preliminary investigation into the relationship between Big-Five personality traits and behavior problems in children. *Psychology in the Schools*, **36**, 451–458.

Farrington, D. (2005*a*) The importance of child and adolescent psychopathy. *Journal of Abnormal Child Psychology*, **33**, 489–497.

Farrington, D. (2005*b*) Childhood origins of antisocial behavior. *Clinical Psychology & Psychotherapy*, **12**, 177–190.

Fontaine, N., Carbonneau, R., Vitaro, F., *et al* (2009) Research review: a critical review of studies on the developmental trajectories of antisocial behaviour in females. *Journal of Child Psychology and Psychiatry*, **50**, 363–385.

Forth, A. (2005) The Hare Psychopathy Checklist – Youth Version. In *Mental Health Screening and Assessment in Juvenile Justice* (eds T. Grisso, G. Vincent & D. Seagrave), pp. 324–336. Guilford Press.

Frick, P. (1998) Callous/unemotional traits and conduct problems: applying the two-factor model of psychopathy to children. In *Psychopathy: Theory, Research and Implications for Society* (eds D. J. Cooke, A. R. Forth & R. D. Hare), pp. 161–187. Kluwer Academic.

Frick, P. (2002) Developmental pathways to conduct disorder: implications for servicing youth who show severe and aggressive antisocial behaviour. *Psychology in the Schools*, **41**, 823–834.

Frick, P., O'Brien, B., Wootton, J., *et al* (1994) Psychopathy and conduct problems in children. *Journal of Abnormal Psychology*, **103**, 700–707.

Harrington, R. & Bailey, S. (2004) Prevention of antisocial personality disorder: mounting evidence on optimal timings and methods. *Criminal Behaviour and Mental Health*, **14**, 75–81.

Heilbrunn, G. (1979) Neurobiologic correlates with defense mechanisms and psychotherapy. *American Journal of Psychotherapy*, **33**, 547–554.

Henggeler, S., Melton, G. & Smith, L. (1992) Family preservation using MST: an effective alternative to incarcerating serious juvenile offenders. *Journal of Consulting and Clinical Psychology*, **60**, 953–961.

James, A. C., Winmill, L., Anderson, C., *et al* (2011) A preliminary study of an extension of a community dialectic behaviour therapy (DBT) programme to adolescents in the looked after care system. *Child & Adolescent Mental Health*, **16**, 9–13.

John, O., Caspi, A., Robins, R., *et al* (1994) The 'Little five': exploring the nomological network of the five-factor model of personality in adolescent boys. *Child Development*, **65**, 160–178.

Johnson, J., Cohen, P., Brown, J., *et al* (1999) Childhood maltreatment increases the risk for personality disorders during early adulthood. *Archives of General Psychiatry*, **56**, 600–606.

Johnson, J., Cohen, P., Smailes E., *et al* (2000) Adolescent personality disorder is associated with violence and criminal behaviour during adolescence and early adulthood. *American Journal of Psychiatry*, **157**, 1406–1412.

Johnson, J., Cohen, P., Kasen, S., *et al* (2008) Psychiatric disorders in adolescence and early adulthood and risk for child rearing difficulties during middle adulthood. *Journal of Family Issues*, **29**, 210–233.

Kasen, S., Cohen, P., Skodol, A., *et al* (1999) Influence of child and adolescent psychiatric disorders on young adult personality disorder. *American Journal of Psychiatry*, **156**, 1529–1535.

Katz, L., Cox, B., Gunasekara, S., *et al* (2004) Feasibility of DBT for suicidal adolescent inpatients. *Journal of the American Academy of Child & Adolescent Psychiatry*, **43**, 276–282.

Kim-Cohen, J., Caspi, A., Taylor, A., *et al* (2006) MAOA, maltreatment, and gene-environment interaction predicting children's mental health: new evidence and a meta-analysis. *Molecular Psychiatry*, **11**, 903–913.

Kjelsberg, D. & Dahl, A. A. (1998) High delinquency, disability and mortality- register study of former adolescent psychiatry. *Acta Psychiatrica Scandinavica*, **98**, 34–40.

Klimstra, T. A., Hale, W. W. & Raaijmoken, Q. A. (2009) Maturation of personality in adolescence. *Journal of Personality, Society & Psychology*, **96**, 898–912.

Kroes, G., Verman, J. W. & Der Bruyn, E. E. (2005) The impact of the Big 5 traits on reports of child behaviour by different informants. *Journal of Abnormal Child Psychology*, **33**, 231–240.

Kuperman, S., Schlosser, S., Lidral, J., *et al* (1999) Relationship of child psychopathology to parental alcoholism and antisocial personality disorder. *Journal of the American Academy of Child & Adolescent Psychiatry*, **27**, 163–170.

Lahey, B. B., Piacentini, J. C., McBurnett, K., *et al* (1988) Psychopathology in the parents of children with conduct disorder and hyperactivity disorder. *Journal of the American Academy of Child & Adolescent Psychiatry*, **27**, 163–170.

Laub, J. & Sampson, R. (2003) *Shared Beginnings, Divergent Lives: Delinquent Boys to Age 70*. Harvard University Press.

Lee, D. A., Scragg, P. & Turner, S. (2001) The role of shame and guilt in traumatic events: a clinical model of shame-based and guilt-based PTSD. *British Journal of Medical Psychology*, **74**, 451–466.

Levy, K., Becker, D., Grilo, C., *et al* (1999) Concurrent and predictive validity of the personality disorder diagnosis in adolescent inpatients. *American Journal of Psychiatry*, **156**, 1522–1528.

Lewis, M. L. (2001) On the development of the personality. In *Handbook of Personality: Theory and Research* (2nd edn) (eds L. A. Pervin & O. P. John), pp. 327–346. Guilford Press.

Littell, J. (2005) Lessons from a systematic review of effects of multisystemic therapy. *Child and Youth Service Review*, **27**, 445–463.

Livesley, W. J., Jang, K. L., Jackson, D. N., *et al* (1993) Genetic and environmental contributions to dimensions of personality disorder. *American Journal of Psychiatry*, **150**, 1826–1831.

McAdams, D. (2008) Personal narratives and the life story. In *Handbook of Personality: Theory and Research* (3rd edn) (eds O. P. John, R. W. Robins & L. A. Pervin), pp. 242–262. Guilford Press.

McAdams, D. & Olsen, B. (2010) Personality development: continuity and change over the life course. *Annual Review of Psychology*, **61**, 517–542.

Meins, E. (1997) *Security of Attachment and the Social Development of Cognition*. Psychology Press.

Millon, T., Millon, C., Davis, R., *et al* (2006) *Millon Adolescent Clinical Inventory Manual (MACI)* (2nd edn). Pearson Education.

Moffitt, T. E. & Caspi, A. (2001) Childhood predictors differentiate life-course persistent and adolescent limited antisocial pathways among males and females. *Development and Psychopathology*, **13**, 355–375.

Moffitt, T. E. & Caspi, A., Harrington H., *et al* (2002) Males on the life-course-persistent and adolescence-limited antisocial pathways: follow-up at age 26 years. *Developmental Psychopathology*, **14**, 179–207.

National Collaborating Centre for Mental Health (2009a) *Borderline Personality Disorder: Treatment and Management (Clinical Guideline CG78)*. National Institute for Health and Clinical Excellence.

National Collaborating Centre for Mental Health (2009*b*) *Antisocial Personality Disorder: Treatment, Management and Prevention (Clinical Guideline CG77)*. National Institute for Health and Clinical Excellence.

Nigg, J. T. & Hinshaw, S. P. (1997) Parent personality traits and psychopathology associated with antisocial behaviors in childhood ADHD. *Journal of Child Psychology & Psychiatry*, **39**, 145–159.

Northoff, G., Bermpohl, F., Schoeeich, F., *et al* (2007) How does our brain constitute defense mechanisms? First person, neuroscience and psychoanalysis. *Psychotherapy & Psychosomatics*, **76**, 141–153.

Olney, J., Farber, N. B., Wozniak, D. F., *et al* (2000) Environmental agents that have the potential to trigger massive apopototic neurodegeneration in the developing brain. *Environmental Health Perspective*, **108** (suppl 3), 383–388.

Pajer, K. (1998) What happens to 'bad' girls? A review of the adult outcomes of antisocial adolescent girls. *American Journal of Psychiatry*, **55**, 862–877.

Rathus, J. H., Miller, A. L. (2002) Dialectical behavior therapy adapted for suicidal adolescents. *Suicide & Life-Threatening Behavior*, **32**, 146–157.

Rice, D. & Barone Jr, S. (2000) Critical periods of vulnerability for the developing nervous system: evidence from humans and animal models. *Environmental Health Perspectives*, **108** (suppl 3), 511–533.

Robins, L. N. (1966) *Antisocial Children Grown Up: A Sociological and Psychiatric Study of Sociopathic Personality*. Williams & Wilkins.

Rosenstein, D. S. & Horowitz, H. A. (1996) Adolescent attachment and psychopathology. *Journal of Consulting and Clinical Psychology*, **64**, 244–253.

Salekin, R. T. & Frick, P. J. (2005) Psychopathy in children and adolescents: the need for a developmental perspective. *Journal of Abnormal Child Psychology*, **33**, 403–409.

Sarkar, J. & Adshead, G. (2006) Personality disorders as disorganisation of attachment and affect regulation. *Advances in Psychiatric Treatment*, **12**, 297–305.

Schore, A. (2001) The effect of early relational trauma on right brain development, affect regulation and infant mental health. *Infant Mental Health Journal*, **22**, 201–269.

Schuppert, H. M., Giesen-Boo, J., van Gemert, T. G., *et al* (2009) Effectiveness of an emotion regulation group training for adolescents: a randomised controlled pilot study. *Clinical Psychology & Psychotherapy*, **16**, 467–478.

Shiner, R. (2005) A developmental perspective on personality disorders. *Journal of Personality Disorders*, **19**, 202–210.

Shiner, R. (2009) The development of personality disorders: perspectives from normal development. *Development and Psychopathology*, **4**, 715–734.

Shiner, R. & Caspi, A. (2003) Personality differences in childhood and adolescence: measurement, development and consequences. *Journal of Child Psychology & Psychiatry*, **44**, 2–32.

Shiner, R. L., Masten, A. S. & Roberts, J. M. (2003) Childhood personality foreshadows adult personality and life outcomes two decades later. *Journal of Personality*, **71**, 1145–1170.

Soldz, B. & Vaillant, G. (1999) The Big 5 and the life course: a 45 year longitudinal study. *Journal of Research into Personality*, **33**, 208–232.

Sowell, E., Thompson, P., Holmes, C., *et al* (1999) In vivo evidence for post-adolescent brain maturation in frontal and striatal regions. *Nature Neuroscience*, **2**, 859–861.

Sroufe, A., Egeland, B., Carlson, E., *et al* (2005) *The Development of the Person: The Minnesota Study of Risk and Adaptation from Birth to Adulthood*. Guilford Press.

Sunderland, M. (2006) *The Science of Parenting: Practical Guidance on Sleep, Crying, Play and Building Emotional Well Being for Life*. Dorling Kindersley.

Tappan, M. (1989) Stories lived and stories told: the narrative structure of late adolescent moral development. *Human Development*, **32**, 300–315.

Trupin, E., Stewart, D. E., Beach, B., *et al* (2002) Effectiveness of a dialectical behaviour therapy program for incarcerated female juvenile offenders. *Child and Adolescent Mental Health*, **7**, 121–127.

Tyrer, P. & Johnson, T. (1996) Establishing the severity of personality disorder. *American Journal of Psychiatry*, **153**, 593–597.

Vaillant, G. (1983) *The Wisdom of the Ego*. Harvard University Press.

Vizard, E., French, L., Hickey, N., *et al* (2004) Severe personality disorder emerging in childhood: a proposal for a new developmental disorder. *Criminal Behaviour & Mental Health*, **14**, 17–28.

Werner, E. (1993) Risk, resilience and recovery: perspectives from the Kauai Study. *Development and Psychopathology*, **5**, 503–515.

Westen, D., Thomas, C., Nakash, O., *et al* (2006) Clinical assessment of attachment and personality disorder in adolescence and adulthood. *Journal of Consulting and Clinical Psychology*, **74**, 1065–1085.

Wolff, S. & Acton, W. P. (1968) Characteristics of parents of disturbed children. *British Journal of Psychiatry*, **114**, 593–601.

Part 2

Management and general treatment approaches

CHAPTER 9

Assessment of personality disorder

Penny J. M. Banerjee, Simon Gibbon and Nick Huband

Summary It is important that personality disorders are properly assessed as they are common conditions that have a significant impact on an individual's functioning in all areas of life. Individuals with personality disorder are more vulnerable to other psychiatric disorders, and personality disorders can complicate recovery from severe mental illness. This chapter reviews the classification of personality disorder and some common assessment instruments. It also offers a structure for the assessment of personality disorder.

Historically, health professions have not always agreed on how best to conceptualise, categorise and define personality disorders. Although there are still many divergent views, there has been an increased consensus following the publication of definitions of personality disorder in ICD-10 (World Health Organization, 1992) and DSM-IV (American Psychiatric Association, 1994). In 2003, the Department of Health, in conjunction with the National Institute for Mental Health in England, produced *Personality Disorder: No Longer a Diagnosis of Exclusion* (National Institute for Mental Health in England, 2003). This document outlined the need for provision of mental health services (both general and forensic) for people with a diagnosis of personality disorder, and emphasised the importance of practitioners having skills in identifying and assessing personality disorder in order to appropriately treat a person's difficulties.

Prevalence and comorbidity of personality disorders

Personality disorders are common conditions (Coid *et al*, 2006*a*) that, by definition, run a prolonged course and are often associated with poor outcome (Stone, 1993; Skodol *et al*, 2005) and increased mortality (Harris & Barraclough, 1998). In a general population study of British households, Coid *et al* (2006*a*) found a weighted prevalence of 4.4% for a diagnosis of any personality disorder. The weighted prevalence for each individual personality disorder varied between 0.06 and 1.9%, with obsessive–compulsive, avoidant, schizoid and borderline subtypes being the most common. Dependent and schizotypal personality disorders were the least prevalent (the study identified no cases of histrionic or narcissistic personality disorder, suggesting that these disorders are particularly rare in the general population). Comorbidity within personality disorders is common; thus, patients with personality disorder are likely to fulfil diagnostic criteria for more than one subtype of personality disorder. In Coid *et al*'s (2006a) sample, 54% had only one personality disorder, 22% had two, 11% had three and 14% had between four and eight personality disorders.

In a non-clinical sample, all personality disorders, except schizotypal, were more prevalent in men than in women (Coid *et al*, 2006a). However, in clinical samples, women with borderline personality disorder may be more likely to seek treatment (Tyrer & Seivewright, 2000). There is an increased prevalence of personality disorder in people who are unemployed, divorced or separated, living in urban areas and from lower socioeconomic groups (Coid *et al*, 2006a). Antisocial personality disorder is common in criminal justice settings. A large systematic review found that 65% of male and 42% of female prisoners had a personality disorder (Fazel & Danesh, 2002). Of those, the majority had antisocial personality disorder (47% of males and 21% of females).

Personality disorder is also frequently comorbid with other mental illness. There are strong associations between cluster B personality disorders (antisocial, borderline, histrionic and narcissistic) and psychotic, affective and anxiety disorders. There is also a strong association between cluster C personality disorders (dependent, obsessive–compulsive and avoidant) and affective and anxiety disorders (Coid *et al*, 2006a). Both psychiatric in- and out-patients have a high prevalence of personality disorder – estimated to be of the order of 50%. In-patients with substance misuse and eating disorders have a particularly high prevalence of personality disorder, thought to be in the region of 70% (Moran, 2002).

The presence of more than one personality disorder in an individual is likely to result in a worse outcome for co-occurring mental illness (Tyrer & Seivewright, 2000; Newton-Howes *et al*, 2006) and may also increase the risk of violence in psychotic illness (Moran *et al*, 2003). It is important that where personality disorder occurs in conjunction with other mental illness this is recognised, as it may require adaptation of either the treatment or the way in which this is delivered (Tyrer & Simmonds, 2003; Dowsett & Craissati, 2007).

Classification of personality disorder

The ICD-10 definition of personality disorder is:

'a severe disturbance in the characterological constitution and behavioural tendencies of the individual, usually involving several areas of the personality, and nearly always associated with considerable personal and social disruption' (World Health Organization, 1992: p. 202).

In DSM-IV it is defined as:

> 'an enduring pattern of inner experience and behavior that deviates markedly from the expectations of the individual's culture, is pervasive and inflexible, has an onset in adolescence or early adulthood, is stable over time, and leads to distress or impairment'(American Psychiatric Association, 1994: p. 629).

Despite minor differences, these two definitions are broadly similar and share several components: the disorder is problematic for either the individual or others; it is pervasive across a number of situations; it is persistent across the lifespan; and it involves a disturbance of both behaviour and emotion. In DSM-IV the disorders can be grouped into three clusters: cluster A (the odd or eccentric disorders); cluster B (the dramatic disorders); and cluster C (the anxious or fearful disorders). There are nine categories of personality disorder in ICD-10 and ten in DSM-IV (Table 9.1).

Dimensional and categorical approaches to personality disorder

Two broad approaches to the classification of personality disorder exist: the categorical and the dimensional.

Categorical classification is largely based on clinical psychiatry and uses clear operational criteria to define the behavioural elements of personality disorder, inferring that each personality disorder represents a qualitatively distinct clinical syndrome. This approach is used in both DSM-IV and ICD-10. Categorical classification has a number of fundamental problems. It focuses largely on the behavioural characteristics while ignoring the underlying psychopathology. As a number of different behavioural criteria can characterise a disorder, this system allows heterogeneity. Categorical systems have arbitrary cut-offs to classify a disorder. Some of the information obtained through a personality profile is lost in a categorical system.

There is minimal empirical support for the perspective that disordered personalities can be captured by distinct categories, compared with the alternative perspective that there should be a quantitative distinction, with personality disorders on a continuum with one another, with mental disorders and with normal personality functioning. A dimensional approach reflects this perspective. It is based on personality traits and views personality along a continuum, with normal variation at one end and personality disorder at the other.

Purpose of personality disorder assessment

Central to any discussion regarding the assessment of personality is the difficulty in describing, conceptualising and categorising any disturbance. Part of this difficulty arises from the disorder itself. For example, who is best placed to report on someone's personality: the person themselves, who may

Table 9.1 ICD-10 and DSM-IV descriptions of personality disorders

DSM-IV	ICD-10
Cluster A: Odd/eccentric	
Paranoid: Interpretation of other's actions as deliberately demeaning or threatening	Paranoid: Excessive sensitivity, preoccupation with conspiratorial explanations of events, persistent tendency to self-reference
Schizoid: Indifference to social relationships and restricted range of emotional experiences and expression	Schizoid: Emotional coldness, detachment, lack of interest in others, eccentricity and introspective fantasy
Schizotypal: Deficit in interpersonal relatedness, with peculiarities of ideation, odd beliefs and thinking, unusual appearance and behaviour	Categorised as a mental disorder (Schizotypal Disorder, F21) rather than a personality disorder
Cluster B: Dramatic	
Antisocial: Pervasive pattern of disregard for and violation of the rights of others	Dissocial: Callous unconcern for others, irritability and aggression, and incapacity to make enduring relationships
Borderline: Pervasive instability of mood, interpersonal relationships and self-image associated with marked impulsivity, fear of abandonment, identity disturbance and recurrent suicidal behaviour	Emotionally unstable borderline type: Impulsivity, with uncertainty over self-image, liability to become involved in intense and unstable relationships, and recurrent threats of self-harm
No direct equivalent	Emotionally unstable impulsive type: Inability to control anger, to plan ahead or think before acts, with unpredictable mood and quarrelsome behaviour
Histrionic: Excessive emotionality and attention-seeking, suggestibility and superficiality	Histrionic: Self-dramatisation, shallow mood, egocentricity and craving for excitement, with persistent manipulative behaviour
Narcissistic: Pervasive grandiosity, lack of empathy, arrogance and requirement for excessive admiration	Not defined
Cluster C: Anxious/fearful	
Avoidant: Pervasive social discomfort, fear of negative evaluation and timidity, with feelings of inadequacy in social situations	Anxious (avoidant): Persistent tension, self-consciousness, exaggeration of risks and dangers, hypersensitivity to rejection and restricted lifestyle because of insecurity
Dependent: Persistent dependent and submissive behaviour	Dependent: Failure to take responsibility for actions, with subordination of personal needs to those of others, excessive dependence, with need for constant reassurance and feelings of helplessness when a close relationship ends
Obsessive–compulsive: Preoccupation with orderliness, perfectionism and inflexibility which leads to inefficiency	Anankastic: Indecisiveness, doubt, excessive caution, pedantry, rigidity and need to plan in immaculate detail

have no insight into how their personality interferes with their functioning, or an informant, who may experience the effects of an individual's adverse personality traits but has no insight into that person's inner subjective world? Another part of the difficulty arises from the definition of each of the personality disorders, in that some personality characteristics appear in the description of more than one personality disorder (e.g. avoidance of contact with others is associated with both schizoid and avoidant personality disorders). Such overlap requires the assessor not only to describe the behaviour, but also to enquire about its meaning or purpose (e.g. a person with schizoid personality traits will avoid contact with others because they have no interest in engaging with them, whereas a person with avoidant personality traits will desire contact but avoid it because of feelings of inferiority and anxiety).

To add to the confusion, personality disorder frequently occurs in combination with mental illnesses and substance use disorders (Coid *et al*, 2006*a*). There may be particular problems in assessing personality disorder in people with intellectual disability (Alexander & Cooray, 2003; Mason, 2007) or severe mental illness (Tyrer *et al*, 1983; Moran *et al*, 2003).

Personality may be briefly assessed as part of a standard psychiatric assessment. However, an increasing number of instruments are being designed specifically for personality assessment. Several factors have contributed to this development. In 1980, the American Psychiatric Association officially recognised personality disorder as a distinct and separate realm of psychopathology by giving it a separate axis within the DSM, Axis II (American Psychiatric Association, 1980). This resulted in increased clinical and research interest in personality disorder and the need for assessment instruments. In the field of psychology, the areas of personality and psychopathology developed along separate paths for decades, but in recent years their relationship has become the focus of much research. It began to be recognised that the knowledge accumulated about normal personality structure and personality measures could be used in the understanding of psychopathology. Assessment and classification of personality disorder are closely linked and therefore it is important to consider both areas before deciding how personality disorder may best be assessed.

In the UK in 1994, the Working Group on Psychopathic Disorder suggested that standardised assessments should be used (Reed, 1994), recommending 'multi-method criteria' for the assessment of severe personality disorder. A postal survey was carried out to evaluate how severe personality disorder was assessed in secure services and how the assessments compared with these recommendations (Milton, 2000). This survey revealed that only 40% of those who responded carried out a formal assessment. Assessments of personality structure and cognitive and emotional styles were more common than the use of structured diagnostic instruments or ratings of interpersonal functioning. This suggests that, even in specialist centres, there is wide variation both in whether assessment of personality disorder occurs and which assessment tools are used.

143

A pragmatic approach to assessing personality disorder

Important factors in the assessment of personality disorder include the setting, purpose and time available for the assessment, as these will influence which of the several assessment methods are the most appropriate. Assessment to provide an accurate diagnosis requires a different emphasis from that used in assessing motivation to participate in treatment or suitability for a particular treatment model. Assessment tools often allow more accurate diagnosis but give less information about other factors, such as how an individual's interpersonal functioning actually affects them, the presence of comorbidity or response to previous treatments.

Assessment conducted in line with the principles of the National Health Service's care programme approach places an emphasis on the following areas (Bennett, 2006: p. 284):

- risk of harm to self and others
- the presence of other mental health difficulties
- the complexity of the individual's personality difficulties
- the level of burden and/or distress placed on other family members or agencies.

History-taking

A good psychiatric history provides the assessor with valuable information about the history of the problematic behaviour. Further understanding of problematic interpersonal functioning can be gained from education, employment and relationship histories. It is important to explore how long problems have been present, variations in the difficulties, any previous treatment and the efficacy of treatment. Other previous or current mental health problems and substance misuse should be explored.

Presentation

Part of the difficulty in assessing for personality disorder is that a person's presentation can vary greatly, depending on their current affect or DSM Axis I (mental illness) symptomatology. It is therefore often helpful to carry out an assessment over several interviews. This allows the interviewer to be more confident that the patient's presentation reflects personality traits rather than their current mental state. It is also important to bear in mind that fluctuation in presentation may itself be a characteristic of personality disorder (e.g. emotional lability in borderline personality disorder).

Clinical interview

Clinical interview offers the opportunity to observe the patient's interaction with the interviewer. The interviewer has the opportunity to reflect not only on the content of the response, but also on the emotional expression and any non-verbal communication. The patient's response to the assessor and the feelings evoked in the assessor also inform the assessor's understanding of the patient's interpersonal functioning and difficulties.

As well as developing an understanding of the individual's problems, it is important to allow them the opportunity to identify which part of their interpersonal functioning causes them most distress and what they wish to change or modify. A joint understanding of the patient's treatment goals helps to build a positive therapeutic alliance. It is important to enquire about high-risk behaviour directed against the self and others, as this affects treatment and management.

Clinical interview has some limitations in the assessment of personality disorder in comparison with assessment of other mental disorders. The interviewer is interested not just in the standardised recording of symptoms and clinical features; in particular, they should assess maladaptive behaviour, its effect on the individual and others, attitudes and relationships with others, and social functioning in all areas of the person's life over a prolonged period. The interviewer must assess both the individual's current functioning and their normal functioning throughout their life. Some individuals, particularly those with cluster B personality disorders, exaggerate their difficulties; others minimise them. In our experience, it is beneficial to supplement a clinical interview with a more structured assessment to gain a fuller understanding of a person's problems.

Other sources of information

In addition to information from clinical interview and structured assessment it is also advantageous to use information from sources other than the patient. Often a patient has difficulty recognising which aspects of themselves are most problematic, and sometimes family or friends are more able to identify these personality traits. Of course, information from an informant may also not be totally reliable; the informant's descriptions may be influenced by their relationship with the patient or their own personality traits. Also, informants will usually be able to provide information on the patient's behaviour, but not on their emotions. Sources such as previous records can add to the assessment and be beneficial in supporting or refuting the problems identified.

Assessment instruments

Personality disorder can be assessed in a number of ways, including self-report, checklists and structured clinical interview. Numerous instruments are available to aid the clinician in making a diagnosis. These differ in terms of both reliability and validity. The validity of an instrument is the degree to which it measures the true concept that it purports to. This usually requires comparison with a gold-standard measure. As there is currently no accepted gold-standard measure of assessment of personality disorder it is difficult to assess the validity of the available instruments. Reliability is the extent of agreement between assessors (interrater reliability) or with subsequent testing (test–retest reliability). Generally, the structured clinical interview is regarded as more robust than self-report questionnaires, as the latter tend to overreport personality pathology compared with a more detailed structured clinical evaluation (Hunt & Andrews, 1992; Clark & Harrison, 2001).

It is beyond the scope of this chapter to give a detailed description of all the available instruments, but Box 9.1 lists those most commonly used. A small number of these are described below in more depth. Readers seeking further information are advised to consult Tyrer & Seivewright (2000) or Livesley (2001).

Box 9.1   Structured personality disorder assessment instruments

Structured categorical (diagnostic) assessments

Observer-rated structured interview

- International Personality Disorder Examination (Loranger *et al*, 1994)
- Diagnostic Interview for DSM-IV Personality Disorders (Zanarini *et al*, 1996)
- Structured Interview for DSM-IV Personality Disorders (Pfohl *et al*, 1997)
- Structured Clinical Interview for DSM-IV Axis I Disorders (First *et al*, 1997)
- Personality Disorder Interview-IV (Widiger *et al*, 1995)

Self-rated questionnaire

- Personality Diagnostic Questionnaire (Hyler, 1994)
- Structured interview – other sources
- Standardised Assessment of Personality (Mann *et al*, 1981)
- Personality Assessment Schedule (Tyrer *et al*, 1979)

Structured dimensional assessments

Observer-rated structured interview

- Schedule for Normal and Abnormal Personality (Clark, 1990)

Self-rated questionnaire

- Personality Assessment Inventory (Morey, 1991)
- Minnesota Multiphasic Personality Inventory-2 (Butcher *et al*, 2001)
- Millon Clinical Multiaxial Inventory-III (Millon *et al*, 2009)
- Eysenck Inventory Questionnaire (Eysenck & Eysenck, 1975)
- NEO Five-Factor Inventory-3 (McCrae & John, 1992; McCrae & Costa, 2004)

Unstructured assessments

Interview based

- Clinical interview
- Psychodynamic formulation

Other

- Rorschach test (Rorschach, 1964)
- Thematic Apperception Test (Morgan & Murray, 1935)

Minnesota Multiphasic Personality Inventory-2 (MPPI-2)

The MPPI-2 (Butcher *et al*, 2001) is a self-report measure of global psychopathology consisting of 567 true/false items giving information about symptoms and interpersonal relationships. It does not strictly describe personality dimensions, but describes different characteristics of personality, their coexistence and differing severity. This instrument takes about 60–90 minutes to complete.

Millon Clinical Multiaxial Inventory-III (MCMI-III)

This is a self-report instrument consisting of 175 items requiring a true/false response. It is designed to help practitioners assess the presence of DSM-IV Axis II disorders as well as a number of other clinical syndromes such as anxiety, alcohol dependence and post-traumatic stress disorder (Millon *et al*, 2009). It takes about 25 minutes to complete.

International Personality Disorder Examination (IPDE)

The IPDE (Loranger *et al*, 1994) is a semi-structured clinical interview developed by the WHO and US National Institute of Health joint programme on psychiatric diagnosis and classification (World Health Organization, 1995). The instrument is set out in a format that attempts to provide an optimum balance between a spontaneous, natural clinical interview and the requirements of objectivity. The questions are arranged under six headings: work, self, interpersonal relationships, affect, reality testing and impulse control. Each question assesses either a criterion or a partial criterion in the DSM-IV or ICD-10 classification. The IPDE examines for the presence or absence of a personality disorder and also results in a dimensional score for each disorder. It takes about 2–4 h to administer.

There is also a self-administered screening questionnaire version of the IPDE (World Health Organization, 1995). This requires less time and expertise, but produces a higher level of false positives. The use of such an instrument allows an interviewer to focus on highlighted areas and screen out individuals with no personality disorder.

NEO Five-Factor Inventory-3 (NEO-FFI-3)

This five-factor model of personality is the result of years of debate and research between scientists such as Cattell, Eysenck and Guilford, and psychometricians (McCrae & John, 1992; McCrae & Costa, 2004). The five factors are neuroticism, extraversion, openness to experience, agreeableness and conscientiousness. It is a dimensional model in which personality disorder can be interpreted as a maladaptive variant of personality. It has been argued that the dimensional approach to the assessment of personality disorder is theoretically superior. However, although this model offers a description of the various personality processes, it does not offer an explanation of the behaviour that a patient presents. The inventory is a self-report checklist that takes about 5–10 minutes to complete.

Personality Assessment Schedule (PAS)

The PAS (Tyrer et al, 1979) is another trait-based approach to the assessment of personality. It is a semi-structured assessment which also uses information from a collateral source; it takes 30–40 minutes to complete. It assesses 24 traits, such as conscientiousness, aggression and impulsiveness, grouped together into five personality styles: normal, passive–dependent, sociopathic, anankastic (compulsive) and schizoid. Several studies have found good interrater reliability (Tyrer et al, 1984) and also validity when compared with other widely used instruments.

Assessment of comorbidity, severity and ability to benefit from treatment

Comorbidity

Patients with one diagnosed personality disorder often have further personality disorders and other dysfunctional personality traits and mental health problems. The presence of comorbidity should be explored in the psychiatric history, and additional assessment instruments should be administered to check for further personality disorders. A structured clinical assessment tool such as the Structured Clinical Interview for DSM-IV Axis I Disorders (SCID-I; First et al, 1997) may increase the identification of comorbid mental health problems.

Severity

The type of personality disorder diagnosed and an understanding of its impact on functioning give an indication of the severity of the disorder. The notion of severe personality disorder is particularly pertinent in specialised personality disorder services and the field of forensic psychiatry. However, there is no standard way of recording this from DSM-IV or ICD-10. It has been noticed in many studies that people with more severe personality disorder tend to have a greater number of personality disorder diagnoses than those with a less severe disorder (Dolan et al, 1995). Disorder severity is also considered greater in those with disorders in more than one cluster. Some individuals have problematic personality traits but do not reach the threshold for a diagnosis of a particular disorder. Nevertheless, they can still experience marked interpersonal dysfunction and often show increased vulnerability under stress.

Tyrer & Johnson (1996) proposed a system for classifying the severity of personality disorder into five levels, ranging from 0 (no personality disorder)

Table 9.2 Classification of personality disorder severity

Level	Diagnosis	Characteristics
0	No personality abnormality	No personality abnormality
1	Personality difficulty	Meeting a probable diagnosis (DSM-IV) and three diagnostic criteria for paranoid, schizoid, histrionic, anankastic and/or anxious personality disorder and two criteria for dissocial, impulsive and/or borderline personality disorder (ICD-10)
2	Simple personality disorder	Either a single personality disorder or, if more than one, all personality disorders are within the same cluster
3	Complex personality disorder	Two or more personality disorders from different clusters
4	Severe personality disorder	Two or more personality disorders from different clusters, which cause gross societal disturbance

Adapted from Tyrer & Johnson (1996).

to 4 (severe personality disorder) (Table 9.2). They define severe personality disorder as the presence of widespread personality abnormalities in more than one cluster and leading to gross societal disturbance.

Treatability

Assessment of personality disorder often precedes decisions about treatability and whether an individual is suitable for a particular intervention. Interventions such as cognitive–behavioural programmes require a certain level of intellectual ability. If a programme or treatment intervention is too intellectually challenging for an individual, they may not be able to benefit from it. It is also likely to have a negative impact on their confidence and self-esteem and possibly exacerbate problem behaviours. Often the clinical interview will give some indication of level of intellectual functioning. It should be borne in mind that this can be influenced by many factors, including current mental state, education and cultural background. A formal assessment is valuable for predicting whether an individual can potentially benefit from a particular treatment.

Many patients with a diagnosis of personality disorder disengage from treatment and services. This has a number of consequences. Studies looking at non-completion of treatment programmes in offender populations, both in the community and in institutions, revealed that non-completers were more likely to reoffend than those who had received no treatment (McMurran & Theodosi, 2007). A number of explanations have been offered for non-completion, including low motivation, resistance and low responsiveness. Howells & Day (2007) proposed the term 'readiness for treatment', which they defined as:

'the presence of characteristics (states or dispositions) within either the client or the therapeutic situation, which are likely to promote engagement in therapy and which, thereby, promote therapeutic change.'

They suggested that readiness is a function of both internal (patient) and external (context) factors. Internal factors include cognition, affect, volition, behaviour and identity. External factors include circumstances, location, opportunity, resources, support and treatment available. Internal factors that suggest a greater level of readiness for treatment include: a positive appraisal of the treatment offered; ability to trust others; a capacity to express emotions and reflect on emotional states; moderate (but not overwhelming) distress; experiencing guilt rather than shame; and a belief that change is possible.

The diagnosis of personality disorder is often seen as pejorative, so an important part of assessment should be the identification of the individual's strengths and protective factors. These can be revealed in the clinical history and by some of the assessment instruments, and they need to be emphasised by both patient and clinician: successful treatment requires the management of problematic functioning, and the building and enhancing of the individual's positive qualities.

Assessment of risk to self and others

People with personality disorders are at increased risk of harming themselves and others (Stone, 1993; National Institute for Mental Health in England, 2003). Although the magnitude and causes of this increased risk are unclear, it should be acknowledged that only a minority represent a risk to others. People with cluster B personality disorders are at greater risk of criminal offending than the general population, but this increased risk is not found in those with cluster A and C personality disorders (Coid et al, 2006a). There is a particularly strong association between antisocial (dissocial) personality disorder and violent offending (Coid et al, 2006b), but given that features of this disorder include anger outbursts, failure to conform to social norms and lack of concern for others, perhaps this is not surprising. Despite the association between cluster B personality disorders and violence, most people with personality disorders, including half of those with antisocial personality disorder, have no history of violent behaviour (Coid et al, 2006b).

Risk is an important part of any psychiatric assessment and risk to both self and others should be evaluated. The depth and breadth of the risk assessment for a person with possible personality disorder will depend on the particular clinical circumstances, but the factors in Box 9.2 should be considered. Many different instruments are available to help the process of assessing risk to others, although there is increasing evidence that structured clinical judgement, using, for example, the Historical, Clinical and Risk Management scale (HCR-20; Webster et al, 1997) may have particular clinical utility (Doyle & Dolan, 2006; Maden, 2007).

Box 9.2   Factors to be considered during assessment

- Demographic factors
- Current social situation
- Current presentation
- Psychosocial stressors
- Previous history of violence and self-harm
- Previous response to treatment/supervision
- Level of social support
- Anger
- Impulsivity
- Substance misuse
- Presence or absence of mental illness

(Doyle & Dolan, 2006)

Psychopathy

Of particular relevance to the assessment of risk of harm to others in people with personality disorder is the Psychopathy Checklist Revised (PCL-R; Hare, 2003). This rating instrument aims to operationalise a clinical concept of psychopathy based on Hare's modification of Cleckley's description of psychopathy (Cleckley 1976). Compared with offenders without psychopathy, those with psychopathy (as assessed by the PCL-R) begin offending at an earlier age, commit more criminal offences, commit more types of offence and are more likely to reoffend (Harris *et al*, 1991; Hart, 1998).

Psychopathy is a clinical concept that, although not included as a category of personality disorder in ICD-10 or DSM-IV, meets the general DSM-IV criteria for personality disorder. It may be thought of as a more severe form of antisocial/dissocial personality disorder in which antisocial behaviour is accompanied by emotional deficits such as callousness and lack of empathy (Hare, 1996). There is increasing evidence that psychopathy may have a particular neurobiological basis (Raine & Yang, 2006).

The PCL-R assesses traits of psychopathic personality on the basis of patient interview and review of previous records. Although clinical judgement is required, trained raters yield reliable scores and the test–retest reliability is also high (Hare, 2003). The result of a PCL-R assessment may have negative implications for the individual, such as exclusion from treatment programmes or harsher disposal by the criminal justice system. It is therefore important that assessment is carried out for a specific purpose and that the full implications of an assessment are shared with the individual before it is undertaken. One of the benefits of the identification of high-risk behaviour is that it helps in setting treatment goals.

Dangerous and severe personality disorder

The criminal justice system in England and Wales has shown increased interest in personality disorder as a result of the government's Dangerous and Severe Personality Disorder (DSPD) programme (DSPD Programme *et al*, 2005). The DSPD programme was set up after a number of high-profile cases in England focused public opinion on the potential risk that individuals with personality disorder present to the public (Feeney, 2003). 'Dangerous and severe personality disorder' is not a clinical diagnosis. Rather, it is a descriptive term, embodying both psychiatric and social references, that is applied to a small number of individuals who are thought to be potentially suitable for this treatment programme. The Department of Health has defined this group as '[people over 18] who have an identifiable personality disorder to a severe degree, who pose a high risk to other people because of serious antisocial behaviour resulting from their disorder' (Department of Health *et al*, 2004). The DSPD is currently being decommissioned, but treatment of individuals in this category is discussed in Chapter 3, this volume.

Being classified as having a personality disorder and being at high risk of harming others may have significant consequences, such as long-term incarceration (Morris *et al*, 2007).

Although the aim of formal risk assessment is to provide a means of identifying and predicting any potential risk that an individual poses to both themselves and others, it should be used in tandem with risk management. This involves the interpretation of assessment tools in monitoring both dynamic and static risk factors and identifying appropriate treatment and/ or supervision for the individual.

Conclusion

Personality disorders are common conditions that have an impact on all areas of an individual's functioning and on any other mental health problems that they have. It is important to make a detailed diagnosis specifying both the personality disorder(s) diagnosed and the maladaptive traits displayed, together with the evidence on which this is based. An accurate description of the disorder is an essential prerequisite to providing appropriate treatment.

Personality disorder is highly comorbid with other conditions and it is important that a systematic attempt is made to evaluate whether the patient has other personality disorders, mental illnesses and substance use disorders.

The eventual aim of assessment is to arrive at a shared understanding with the patient about their difficulties so that patient and professional can work collaboratively on mutually agreed treatment goals. Part of this assessment should focus on the patient's strengths and protective factors.

References

Alexander, R. & Cooray, S. (2003) Diagnosis of personality disorders in learning disability. *British Journal of Psychiatry*, **182** (suppl. 44), s28–31.

American Psychiatric Association (1980) *Diagnostic and Statistical Manual of Mental Disorders (3rd edn) (DSM-III)*. APA.

American Psychiatric Association (1994) *Diagnostic and Statistical Manual of Mental Disorders (4th edn) (DSM-IV)*. APA.

Bennett, L. (2006) Community mental health teams and the assessment of personality functioning. In *Personality Disorder and Community Mental Health Teams: A Practitioner's Guide* (eds M. J. Sampson, R. A. McCubbin & P. Tyrer), pp. 283–300. John Wiley & Sons.

Butcher, J. N., Dahlstrom, W. G., Graham, J. R., *et al* (2001) *Manual for the Restandardized Minnesota Multiphasic Personality Inventory: MMPI-2*. University of Minnesota Press.

Clark, L. A. (1990) Toward a consensual set of symptom clusters for assessment of personality disorder. In *Advances in Personality Assessment, Vol. 8* (eds J. Butcher & C. Spielberger), pp. 243–266. Lawrence Erlbaum.

Clark, L. & Harrison, J. (2001) Assessment instruments. In *Handbook of Personality Disorders Theory Research and Treatment* (ed. W. J. Livesley), pp. 277–306. Guilford Press.

Cleckley, H. (1976) *The Mask of Sanity* (5th edn). Mosby.

Coid, J., Yang, M., Tyrer, P., *et al* (2006a) Prevalence and correlates of personality disorder in Great Britain. *British Journal of Psychiatry*, **188**, 423–431.

Coid, J., Yang, M., Roberts, A., *et al* (2006b) Violence and psychiatric morbidity in the national household population of Britain: public health implications. *British Journal of Psychiatry*, **189**, 12–19.

Department of Health, Home Office & HM Prison Service (2004) *Dangerous and Severe Personality Disorder (DSPD) High Security Services: Planning and Delivery Guide*. Home Office.

Dolan, B., Evans, C. & Norton, K. (1995) Multiple axis-II diagnoses of personality disorder. *British Journal of Psychiatry*, **166**, 107–112.

Dowsett, J. & Craissati, J. (2007) *Managing Personality Disordered Offenders in the Community: A Psychological Approach*. Routledge.

Doyle, M. & Dolan, B. (2006) Predicting community violence from patients discharged from mental health services. *British Journal of Psychiatry*, **189**, 520–526.

DSPD Programme, Department of Health, Home Office, *et al* (2005) *Dangerous and Severe Personality Disorder (DSPD) High Secure Services for Men: Planning & Delivery Guide*. Home Office (http://www.pdprogramme.org.uk/assets/resources/122.pdf).

Eysenck, H. J. & Eysenck, S. B. G. (1975) *Manual of the Eysenck Personality Questionnaire*. Hodder & Stoughton.

Fazel, S. & Danesh, J. (2002) Serious mental disorder in 23 000 prisoners: a systematic review of 62 surveys. *Lancet*, **359**, 545–550.

Feeney, A. (2003) Dangerous severe personality disorder. *Advances in Psychiatric Treatment*, **9**, 349–358.

First, M. B., Spitzer, R. L., Williams, J. B. W., *et al* (1997) *Structured Clinical Interview for DSM-IV Axis I Disorders (SCID–I)*. American Psychiatric Association.

Hare, R. D. (1996) Psychopathy and antisocial personality disorder: a case of diagnostic confusion. *Psychiatric Times*, **13**(2), 1 February (http://www.psychiatrictimes.com/display/article/10168/51816).

Hare, R. D. (2003) *The Hare Psychopathy Checklist – Revised* (2nd edn). Multi-Health Systems.

Harris, E. C. & Barraclough, B. (1998) Excess mortality of mental disorder. *British Journal of Psychiatry*, **173**, 11–53.

Harris, G. T., Rice, M. T. & Cormier, C. A. (1991) Psychopathy and violent recidivism. *Law and Human Behaviour*, **15**, 625–637.

Hart, S. D. (1998) Psychopathy and risk for violence. In *Psychopathy: Theory, Research and Implications for Society* (eds D. Cooke, A. E. Forth & R. D. Hare), pp. 355–375. Kluwer.

Howells, K. & Day, A. (2007) Readiness for treatment in high risk offenders with personality disorders. *Psychology, Crime and Law*, **13**, 47–56.

Hunt, C. & Andrews, G. (1992) Measuring personality disorder: the use of self-report questionnaires. *Journal of Personality Disorders*, **6**, 125–133.

Hyler, S. E. (1994) *Personality Diagnostic Questionnaire-4 (PDQ-4)*. New York Psychiatric Institute.

Livesley, J. (ed.) (2001) *Handbook of Personality Disorders: Theory, Research and Treatment*. Guilford Press.

Loranger, A. W., Sartorius, N., Andreoli, A., *et al* (1994) The International Personality Disorder Examination: the World Health Organization/Alcohol, Drug Abuse, and Mental Health Administration international pilot study of personality disorders. *Archives of General Psychiatry*, **51**, 215–224.

Maden, A. (2007) *Treating Violence – A Guide to Risk Management in Mental Health*. Oxford University Press.

Mann, A. H., Jenkins, R., Cutting, J. C., *et al* (1981) The development and use of standardized assessment of abnormal personality. *Psychological Medicine*, **11**, 839–847.

Mason, J. (2007) Personality assessment in offenders with mild and moderate intellectual disabilities. *British Journal of Forensic Practice*, **9**, 31–39.

McCrae, R. & Costa, P. (2004) A contemplated revision of the NEO Five-Factor Inventory. *Personality and Individual Differences*, **36**, 587–596.

McCrae, R. M. & John, O. P. (1992) An introduction to the five-factor model and its applications. *Journal of Personality*, **60**, 175–215.

McMurran, M. & Theodosi, E. (2007) Is offender treatment non-completion associated with increased reconviction over no treatment? *Psychology, Crime and Law*, **13**, 333–343.

Millon, T., Davis, R., Millon, C., *et al* (2009) *The Millon Clinical Multiaxial Inventory-III (MCMI-III)*. PsychCorp.

Milton, J. (2000) A postal survey of the assessment procedure for personality disorder in forensic settings. *Psychiatric Bulletin*, **24**, 254–257.

Moran, P. (2002) *The Epidemiology of Personality Disorders*. Department of Health.

Moran, P., Walsh, E., Tyrer, P., *et al* (2003) Impact of comorbid personality disorder on violence in psychosis: report from the UK700 trial. *British Journal of Psychiatry*, **182**, 129–134.

Morey, L. C. (1991) *Personality Assessment Inventory – Professional Manual*. Psychological Assessment Resources.

Morgan, C. D. & Murray, H. A. (1935) A method for investigating fantasies: the Thematic Apperception Test. *Archives of Neurology and Psychiatry*, **34**, 298–306.

Morris, A., Gibbon, S. & Duggan, C. (2007) Sentenced to hospital – a cause for concern? *Personality and Mental Health*, **1**, 74–79.

National Institute for Mental Health in England (2003) *Personality Disorder: No Longer a Diagnosis of Exclusion. Policy Implementation Guidance for the Development of Services for People with Personality Disorder*. Department of Health.

Newton-Howes, G., Tyrer, P. & Johnston, T. (2006) Personality disorder and the outcome of depression: meta-analysis of published studies. *British Journal of Psychiatry*, **188**, 13–20.

Pfohl, B., Blum, N. & Zimmerman, M. (1997) *Structured Interview for DSM-IV Personality (SIDP-IV)*. American Psychiatric Press.

Raine, A. & Yang, Y. (2006) The neuroanatomical basis of psychopathy: a review of brain imaging findings. In *Handbook of Psychopathy* (ed. C. Patrick), pp. 278–295. Guilford Press.

Reed, J. (1994) *Report of the Department of Health and Home Office Working Group on Psychopathic Disorder*. Home Office.

Rorschach, H. (1964) *Psychodiagnostics*. Grune & Stratton.

Skodol, A. E., Gunderson, J. G., Shea, T. M., *et al* (2005) The collaborative longitudinal personality disorders study (CLPS): overview and implications. *Journal of Personality Disorders*, **19**, 487–504.

Stone, M. H. (1993) Long-term outcome in personality disorders. *British Journal of Psychiatry*, **162**, 299–313.

Tyrer, P. & Johnson, T. (1996) Establishing the severity of personality disorder. *American Journal of Psychiatry*, **153**, 1593–1597.

Tyrer, P. & Seivewright, H. (2000) Outcome of personality disorder. In *Personality Disorders: Diagnosis, Management, and Course* (2nd edn) (ed. P. Tyrer), pp. 105–125. Butterworth-Heinemann.

Tyrer, P. & Simmonds, S. (2003) Treatment models for those with severe mental illness and comorbid personality disorder. *British Journal of Psychiatry*, **182** (suppl. 44), s15–18.

Tyrer, P., Alexander, M. S., Cicchetti, D., *et al* (1979) Reliability of a schedule for rating personality disorders. *British Journal of Psychiatry*, **135**, 168–174.

Tyrer, P., Strauss, J. & Ciccheti, D. (1983) Temporal reliability of personality in psychiatric patients. *Psychological Medicine*, **13**, 393–398.

Tyrer, P., Cicchetti, D., Casey, P., *et al* (1984) Cross-national reliability of a schedule for assessing personality disorders. *Journal of Nervous and Mental Diseases*, **172**, 718–721.

Webster, C. D., Douglas, K. S., Eaves, D., *et al* (1997) *HCR-20: Assessing Risk for Violence, Version 2*. Mental Health, Law and Policy Institute, Simon Fraser University.

Widiger, T. A., Mangine, S., Corbitt, E. M., *et al* (1995) *Personality Disorder Interview-IV: A Semistructured interview for the Assessment of Personality Disorders*. Psychological Assessment Resources.

World Health Organization (1992) *International Classification of Diseases and Health Related Problems – Tenth Revision (ICD-10)*. WHO.

World Health Organization (1995) *International Personality Disorder Examination (IPDE Manual)*. American Psychiatric Publishing.

Zanarini, M. C., Frankenburg, F. R., Sickel, A. E., *et al* (1996) *The Diagnostic Interview for DSM-IV Personality Disorders (DIPD-IV)*. McLean Hospital.

155

Diagnosis and classification of personality disorder: difficulties, their resolution and implications for practice

Jaydip Sarkar and Conor Duggan

Summary There are many difficulties associated with the diagnostic guidelines for personality disorder in the current international classificatory systems such as ICD-10 and DSM-IV. These lead not only to significant overlap with DSM Axis I disorders, resulting in high rates of diagnoses of comorbidities and multiple personality disorders, but also to lack of adequate capture of core personality pathology. The current classifications are also unhelpful in treatment selection, presumably the prime reason for assessing individuals in the first place. In this chapter we highlight various deficits and inadequacies related to the nosology of the current systems and suggest some strategies for dealing with these. We offer an integrated model of assessing and diagnosing personality disorders. We attempt to demonstrate how using a more integrated approach minimises or even eliminates some of the key problems highlighted in the current systems.

Criteria for diagnosis of personality disorders have been established in the two international classificatory systems, ICD-10 (World Health Organization, 1992) and DSM-IV (American Psychiatric Association, 1994). Both systems are atheoretical, i.e. based not on any causative explanatory paradigm but on expert consensus. Their approach to diagnostic classification has problems that are so serious that, in our experience, many practitioners question the value of making a diagnosis of personality disorder at all.

Given that both ICD-10 and DSM-IV are in the process of revision, we begin with deficiencies of the current systems that have been identified as being especially important. First, the current systems are neither theoretically sound nor empirically validated (Livesley, 2007; Tyrer *et al*, 2007). Second, they pose problems not only of overlap (an individual might satisfy several personality disorder diagnoses) but also of inadequate capture of important clinical aspects of personality pathology (e.g. passive–aggressive and sadistic traits) (Westen & Arkowitz-Westen, 1998). Furthermore, they are not sufficiently discriminating, so a substantial number of individuals are classified as having a 'personality disorder not otherwise specified' (Verheul & Widiger, 2004). Third, clinical assessments of personality disorder have been shown to be very unreliable and self-report inventories have been shown to generate too much psychopathology (Zimmerman, 1994). Although semi-structured instruments show an acceptable level of reliability, their administration is cumbersome and often requires considerable training. Consequently, their utility for many practitioners is limited. Moreover, the concurrent validity between these instruments is poor: someone who meets criteria for a personality disorder with one instrument might not do so with another. This is clearly unsatisfactory. Finally, and most importantly, the current classificatory scheme is unhelpful in treatment selection (Sanderson & Clarkin, 2002; Livesley, 2007). As treatment selection is usually the reason for assessing the individual in the first place, this failure to follow up quite detailed assessments with a coherent treatment plan can be disheartening for both patient and clinician.

These shortcomings relate predominantly to differences between two schools of thought on classification: the categorical and the dimensional. These differences are due to philosophical and theoretical approaches that distinguish the biological and the social sciences: medical systems belong to the former school and psychology to the latter.

The categorical approach

Both ICD-10 and DSM-IV identify categories of personality disorder. In keeping with their medical origins, the two schemes promulgate a system for diagnosing personality disorder that is categorical in nature: people are thought either to have a personality disorder or not to have one. The categorical approach has a two-component structure – generic criteria to make a diagnosis of personality disorder, and specific criteria for the different types of the disorder. The generic criteria (Box 10.1)

Box 10.1   Generic criteria for a diagnosis of personality disorder

Characteristic features:

- maladaptive thinking, feeling, behaving and social functioning
- developmental origin, tend to be lifelong, relatively inflexible
- clinically significant distress to self and others
- thinking, feeling, behaviour and social functioning deviate markedly from cultural norms
- not due to any other mental or medical condition

seek to separate personality disorder (DSM Axis II disorders) from other mental disorders (DSM Axis I disorders), whereas the disorder-specific criteria attempt to distinguish different types of personality disorder (e.g. borderline and narcissistic) from one another.

Disorder-specific criteria

The trait is adopted as the basic descriptive unit, and is defined in DSM-IV-TR as '[behavioural] patterns of perceiving, relating to, and thinking about the environment and oneself' (American Psychiatric Association, 2004: p. 630). There is much confusion as to how a trait should be defined and/or described. Each trait within the classificatory systems consists of various behavioural and phenomenological markers that are used as diagnostic criteria. In some cases a single phenomenon (e.g. suspiciousness in paranoid personality disorder) with various manifestations as additional criteria (e.g. suspects others, doubts loyalty, reads hidden meanings) is described; in others a wide range of features are encompassed. For example, borderline personality disorder uses impulsivity, emotional reactivity and cognitive dysregulation as features, with behavioural markers as criteria. Impulsivity is manifested by drug misuse, binge drinking, self-harm, promiscuity and so on. In all, up to 79 diagnostic criteria have to be evaluated in DSM-IV-TR in order to assess the extent of personality disorder in a patient, and these are then grouped into prototypes of the disorders (Livesley, 2007).

Cluster of disorders

In DSM-IV, personality disorder diagnoses are clustered into three groups on the basis of similarity of symptoms (Box 10.2). Such clustering is not used in ICD-10. Cluster A includes odd and eccentric individuals who tend to live in their own internal world and shun human contact as much as possible. Individuals with cluster B features display dramatic, impulsive and over-emotional behaviour and act in ways that result in unstable relationships with others or even exclusion from their social group. Those with cluster C features are anxious, seemingly avoidant of others, although they desire and cherish human proximity and feel severe stress when they cannot have the perceived support of others.

Box 10.2 The cluster of personality disorders in DSM-IV

- Cluster A: odd and eccentric – paranoid, schizotypal and schizoid personality disorders
- Cluster B: dramatic, emotional – borderline, antisocial, narcissistic and histrionic personality disorders
- Cluster C: anxious, fearful – avoidant, obsessive–compulsive, and dependent personality disorders

Critique of categorical systems

There are major problems with our current nosology – especially with the DSM system, which will be the main focus of the remainder of this chapter. Establishing diagnoses and clusters in a categorical manner may lead to greater agreement and communication between clinicians (increased reliability), but it does not enhance the fundamental understanding of disorders (no increase in validity).

One of the supposed advances of DSM-III (American Psychiatric Association, 1980) was the introduction of the multiaxial system, which separated the newly classified Axis I disorders (which were considered to be transient disorders of state) from Axis II disorders (deemed to be more enduring and dependent on the abnormal traits that the individual possessed). Part of the rationale for this system was that it would force clinicians to consider assessing personality disorder, even in patients with an Axis I condition. By so doing, it was hoped that clinicians would take personality disorder more seriously in their clinical practice and that research into personality disorder would also be promoted (Millon & Frances, 1986). However, many conceptual difficulties remained and have yet to be resolved.

First, the distinction between Axis I and Axis II disorders is not borne out by empiricism. This is because the level of comorbidity is so high, especially for some disorders (e.g. borderline personality disorder with depression, antisocial personality disorder with substance misuse), that the distinction is vitiated.

Second, symptoms specific to personality disorders are continuously distributed across both clinical and healthy samples (Livesley *et al*, 1994). Consequently, diagnostic 'disorders' reflect an arbitrary threshold and not true disorders (Blackburn, 2000).

Third, personality disorder diagnoses often show poor psychometric properties such as validity and reliability (Blais *et al*, 1998) because current criteria have been selected by clinical consensus rather than empirical analysis (Livesley, 2007). The ICD has a lower threshold for making a diagnosis (Tyrer & Johnson, 1996) but the DSM, a more rigid system advocating a checklist approach, identifies a higher number of personality disorders: 11 by DSM-IV as opposed to 8 by ICD-10.

Fourth, and related, the diagnoses have limited clinical utility, not helping practitioners to choose between pharmacological or psychotherapeutic interventions (Sanderson & Clarkin, 2002; Tyrer & Bateman, 2004).

Fifth, owing to 'loose' taxonomic criteria, the nomenclature and number of personality disorders have changed with each new edition of the DSM and ICD, further undermining practitioner confidence. With the revision of DSM-III–R to DSM-IV, some personality disorders (e.g. sadistic and self-defeating) disappeared entirely, whereas others (e.g. passive–aggressive) were removed to the appendix. The disappearance of sadistic personality disorder was largely a consequence of political pressure from feminists who wished to remove what they considered to be a psychiatric loop-hole that might exculpate some extreme (male) offenders (Stone, 1998).

The categorical approach has been popular because it is simple to operate and fits with a medical model of disease, establishing clear boundaries between normal and abnormal functioning. In a social welfare system of democratic governance this is important in terms of resource allocation, prioritising of services and identifying suitable individuals for receipt of interventions. The deficits of the categorical system are probably central to the belief among many clinicians in the UK that personality disorder is not a 'real' disorder and that those with personality disorder are so different from people with mental illness that generic mental health services can and should exclude them. Such beliefs and attitudes have led to a crude form of resource allocation within mental health services in the UK that has often tended to 'reserve' services for people with chronic and severe forms of psychoses and mood disorders, most often excluding as untreatable those with personality disorder (Department of Health, 2003).

The dimensional approach

If the individual, interpersonal and group aspects of personality functioning are emphasised in a diagnostic system, personality will be seen to involve a number of different capacities – dimensions, domains or traits – operating at different times and in different settings. Allport first emphasised the role of 'traits' in the make-up of personality as the 'dynamic organization [...] of those psychophysical systems that determine characteristics of behaviour and thought' (Allport, 1955). The most influential model of normal personality was proposed by Eysenck. It focuses on the individual's intra-personal characteristics rather than social interactions and describes personality in terms of three dimensions of higher-order traits or 'superfactors': psychoticism, extraversion and neuroticism – the PEN model (Eysenck, 1990). A modern extension of this model has five dimensions: neuroticism, extraversion, agreeableness, openness and conscientiousness – the so-called 'big five' or the five-factor model of personality (McCrae & Costa, 1987). These dimensions can be measured reliably and, with the exception of openness, all the factors have been replicated across cultures and shown to be moderately heritable (Bouchard & Loehlin, 2001).

There is overwhelming empirical support for a dimensional representation of normal personality (Widiger & Frances, 1994; Clark et al, 1997; Livesley, 2007). Many dimensional or trait models of personality exist but most of these collapse into three (extraversion, neuroticism, psychoticism: Table 10.1), four (emotional dysregulation, dissocial behaviour, inhibitedness, compulsivity: discussed below) or five (neuroticism, extraversion, agreeableness, openness and conscientiousness) basic structures.

Personality disorder within a dimensional model of understanding might represent an extreme position on a personality continuum (Blackburn,

Table 10.1 Tri-dimensional model reflected in most personality theories

Proponent	Extraversion	Neuroticism	Psychoticism
Gray	Behavioural activation Impulsivity Positive affect	Behavioural inhibition Anxiety Negative affect	Fight v. flight Aggression
Atkinson	Approach motivation Need for achievement Joy of success	Avoidance motivation Fear of failure Pain of failure	
Barratt	Action orientation	Anxiety	
Cloninger	Behavioural activation Novelty-seeking	Behavioural inhibition Harm avoidance	Behavioural maintenance Reward dependence
Davidson	Approach (Non-)depression (presence or absence of depression)	Avoidance Inhibition Depression	
Depue	Behavioural facilitation Mania Positive emotionality	Behavioural inhibition	
Dollard & Miller	Approach	Avoidance	
Eysenck	Extraversion Arousal Positive affect	Neuroticism Activation Negative affect	Psychoticism Anger
Fowles	Behavioural activation Impulsivity Positive affect	Behavioural inhibition Aversion	Non-specific arousal
Kagan		Behavioural inhibition	
Newman	Impulsivity Positive affect	Anxiety Negative affect	
Revelle	Approach Instigation of behaviour	Avoidance Inhibition of behaviour	Aggression
Simonov	'Strong' type (choleric) v. 'weak' type (melancholic)		
Tellegen	Positive affectivity Positive affect	Negative affectivity Negative affect	Constraint avoidance
Thayer	Energetic arousal	Tense arousal	
Watson & Clark	Positive affectivity	Negative affectivity	
Zuckerman	Extraversion Positive affect	Neuroticism	Psychoticism Impulsivity Sensation-seeking Aggression/anger

Sources: Eysenck, 1990; Revelle, 1997.

2000). Although this has an intuitive appeal, Livesley (2007) has argued that for a disorder to be present, then more is required than an extreme position on a continuum. Instead, he argues that it is the failure to accomplish one or more of certain life tasks that needs to be present for personality to be regarded as disordered. We will return to this when we come to discuss the general features of personality disorder.

Critique of dimensional systems

There are advantages to using a dimensional approach. First, it would fit with other accounts of chronic developmental disorders, which assess both vulnerability and resilience factors, and reframe personality disorder as a disability rather than a disease (Fulford, 1989; Chapter 11, this volume). Second, it would help to limit the reductionist and rather stigmatising approach to personality disorder, whereby those with the disorder are seen as having a 'lifelong' condition that is impervious to change. Third, treatment selection would be informed by the existing evidence base: some degrees of disordered personality dimensions will, and clearly do, ameliorate both with time and the appropriate interventions. However, dimensional schemes are simply too complex for everyday use, as substantial knowledge and clinical ability are required to identify the wide range of traits, many of which fall below a threshold for determining abnormality (First, 2005). When assessment of abnormal personality is required, much time and effort might be spent in assessing the normal aspects while clinically useful constructs such as suspiciousness, insecure attachment, self-harm and narcissism are overlooked.

An integrated diagnostic system for personality disorders

John Livesley has been one of the most influential critics of the current psychiatric nosology and of the DSM in particular. What we find particularly attractive about his suggested revisions is his attempt to integrate into the existing system solutions to many of the criticisms targeted at it. This integration is crucial for two reasons. First, if one were to replace DSM-IV (or ICD-10) with a completely different classificatory system, it would be impossible to draw inferences from research knowledge which is based on the current systems. We would in effect know nothing about the epidemiology of personality disorders, their naturalistic course or their treatment. Second, at a pragmatic level, there would be no reason for the body of practitioners to switch suddenly from one classificatory approach to another, especially as many of the advantages of any new system would be largely theoretical and await empirical verification. Therefore, why would anyone wish to change? Hence, it would be far better to integrate any new system into the existing DSM, as there is too much now invested in the latter to allow its complete replacement.

Here, we provide a brief distillation of the work of Livesley and his colleagues, but we would strongly recommend the interested reader to refer to their many original contributions (Livesley *et al*, 1994, 1998, 2003; Livesley, 2003, 2005, 2007). Although much of Livesley's work focuses on the arguments for a dimensional rather than a categorical classification, this will not be our main focus. Rather, we wish to concentrate on Livesley's general approach and on certain of his crucial changes of emphasis that address many of the criticisms described above.

Livesley's work re-directs the clinician to the two-step approach that the DSM recommends – application first of the general criteria (Box 10.1) and then of the specific criteria – which appears to have been lost in current clinical practice. What happens currently is a 'bottom-up' approach: first, individual personality traits are assessed and then these are grouped into the various categorical disorders. In contrast, Livesley recommends a 'top-down' approach whereby the first decision to be made is whether the individual has a personality disorder or not. If the answer to this question is in the affirmative, two further tiers of investigation of increasing specificity may be applied if required. The important point is that the process is hierarchical, proceeding from the general to the specific, rather than the other way round. We will now briefly expand on this process, as described by Livesley (2007).

A three-step, top-down approach

In defining the general features of personality (and personality disorder), Livesley takes an evolutionary perspective and suggests that there are three life tasks that individuals need to carry out as evidence that they are adapted to their environment. Failure or difficulty in meeting one or more of these tasks is a general sign of personality disorder. The three areas and corresponding potential failures are:

- achieving a coherent sense of self (intrapersonal failure)
- developing intimacy in personal relationships (interpersonal failure)
- behaving prosocially (social group failure).

It is important to recognise that these general features of personality disorder, unlike the secondary domains and primary traits that we shall describe further below, are purely social constructs. Livesley proposes that with a few simple screening questions focused on each of these three 'general' areas, it ought to be possible to decide whether or not someone has a personality disorder (Fig. 10.1, step 1). These questions might be along the lines of 'Do you have a clear sense of yourself and what you wish to accomplish in your life?' (the intrapersonal domain); 'Do you find it difficult either being too close or being very detached from important people in your

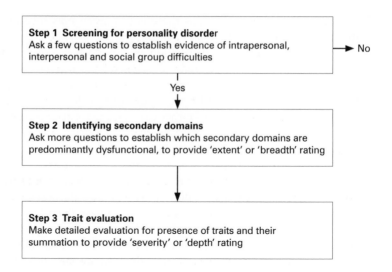

Fig. 10.1 A three-step, top-down evaluation model for personality disorder.

life, so that relationships are inevitably problematic?' (the interpersonal domain); 'Do you find it difficult to conform to the expectations that your family, friends or society at large have of you, so that you are quite often at odds with them?' (the prosocial domain). It is possible that answers to the last two questions may not be honest, but it is likely that other sources of information (such as key informants or documentary evidence from statutory agencies) may be available to inform one's conclusions.

Proceeding from these general features of personality to the two lower levels in the hierarchy, Livesley commences his discussion of secondary domains by drawing attention to one of the most robust findings in the field of personality disorder. That is, when individual personality traits are subjected to factor analysis, four domains invariably emerge, so that 'the robustness of the 4 factor model across clinical and nonclinical samples, cultures, and measurement instruments suggests that it reflects the biological organisation of personality' (Livesley, 2007). This is where 'nature is carved at its joints', as these four domains of phenotypes are closely correlated to four genetic factors. Indeed, Livesley defines a secondary domain as 'a cluster of traits influenced by the same general genetic factor' (Livesley, 2007). Livesley labels these four domains emotional dysregulation, dissocial behaviour, inhibitedness and compulsivity (Table 10.2). These dimensions correspond to Mulder & Joyce's (1997) nomenclature of the four 'As' of personality: asthenic, antisocial, asocial and anankastic.

It is important to recognise that some of these higher-order categories/domains comprise entities that encompass a broader array of traits than is implied by the domain name. For instance, Mulder & Joyce's antisocial secondary domain includes not only simple rule-breaking and criminal behaviour but also features of suspiciousness, paranoia and narcissism. The asthenic domain includes not only those with anxious dependent traits but also traits of emotional dysregulation. The asocial domain similarly includes both anxious avoidant and schizoid traits. Finally, the anankastic domain comprises obsessive–compulsive personality traits. We recognise that these four higher-order categories or domains do not map easily onto the three clusters in DSM-IV (Box 10.2). The antisocial domain, for instance, includes features not only of personality disorders in cluster B but also of those in cluster A. The asthenic domain includes features of both cluster B (emotional dysregulation) and cluster C (anxious avoidant). The asocial domain comprises traits that occur in both cluster A (schizoid) and cluster C (avoidant). Step 2 of the evaluation (Fig. 10.1) would involve categorising someone with a personality disorder into one (or more) major domain of dysfunctions. This would allow clinical 'clustering'.

Livesley (2007) argues that the four secondary domains are composed in turn of a number of primary traits, which he defines as 'a cluster of behaviours influenced by the same general and specific factors'. These primary traits are 'the fundamental building blocks of personality and hence the basic unit for describing and explaining personality disorder'. Through factor and behavioural genetic analysis, Livesley identifies 30 such primary traits, divided unequally between the four secondary domains (Table 10.2). Step 3 of the evaluation would involve detailed

Table 10.2 The mapping of Livesley's secondary domains and primary traits and Mulder & Joyce's four 'As' of personality

	Livesley	
Secondary domain	Associated primary traits	Mulder & Joyce
Emotional dysregulation (12 traits)	Anxiousness; emotional reactivity; emotional intensity; pessimistic anhedonia; submissiveness; insecure attachment; social apprehension; oppositional; need for approval; self-harming ideas; cognitive dysregulation; self-harming acts	Asthenic
Dissocial behaviour (9 traits)	Narcissism; exploitativeness; sadism; conduct problems; hostile dominance; sensation-seeking; impulsivity; suspiciousness; egocentrism	Antisocial
Inhibitedness (7 traits)	Low affiliation; avoidant attachment; attachment need; inhibited sexuality; self-containment; lack of empathy; inhibited emotional expression	Asocial
Compulsivity (2 traits)	Orderliness; conscientiousness	Anankastic

Adapted from Livesley (2007) with kind permission of the author and Guilford Press.

Table 10.3 Recommended evaluation scheme for the four[a] secondary domains

	Asthenic	Antisocial	Asocial/anankastic
Impulses	Alternating high or low	High, with sensation-seeking	Inhibited
Affects	Increased intensity, reactivity and instability: range of affects	Increased expression of hostility and suspiciousness	Inhibited emotional expression, unempathic
Cognitions	Dysregulated, thoughts of self-harm	Egocentric and self-aggrandising views, exploitative and rule-breaking ideas	Poor narrator, unexpressive, limited theory of mind
Behaviours	Alternating oppositional and submissive, self-harm, chaotic interpersonal relationships	Conduct problems, sadistic	Low affiliation, self-contained, avoidant, orderliness

a. As the anankastic domain has only two traits, we have combined it with the asocial domain.

assessment of the particular dysfunctional domain and would provide behavioural and phenomenological markers (Table 10.3).

Advantages of an integrated system

As already stated, we believe that an integrated classification system such as that offered by the three-step, top-down evaluation model outlined in Fig. 10.1 meets many of the objections levelled at the DSM system in particular.

First, both the primary traits and the secondary domains are empirically derived and so can be tested with a rigour that is currently impossible.

Second, they make clinical sense, with a focus on the personality traits rather than on behaviour. An obvious example is the antisocial higher-order factor, which includes many traits that are recognised by clinicians, such as suspiciousness, narcissism and hostile dominance, in the presentation in addition to rule-breaking behaviour and conduct disorder. This moves the description of antisocial personality disorder away from simple criminality to encompass broader features of dissocial personality disorder.

Third, the top-down and hierarchical structure provides the evaluation model with a flexibility in application that current systems lack. For instance, if the question is 'Does the individual have a personality disorder?', the answer is provided by screening for three general criteria of personality disorder (i.e. the ability to form an intimate relationship, to act prosocially and to have a sense of identity). If the answer is 'No' to any one or more of these criteria, the four secondary domains can be examined with a few further screening questions to discern the predominant features in each (Table 10.3). It is only when more detailed information is required to identify the specific primary traits that a detailed inquiry has to be made. Even then, Livesley's proposal is parsimonious, as it requires the assessment of only 30 traits, compared with the 79 in DSM-IV-TR: a reduction of 62% (Livesley, 2007).

Fourth, the three-step, top-down model is arguably more comprehensive than the current system, so that fewer individuals are placed in the 'not otherwise specified' category, a problem with the current system (Verheul & Widiger, 2004).

Finally, and perhaps most importantly, as the four secondary domains differ aetiologically, they should have differing courses and implications for treatment. Detailed consideration of treatment implications is beyond the scope of this chapter and will not be addressed here.

Implications of an integrated diagnostic system

Severity or 'depth' of personality disorders

Notwithstanding the above, empirically based thresholds or cut-offs will be required to identify 'cases' and 'severity' of disorder for clinical decisions to be binary – 'to treat or not to treat'. A categorical diagnosis could be made by treating primary traits as equivalent to current diagnostic criteria and applying a severity rating determined by measuring each trait (diagnostic criteria/item) on a 3-point Likert scale, with trait rating summed to provide a dimensional assessment of each disorder. Trait rating should be weighted depending on the contribution that each trait makes to a domain, with higher-level traits given more weight.

A similar strategy exists in psychiatry for diagnostic assessment of intellectual disability: in addition to a continuous-variable distribution of IQ scores, cut-offs exist to separate those with more severe forms of the disorder from those with less severe forms. It is also applied to medical syndromes (e.g. anaemia, hypertension, chronic renal failure), where clinicians place consensual cut-offs separating the pathological from the normal. The thresholds are decided on the basis of clinical experience of the degree of disability implied by scoring above or below the cut-offs. Using such a system for personality disorder, instead of a diagnosis stating that a person does or does not have a personality disorder, they may be considered to have a degree of personality disorder – ranging from personality difficulties to mild, moderate or severe personality disorder.

Extent or 'breadth' of personality disorder

A hidden facet of current classificatory systems is that personality disorder diagnoses differ in the 'breadth and depth' of the disorder. For example, borderline and antisocial personality disorders encompass a wide range of features, whereas paranoid and obsessive–compulsive personality disorders are little more than single-trait disorders (Livesley, 2007). A benefit of an integrated approach might be that 'broader' personality disorders will 'trump' 'narrower' personality disorders, for example asthenic 'trumps' anankastic, and this will help with the conundrum of multiple diagnoses of personality disorder and of 'personality disorder not otherwise specified'. Such an approach is already in operation for mental illness diagnoses, where a diagnosis of psychosis often 'trumps' other illnesses such as anxiety and mood disorders (Sarkar *et al*, 2005).

'Episodes of personality disorder'

An important consideration that has bedevilled much of the thinking in personality disorder is the immutability that is built into its definition (i.e. that it is lifelong). Increasingly, however, follow-up studies have challenged this proposition (e.g. Paris, 2003; Skodol *et al*, 2005; Zanarini *et al*, 2005). Attention has been focused almost exclusively on the course of borderline personality disorder, with these studies (that by Zanarini *et al* in particular) showing not only that people with borderline personality disorder can lose their traits, but also that if they do so they continue to remain well.

This interpretation has its critics (e.g. Widiger, 2005), who claim that although some of the superficial features of borderline personality disorder might well disappear (e.g. self-harming behaviour), certain core features remain. This makes sense to us. Thus, people with personality disorder might be thought of as having a continuing underlying diathesis that makes them prone to decompensate if the appropriate triggering events are present. For some, their trait summation might cross an established threshold or cut-off, such that they become 'personality disordered' during a period of heightened stress and then recover. This conceptualisation has the capacity to explain the acquisition of personality disorders in adulthood and diagnostic labels such as 'disorders of extreme stress not otherwise specified' (DSM-IV) or 'enduring personality change after a catastrophic experience' (ICD-10). Taking this to its ultimate conclusion, Tyrer & Bajaj have concluded that there are some individuals who are so vulnerable that only the management of their environment (so that no triggering events occur, or if they do, they occur only very rarely) is necessary for them to remain stable: so-called nidotherapy (Chapter 20, this volume).

Clinical prediction and treatment planning

As the four secondary domains represent aetiologically different facets of disorder, each is likely to be associated with a differential course, response to treatment and prognosis. The borderline domain is more responsive to treatment and also has a better long-term outcome without treatment than the other constellations (Paris, 2003). The secondary-domain dysfunctions provide broad goals that can guide focused targets for treatment, establish collaboratively agreed therapeutic contracts and inform more frequent use of generic strategies. Thus, the asthenic domain will require interventions to regulate affect and to contain thoughts and actions of self-harm as broad treatment goals and develop targeted management strategies. The antisocial domain will require structure and boundaries as broad goals to contain exploitativeness and deception traits, and a focus on sensation-seeking and impulsivity as key treatment targets. The asocial domain will require broad emphasis on promoting safety in attachments, with emotional expression as a treatment target. The anankastic domain will have as its broad treatment goal the capacity to tolerate uncertainty and unpredictability in the patient's ordered world and will use conscientiousness to facilitate engagement in prosocial behaviour.

Harmful dysfunction

One final point to note is the increasing interest in the interplay between genetic vulnerability (as a hard-wired process) and environmental adversity in producing personality disorder in an individual, with the realisation that this is much more complex and fluid than was earlier believed. In this regard, personality disorder is not dissimilar to medical disorders that lead to a wide range of harmful dysfunctional states for the individual and for others. For instance, the new science of epigenetics points the way to a much more complex process than the simple determinism that previously prevailed, so that certain deleterious genes become activated only in the presence of an abnormal environment. This more sophisticated view of gene–environment interaction offers an opportunity to intervene at certain strategic times (Caspi & Moffitt, 2006). This will only be achieved, however, if a good nosology provides a firm foundation to direct that process.

Conclusion

There are problems with the diagnosis of personality disorders using current classificatory systems which, in our view, neither an entirely categorical nor an entirely dimensional approach will be able to rectify. We believe that the best way forward is to incorporate aspects of both approaches into the integrated diagnostic system that we have outlined here. The strength of this approach would be to align prototypical data (descriptive behavioural and phenomenological information) with genotypically grounded empirical data. We have adapted Livesley's dimensional approach and revealed how this can explain certain seemingly irreconcilable difficulties within current classificatory systems related to severity of personality disorder, adult onset, the 'not otherwise specified' category and multiple comorbidities of personality disorders. It remains to be seen whether the DSM-5 and ICD-11 task groups take up these challenges. We are confident that adopting such an approach by the busy clinician will repay the time and effort invested in it.

References

Allport, G. (1955) *Becoming: Basic Considerations for a Psychology of Personality.* Yale University Press.

American Psychiatric Association (1980) *Diagnostic and Statistical Manual of Mental Disorders (3rd edn) (DSM-III).* APA.

American Psychiatric Association (1994) *Diagnostic and Statistical Manual of Mental Disorders (4th edn) (DSM-IV).* APA.

American Psychiatric Association (2004) *Diagnostic and Statistical Manual of Mental Disorders (4th edn, text revision) (DSM-IV-TR).* APA.

Blackburn, R. (2000) Treatment or incapacitation? Implications of research on personality disorders for the management of dangerous offenders. *Legal and Criminal Psychology,* **5**, 1–21.

Blais, M. A., Benedict, K. B. & Norman, D. K. (1998) Establishing the psychometric properties of the DSM-III–R personality disorders: implications for DSM-V. *Journal of Clinical Psychology,* **54**, 795–802.

Bouchard, T. J. Jr & Loehlin, J. C. (2001) Genes, evolution, and personality. *Behavior Genetics,* **31**, 243–273.

Caspi, A. & Moffitt, T. E. (2006) Gene–environment interactions in psychiatry: joining forces with neuroscience. *Nature Reviews Neuroscience,* **7**, 583–590.

Clark, L. A., Livesley, W. J. & Morey, L. (1997) Personality disorder assessment: the challenge of construct validity. *Journal of Personality Disorders,* **11**, 205–231.

Department of Health (2003) *Personality Disorder: No Longer a Diagnosis of Exclusion.* Department of Health.

Eysenck, H. J. (1990) Biological dimensions of personality. In *Handbook of Personality: Theory and Research* (eds L. A. Pervin &, O. P. John), pp. 244–276. Guilford Press.

First, M. B. (2005) Clinical utility: a prerequisite for the adoption of a dimensional approach to DSM. *Journal of Abnormal Psychology,* **114**, 560–564.

Fulford, K. W. (1989) *Moral Theory and Medical Practice.* Cambridge University Press.

Livesley, W. J. (2003) Diagnostic dilemmas in the classification of personality disorder. In *Advancing DSM: Dilemmas in Psychiatric Diagnosis* (eds K. Phillips, M. First & H. A. Pincus), pp. 153–189. American Psychiatric Press.

Livesley, W. J. (2005) Behavioural and molecular genetic contributions to a dimensional classification of personality disorder. *Journal of Personality Disorders,* **19**, 131–155.

Livesley, W. J. (2007) A framework for integrating dimensional and categorical classifications of personality disorder. *Journal of Personality Disorders,* **21**, 199–224.

Livesley, W. J., Schroeder, M. L., Jackson, D. N., *et al* (1994) Categorical distinctions in the study of personality disorder: implications for classification. *Journal of Abnormal Psychology,* **103**, 6–17.

Livesley, W. J., Jang, K. L. & Vernon, P. A. (1998) The phenotypic and genetic structure of traits delineating personality disorder. *Archives of General Psychiatry,* **55**, 941–948.

Livesley, W. J., Jang, K. L.,& Vernon, P. A. (2003) Genetic basis of personality structure. In *Handbook of Psychology. Volume 5: Personality and Social Psychology* (eds T. Millon, M. J. Lerner & I. B. Weiner), pp. 59–83. John Wiley & Sons.

McCrae, R. R. & Costa, P. T. (1987) Validation of the five-factor model of personality across instruments and observers. *Journal of Personality and Social Psychology,* **52**, 81–90.

Millon, T. & Frances, A. J. (1986) Editorial. *Journal of Personality Disorders,* **1**, i–iii.

Mulder, R. T. & Joyce, P. R. (1997) Temperament and the structure of personality disorder symptoms. *Psychological Medicine,* **27**, 1315–1325.

Paris, J. (2003) *Personality Disorders over Time: Precursors, Course, and Outcome.* American Psychiatric Press.

Revelle, W. (1997) *Three Fundamental Dimensions of Personality.* The Personality Project (http://personality-project.org/perproj/theory/big3.table.html).

Sanderson, C. & Clarkin, J. F. (2002) Further use of the NEO-PI-R personality dimensions in differential treatment planning. In *Personality Disorders and the Five Factor Model of Personality* (2nd edn) (eds P. T. Costa & T. A. Widiger), pp. 351–375. American Psychological Association Books.

Sarkar, J., Mezey, G., Cohen, A., *et al* (2005) Comorbidity of post-traumatic stress disorder and paranoid schizophrenia: a comparison of offender and non-offender patients. *Journal of Forensic Psychiatry and Psychology*, **16**, 660–670.

Skodol, A. E., Gunderson, J. G., Shea, M. T., *et al* (2005) The Collaborative Longitudinal Personality Disorders Study (CLPS). *Journal of Personality Disorders*, **19**, 487–504.

Stone, M. H. (1998) The personalities of murderers: the importance of psychopathy and sadism. In *Psychopathology and Violent Crime* (ed. A. E. Skodol), pp. 29–52. American Psychiatric Press.

Tyrer, P. & Bateman, A. W. (2004) Drug treatment for personality disorders. *Advances in Psychiatric Treatment*, **10**, 389–398.

Tyrer, P. & Johnson, T. (1996) Establishing the severity of personality disorder. *American Journal of Psychiatry*, **153**, 1593–1597.

Tyrer, P., Coombs, N., Ibrahimi, F., *et al* (2007) Critical developments in the assessment of personality disorder. *British Journal of Psychiatry*, **190** (suppl. 49), s51–59.

Verheul, R. & Widiger, T. A. (2004) A meta-analysis of the prevalence and usage of the personality disorder not otherwise specified (PDNOS) diagnosis. *Journal of Personality Disorders*, **18**, 309–319.

Westen, D. & Arkowitz-Westen, L. (1998) Limitations of Axis II in diagnosing personality pathology in clinical practice. *American Journal of Psychiatry*, **155**, 1767–1771.

Widiger, T. A. & Frances, A. J. (1994) Toward a dimensional model for the personality disorders. In *Personality Disorders and the Five-Factor Model of Personality* (eds P. T. Costa & T. A. Widiger), pp. 19–39. American Psychiatric Association.

Widiger, T. A. (2005) CIC, CLIPS and MSAD. *Journal of Personality Disorders*, **19**, 586–593.

World Health Organization (1992) *The ICD-10 Classification of Mental and Behavioural Disorders: Clinical Descriptions and Diagnostic Guidelines*. WHO.

Zanarini, M. C., Frankenberg, F. R., Hennen, J., *et al* (2005) The McLean Study of Adult Development (MSAD): overview and implications of the first six years of prospective follow-up. *Journal of Personality Disorders*, **19**, 505–523.

Zimmerman, M. (1994) Diagnosing personality disorders: a review of issues and research methods. *Archives of General Psychiatry*, **51**, 225–245.

CHAPTER 11

Murmurs of discontent: treatment and treatability of personality disorder

Gwen Adshead

Summary   In this chapter, I suggest that the term 'untreatable' should not ever be used in relation to personality disorder. Instead, mental healthcare professionals can use an approach used in medicine for other heterogeneous disorders. It is possible to assess the severity of a personality disorder in terms of its type, spread and comorbidity with other disorders; and then determine what therapies are appropriate. It is also important that therapies are offered even in palliative cases; and that lack of trained therapists does not lead to lack of treatment.

> 'They answered, as they took their Fees,
> "There is no Cure for this Disease".'
>
> From 'Henry King', Hilaire Belloc

Some clinicians still make the global generalisation that personality disorder is not 'treatable' by psychiatrists. To some extent, this is a relic of the Mental Health Act 1983 for England and Wales, in which a legal concept of 'treatability' limited the involuntary hospital admission of patients with certain types of mental disorder. The aim of the treatability criterion for such detention was to protect citizens from detention simply on the grounds of deviance or social dissent; it perhaps was also a tacit acknowledgement that it may not be sensible to detain a group of patients that psychiatrists do not like (Lewis & Appleby, 1988).

The amended Mental Health Bill for England 2007 removed the treatability criterion for detention; so, instead of a legal concept of 'treatability', the amended Mental Health Act requires that 'appropriate medical treatment' is available. Medico-legal debates may therefore arise as to whether the treatment being provided is 'appropriate' for the patient detained.

However, 'treatability' (and its confusing sister, 'untreatable') are still words with medical significance. In this chapter, I will look at them in more

---

Box 11.1 Clinical vignette

Kieran is a young man who has been self-harming for several years, since his late teens. He regularly presents at different emergency departments around the country, always using different names and giving different accounts of himself. He is also regularly in trouble with the criminal justice system for shoplifting. He attends out-patient appointments with his psychiatrist, and takes prescribed antidepressant medication. Recently, his self-harming behaviour has been getting much worse, and his family want him to be admitted to hospital, involuntarily if necessary. The general practitioner and approved social worker are unsure how best to proceed, as the consultant psychiatrist refuses to admit Kieran, saying: 'He's not ill, he's got a personality disorder'.

---

detail, and examine their strengths and limitations in relation to personality disorder. I will argue that treatability is linked to resources and training, as well as psychopathology, and that different understandings of personality disorder may alter ideas about treatability.

Personality disorder: 'not an illness'?

Box 11.1 outlines the case of Kieran. Reading this clinical vignette, we might ask, is Kieran ill? To answer this in full requires a much longer chapter. Here, I can only briefly set out some of the arguments about the nosological status of personality disorder in terms of illness and disease.

The debate about personality disorder's status as a mental illness needs to be seen in the context of the more general debate about the extent to which mental distress of any sort can be understood as a disease, an illness, a disability or a disorder. The status of mental disorder as illness or disease is still a potent source of debate (Box 11.2), and the arguments remain much as they were when reviewed by Fulford in 1989. Much of

---

Box 11.2 Concepts of health disorders

The following are much debated (for a review see Fulford, 1989):

- illness: subjective experience, includes suffering?
- disease: the pathological processes underlying illness?
- dysfunction: failure of normal action?
- disability: a chronic dysfunctional state?
- disorder: all of the above?
- relevance of statistical deviance from norms?

---

the debate has centred on the tension between what are called descriptive and normative accounts. Descriptive accounts of disorders claim that it is possible to describe and classify disease and/or illness without making some sort of value (or normative) judgement about the concept. Normative accounts claim the reverse: that there is no 'objective' account of a disorder that does not contain some reference to an established value or norm.

Theorists such as Boorse (1975) have argued that the term 'disease' describes the pathological processes that give rise to 'illness' as experienced by the patient. 'Diseases' then are those processes that can be described objectively, whereas 'illness' is more subjective, and necessarily involves a normative (value judgement) component.

This distinction between disease and illness has been highly influential, although still leaving room for debate: for example, whether, and to what extent, the terms 'illness' and 'disease' may actually be synonymous. The arguments become even more complex when applied to mental disorders. Most readers will be familiar with claims that all diagnosis of mental disorder is really 'only' or 'just' a type of value judgement (an argument put most forcefully by Thomas Szasz). Boorse himself acknowledged that his formulation makes it difficult for any mental disorder to be a disease, although there might be many mental illnesses. Scadding (1988) has argued that there may be different overlapping accounts of diseases (syndromal, pathological, aetiological), but that the key feature of a disease relates to the extent to which it puts an organism at 'biological disadvantage'. This notion of biological disadvantage has been used to justify mental disorder's claim to have equal disease status with physical disorder (e.g. Kendell, 1975).

Wakefield (1992) has argued that it may be helpful to understand mental disorder as 'harmful dysfunction': a combination of a normative illness account and a descriptive account of loss of function, as determined by evolution. Other theorists have argued that the evaluative/normative aspect of diagnosis is an essential feature of both physical and mental disorders (e.g. Fulford, 1989; Engelhardt, 1999), and mental disorders therefore need not be seen as something conceptually different from physical disorders. The fact that value judgements may be part of diagnosis does not mean that there cannot be agreement between clinicians, or that the disorder is less 'real' (Fulford, 2000).

Few of these theorists have applied their analysis to personality disorder. Formalised diagnostic criteria such as the DSM and ICD have tended to equate its symptoms with negatively evaluated behaviours such as self-harm or violence to others. This causes conceptual problems because usual accounts of illness, and illness behaviour, define 'symptoms' as actions or experiences which are not willed, desired or chosen by the patient. However, negatively evaluated behaviour is so evaluated precisely because it is perceived to be chosen or willed by the patient, and behaviours or experiences that are willed or chosen are not symptoms.

Clearly, it is impossible for anyone to claim with confidence that some behaviours are totally wilful and others are not. Framing of certain behaviours as wilful and/or 'deliberate' appears to reveal clinician bias, arguably due to lack of knowledge, skills and resources. Indeed, the term 'deliberate' in 'deliberate self-harm' is now considered pejorative, and clinicians and patient groups alike are abandoning its use in favour of simply 'self-harm'. If substance misuse or eating disorders are not considered 'deliberate', for example, why should self-harm be?

Behaviours and symptoms cannot always be synonymous, especially in the domain of negatively evaluated behaviour. Therefore, a theoretical approach that classifies or understands personality disorder predominantly in terms of behaviour leads to two problems. Either any negatively evaluated behaviour such self-harm or violence to others is seen as actually willed 'badness' (leaving aside for a moment what that might mean), and people with personality disorders are equated with people who behave badly; or it may be then argued that 'bad' behaviour is not a feature of illness, and therefore people with personality disorder are not ill (e.g. Eldergill, 1999).

There are real philosophical objections, and empirical difficulties, with both positions, which I cannot explore in detail here. One principal objection is that some types of 'bad' behaviour seem to occur more frequently in those with some types of mental illness, as demonstrated by the risk and mental disorder literature. However, the majority of those who have personality disorders do not behave badly; just the ones that come to medical attention, especially in forensic psychiatry.

Another objection is the (albeit limited) evidence that some aspects of 'bad' behaviour have a neurological substrate, and are influenced by poor arousal and affect control. People with personality disorders may not be 'choosing' to behave badly; although whether this would be sufficient to justify personality disorder's definition as an 'illness' is a moot point (Morse, 2006). It might be argued that the sadness and anxiety that characterise many personality disorders (such as those in cluster C) appear not to have attracted the same degree of rejection as the perceived 'badness' found in cluster B and A disorders: another sign of clinician bias in dealing with those with personality disorder. Other clinicians have noted the degree of subjective suffering experienced by patients with personality disorder, which would normally be understood as a necessary (although not sufficient) feature of an illness (Norton, 1996).

Focusing on negatively evaluated behaviours as symptoms distracts attention from other ways of conceptualising 'personality disorder' (see Chapter 10, this volume). More recent accounts (including the DSM; First *et al*, 2002) emphasise the significant failure of interpersonal functioning seen in personality disorder, which arises as a result of a variety of psychological deficits (Blackburn, 1998). Some psychiatrists have argued strongly that personality disorder is an illness on the grounds of resulting biological disadvantage to the individual (Gunn, 1992, 1999). Many studies have noted that patients with personality disorder frequently also have other concurrent mental illnesses, such as anxiety, mood disorders and schizophrenia. Taylor (1999) has argued that personality disorder can claim to be an illness in so far as it reduces individual variance: people with personality disorder are more like each other than not.

A possible solution to the problems described above may lie in Talcott Parsons' notion of the 'sickness role'. People who are ill are expected to avoid behaving in ways that exacerbate their condition, accept the idea they need help, want to get better and seek competent help to do so (Mechanic, 1978). However, many people with personality disorders, although claiming to be ill and in need, do not behave in the ways expected of a sick person. Perhaps we could understand this failure to fulfil sick role expectations as a type of psychological disability – an incapacity to obtain care effectively – which would undoubtedly convey a biological disadvantage in the long term. This incapacity may be understood as a characteristic adaptation to a stressful and uncaring upbringing during the earliest and most critical phases of personality development (Henderson, 1974; Vaillant, 1994). These coping responses were adaptive in a survivor's world, when the survivor was a child, but are maladaptive in the adult social world, and are therefore manifest as the behavioural and affective signs of 'personality disorder' (Paris, 2003; Carlson et al, 2009).

Fulford (1989) has argued that it might be helpful to understand personality disorders as disabilities, rather than illnesses. Accounts of disability usually emphasise the chronic nature of the patient's problems; they also emphasise the interpersonal aspects of function and dysfunction for the disabled. Some readers may remember an advertising campaign for the disabled which ran the slogan, 'Our biggest handicap is other people's attitudes'. Such an interpersonal view is found in American legal definitions of disability (Silver, 1999) it and may be a useful way to understand the difficulties faced by people with disabilities in terms of making choices and being agents of their own destiny (Agich, 1993).

The status of personality disorder as an illness therefore remains contentious, especially while it is defined predominantly in terms of behaviour. Scadding (1988) has argued that most accounts of mental disorder are at a syndromal or symptom level, and that illness claims are stronger when there is an aetiological account. Aetiological models have only recently been developed for personality disorder. These models draw on research from longitudinal follow-up studies of child development and the impact of traumatic events on the personality functioning of adults. Both retrospective and longitudinal studies suggest that abuse or hostility from carers is a potent risk factor for the development of a personality disorder in adulthood (Modestin et al, 1998; Johnson et al, 1999; Carlson et al, 2009). Studies of the effects of exposure to traumatic and frightening events in adulthood also indicate that such events may cause change and damage to the personality (as found in the diagnosis of 'enduring personality change after trauma', defined in ICD-10; World Health Organization, 1992).

> **Box 11.3** Personality disorder and concepts of health
>
> Is personality disorder:
>
> - an illness (suffering; biological disadvantage)?
> - a pejorative label, used to describe 'bad' behaviour?
> - caused by a disease process (amygdala dysfunction, abnormal arousal patterns)?
> - acquired as a result of adverse or traumatic environmental experience?
> - another term for 'deviant' or 'criminal', and nothing to do with health?
> - a complex manifestation of multiple disabilities?
> - all/none/some of the above?

If external events in both childhood and adulthood can shape adult personality functioning, then it is possible to understand personality disorder as an acquired, rather than an innate condition. It can no longer be considered a disorder 'of exclusion' (National Institute for Mental Health in England, 2003a) Although this argument will not deal with all the conceptual difficulties surrounding the disease/illness status of personality disorder (Box 11.3), it does at least challenge the argument that some people are just 'born' with personality disorder (a sort of psychiatric version of St Augustine's notion of original sin) and can therefore be rejected by services for the 'properly' mentally ill.

Treatment and treatability: general medical considerations

I want now to think about what it means to be able to treat a disorder, any clinical disorder. Treatments may have different purposes, not all of which aim at cure. I would like to suggest that 'treatability' of any medical condition is a function of seven factors operating simultaneously (Box 11.4). No one factor will determine a condition's treatability and, especially, its 'untreatability'.

We can apply this model to any condition. I will take as an example the treatment of cancer, partly because it is a disorder that sometimes attracts fear and stigma as well as sympathy and partly because, 20 or 30 years ago, 'cancer' was also treated as a somewhat unitary diagnostic identity with a gloomy prognosis.

The type of cancer is a crucial factor in looking at treatability and prognosis, since it is well-established that different types may be more or less treatable. The treatability of the cancer will depend on its anatomical context (site) and nature (e.g. histological grading, differentiation). The spread of the cancer affects its treatability: more extensive spread may make

Box 11.4   The seven-factor model of treatability

Factor 1: The nature and severity of pathology: site, histology, grade
Factor 2: The involvement of other bodily systems: spread, impact on function
Factor 3: The patient's previous health, comorbid conditions, risk factors
Factor 4: The timing of intervention: diagnosis, early/late identification, action
Factor 5: The experience and availability of staff
Factor 6: Availability of specialist units for special conditions
Factor 7: State of knowledge, cultural attitudes

some types of treatment more difficult. Premorbid health is a relevant factor in assessing treatability, in so far as it reveals risk and resilience factors that may affect the course of the disorder.

The timing of any treatment for cancer influences treatability, given that there is evidence supporting early rather than late intervention. This in turn relates to the process of diagnosis and identification of the problem. In many cases, symptoms are not understood as being those of cancer, or are thought to be caused by another condition. Such uncertainty about identification of symptoms and diagnosis can lead to delay, which in turn affects treatment response.

Once detected, treatability is affected by the availability of specialist staff and services familiar with the specific problems posed by the particular type of cancer. For example, there is good evidence that the treatability (and prognosis) of breast cancer is influenced by the availability of specialist breast cancer surgeons. Such specialists are backed up by specialist teams, with access to specialist facilities and equipment. Even where there is little prospect of cure, specialist palliative care teams can offer therapy to improve quality of life and support to those who care for and support the patient.

The status of scientific knowledge keeps altering the nature and extent of treatable conditions in cancer services. Better understanding of genetic risk factors for tumour growth has led to the development of new treatments that prolong life in ways previously unthinkable. We know now, for example, that breast cancer is several diseases, not one: and there are different genetic risk profiles for developing different types, each of which requires a different therapeutic approach. The absence of randomised controlled trials does not prove that there is no benefit to treatment, and pioneering research work may often still be based on systematic clinical observations.

Application of the seven-factor model to personality disorder

I hope it will already be apparent that there are parallels between the treatment of cancer and the treatment of personality disorder.

Factor 1: Nature and severity

In relation to diagnosis, a simple statement that 'this patient has a personality disorder' is unhelpful. Most individuals can be diagnosed as having more than one personality disorder, indicating a range of difficulties. It is important to identify the predominant pattern of traits, because this is therapeutically relevant. At present, more therapeutic options appear possible for borderline personality disorder than for other personality disorders, and high degrees of antisocial personality traits reduce the likelihood of therapeutic engagement.

Whatever the limitations of the current typologies (dimensional or categorical), it is clear that not all personality disorders are the same. It is also clear that there are degrees of severity. Contrary to what is sometimes claimed, the term 'severe personality disorder' is not simply a recent political invention. It has been in use for almost 50 years (e.g. Craft *et al*, 1964; Department of Health, 1996; Tyrer & Johnson, 1996).

Equally, it is likely that there are both 'mild' and 'moderate' degrees of personality disorder, characterised by significant interpersonal dysfunction, but without the more extreme behavioural manifestations. These conditions may be made worse by the presence of other factors, such as Axis I disorders, or new stressors. Such a dimensional approach provides a better description of the clinical complexities observed in practice. The evidence to date suggests that mild and moderate degrees of personality disorder are treatable with appropriate therapeutic interventions (National Collaborating Centre for Mental Health, 2009a,b).

Factor 2: The degree of spread

In the case of personality disorder, 'spread' would be represented by the extent to which other psychological, healthcare and social systems are involved in the patient's case and the impact the disorder has on the individual's functioning in different areas of life (Remington & Tyrer, 1979). Different degrees of involvement of different systems could be seen as a measure of severity: an individual whose personality disorder has led to the involvement of the healthcare, social and criminal justice systems is likely to be less treatable than one who has been involved only with healthcare providers. Severity may also be indicated by the frequency, variety and harmfulness of any risk behaviours. Such an approach is supported by the literature on the additive nature of risk factors in mental disorder (Swanson, 1994). The emphasis is on understanding abnormal behaviours as manifestations of interpersonal dysfunction, just as abnormal gait may be a behavioural manifestation of metastatic disease.

Factor 3: Comorbid conditions

The treatability of any disorder is likely to be reduced if there are comorbid conditions. This is frequently the case for personality disorder, where comorbidity with mood disorders and substance misuse are especially common. Treatability is also likely to be affected by developmental history, and the presence of risk and resilience factors. For example, most therapists assessing the treatability of personality disorder will look at the history of interpersonal relating from early childhood, arguing that treatment is more likely to be successful if there is any history of an enduring positive attachment to another person (Dozier & Tyrrell, 1998).

Factor 4: Identification, diagnosis and timing

Clearly, personality disorder will be not be 'treatable' if it is not identified as a disorder: hence, the relevance of the illness debate discussed above. There are empirical questions to be answered here: if two individuals with similar presentations are assessed, and both are understood as having a personality disorder, but only one is treated, what difference does that make to subsequent treatability? Do early interventions prevent later pathology? On-going studies of adolescents with personality disorder may provide information about this.

There is also an empirical question about whether the process of rejection by services, failure to identify pathology and failure to offer interventions itself affects the treatability of the condition. Does each negative encounter make the condition worse? Service users with personality disorder say that this is their experience (Castillo, 2000; Barlow *et al*, 2007).

Factors 5 and 6: Specialist knowledge and staff

Factors 5 and 6 relate to the provision of specialist staff and facilities. Clinicians who either do not accept personality disorder as a pathological condition, or who have no experience in treating it even if they do, may well be justified in saying that personality disorder is untreatable by them or in their units. The issue here is that factors outside the patient may make them untreatable, rather than some innate feature of their condition. Given what we know about adverse early childhood experience in personality disorder, and the difficulties in constructive help-seeking that is often a feature, it is unlikely that many individuals with personality disorders will be 'treatable' in facilities that require them to be obedient, compliant, passive and grateful. (This point is legally relevant in relation to detention: it is not lawful to detain someone under the Mental Health Act 1983 if they cannot receive appropriate treatment because there are no such programmes available or staff to deliver them.)

A claim that treatability may be a function of service availability is further supported by evidence that, where specialist staff and facilities are provided, therapeutic benefits are possible in some types of personality disorder (National Collaborating Centre for Mental Health, 2009*a,b*). The case is then no different from that of some types of cancer, where effective therapeutic interventions can only be offered by certain specialist units. No one would now argue with the suggestion that some medical conditions are more effectively treated in a unit that has experience and proven success in treatment. The fact that a complex condition is not treatable in a local general service does not mean it is not treatable at all.

However, the provision of specialist staff and services raises the question of resource allocation in the treatment of mental disorders, and whether such treatment can be afforded by a recession-hit National Health Service. Resource allocation in medicine generally is a complex ethical decision-making process; allocation of resources for the treatment of mental disorders still tends to favour the needs of those with chronic psychotic disorders, who may be seen as more deserving, more conventionally 'ill' and easier to treat with medication, which is cheap. Resources for the treatment of personality disorder tend to become available as a means of controlling violence towards third parties, which reinforces the conflation of a personality disorder diagnosis with violence. Even in the context of violence, resources are not concentrated on patients with personality disorders who are violent towards partners or children, but rather on the minority who are more generally violent, often in bizarre ways.

It is hard but not impossible to quantify exactly the resources needed. Some estimate might be made based on primary care prevalence figures and use of services at all levels. There is evidence that, where specialist therapy for personality disorder is offered and completed, the costs involved are offset by the subsequent reduction in service usage (Dolan *et al*, 1996). The interesting question is why there is so much less provision for personality disorder services, when the prevalence of the disorders is so much higher than that of psychotic disorders. In terms of the ethical debate about treating personality disorder, there is also a real question about whether we can afford not to treat this condition, especially in people who are parents and who may be putting the next generation at risk (Adshead *et al*, 2004).

Factor 7: The state of the art (and science)

Factor 7 involves the state of scientific knowledge, and its influence on both the evidence base and cultural attitudes towards personality disorder. There has been a real increase in the scientific study of personality disorder over the past 20 years (Bateman & Fonagy, 2012*a,b*), but there is still extensive empirical ground to make up. Basic knowledge about the natural history, course and prognosis are still lacking: a review published 20 years ago raises many questions to which there are still no answers (Tyrer *et al*, 1991). Given such a lack of evidence, it seems illogical (not to say irrational) to state categorically that personality disorder is not an illness because it does not have an established course or prognosis (Ferguson & Milton, 2000).

An evidenced-based position supports two claims about personality disorder that are important in considering treatability. First, the evidence that personality disorder may in part be an acquired condition justifies clinicians taking time to think in more complex ways about individuals with personality disorders. Second, there is good evidence that some types of personality disorder, probably of mild-to-moderate severity, do respond to appropriate treatment delivered by clinical teams with experience and training. There can therefore be no justification for global assertions that personality disorder is untreatable, a view which is still taught to trainees, asserted in journals and stated as expert evidence in court.

There is equally no evidence that all personality disorder is treatable, if the clinician's attitude is right and there are enough facilities. A grandiose attitude to the management of personality disorder may be as damaging as a nihilistic one (Cawthra, 2000). Just as in other medical domains, there are likely to be many cases where the damage is so great, and the interpersonal systems failure so profound, that no treatment is going to bring about improvement for the individual. To date, we have no evidence that therapies are available that can ameliorate severe personality disorder with predominant antisocial and narcissistic traits (National Collaborating Centre for Mental Health, 2009a,b).

However, people with severe personality disorders arguably may still require interventions that are therapeutic, or at least, not anti-therapeutic. Their needs resemble those of patients in palliative care, to whom interventions are still offered, if only in terms of a supportive environment and support for staff who are involved in their daily care. Alternatively, if one understand individuals with severe personality disorders as individuals with severe disability (picking up on Fulford's argument), therapeutic interventions could be aimed at damage limitation, quality of life and the management of despair and grief at what has been lost and cannot be repaired.

Treatability is increasingly parsed into component parts, to maximise the effectiveness of interventions. The risk–need–responsivity (RNR) model is probably the most influential model for the assessment and treatment of offenders (Andrews & Bonta, 2006). It takes a general personality and social learning perspective of criminal conduct and, although developed for offenders, the principles of the approach can be adapted for use with anyone with personality disorder. Its three core principles can be outlined as follows.

The risk principle involves matching the level of service to the patient's risk behaviours, such as self-harm, violence, eating disorder, impulsivity. The higher the level of risk, the more enhanced and complex is the appropriate service structure.

The need principle involves assessment of specific psychological needs and targeting them in treatment: for example, the criminogenic needs of an offender with antisocial personality disorder, the attachment needs of someone with borderline personality disorder engaging in self-harm; and the esteem needs of an individual with histrionic personality disorder and anorexia nervosa. Needs can themselves be subdivided into major and minor. Major needs relate to core personality deviance, while minor needs refer to those that are not directly related to risk behaviours.

The responsivity principle involves maximising the patient's ability to learn from an intervention by tailoring the intervention to their learning style, motivation, abilities and strengths. This presupposes that services will adapt treatment to meet the patient's requirements, and not that the patient will adapt to the treatment available. Many patients, as noted above, have been labelled 'untreatable' because services could not tailor treatment delivery in a manner that benefitted the patient. An analogy in cancer treatment might be a service that could offer only radiotherapy for a cancer that responds only to chemotherapy: an unlikely scenario.

General responsivity calls for the use of the most effective social learning strategies regardless of the type of disorder, e.g. regulation of arousal and affect through appropriate use of reinforcement and disapproval, problem-solving, boundaries and consistency. Specific responsivity is a 'fine tuning' of the intervention, taking into account the patient's strengths (e.g. skills that are enhanced as part of a positive psychological approach), learning style (e.g. visual, verbal, kinaesthetic), motivation (capacity, willingness and support required to make changes) and biosocial characteristics (e.g. gender, ethnicity).

Conclusion

'If you can meet with triumph and disaster,
and treat those two impostors just the same.'

From 'If', Rudyard Kipling, 1895

My argument here is that the assessment of treatability of personality disorder is a complex process, which is multifactorial and operational in nature. The approach outlined above is clearly only a preliminary account, which could be further developed. Such an approach might generate ways of rating treatability, which could then be assessed empirically for validity and reliability in different clinical settings.

I have outlined some of the factors I consider to be central to providing a good-quality assessment of treatability; no doubt there are others that will be relevant. For example, I have not discussed the question of repeat assessment, which would take account of both temporal change and the interpersonal nature of the dysfunction to be assessed. One-off assessments alone may be highly unreliable (Bass & Murphy, 1995). Motivation is important, since individuals with personality disorder (like any other patient group) will be more or less willing to engage in treatment, depending on circumstances. For example, a period of crisis may not be the best time to start some types of treatment; and different treatment techniques may be more or less appropriate at different times. Sequencing of treatment to improve mentalisation may be crucial, but this is not yet empirically well researched.

I will close by thinking briefly about the implications of this discussion for services. The key message is that not all patients with personality disorder are the same. Different psychiatric services are likely to meet different types of personality disorder, of different levels of severity, and may therefore need to develop different therapeutic approaches. Clearly, specialist services for personality disorder will be able to offer interventions that cannot be offered in primary care. However, it may be a mistake to generalise from those specialist services to more general ones.

Three different service providers may have specific roles to play. First, specialist psychological therapy services will be important providers not just of highly specialist interventions such as out-patient and in-patient therapeutic communities, but also of advice, consultation and supervision to adult mental health and primary care (Department of Health, 1996). These need to include medical psychotherapists who are familiar with Axis I disorders and managing comorbidity, as well as other psychological therapists from different disciplines.

Second, child and adolescent services will be involved with young people, whose personality disorder may be more amenable to treatment (which can be empirically studied). They will also see a group of adults with personality disorders who are dangerous only to their children. Such individuals arguably also suffer from severe and dangerous personality disorder, but are rarely offered any sort of intervention.

Third, secure forensic services will probably see the people with the most severe and dangerous personality disorder. They will therefore need additional resources in terms of psychological therapists, medical and non-medical, of all theoretical schools. This is especially necessary for the development of therapeutic strategies for men and women who may have to reside in some sort of secure care for the rest of their lives. As my late and much missed predecessor Murray Cox once said, 'If no one ever left Broadmoor, you would need more staff not less'.

We need to be developing better education and training in basic psychological knowledge and techniques for junior medical staff and other members of multidisciplinary teams managing people with personality disorder. Although in theory all psychiatric trainees should be trained in communicating with difficult or challenging people, in fact many do not get such training; and there is no specific professional examination of these skills. This is of particular importance when people with personality disorders come from different cultural and ethnic backgrounds than their doctors.

Provision of education and support to help staff understand the professional demands of working with personality disorder is essential. Staff value time for reflection on the demands of this work and on the effect that patients' interpersonal difficulties have on them (Krawitz, 2001). Such supervisory time makes therapeutic interventions more possible (Norton, 1996) and is considered mandatory for any staff offering specialist treatment for personality disorder (National Institute for Mental Health in England, 2003*b*). This is not to say that all problems will vanish; only that they may be more manageable and that the nature and frequency of professional boundary violations may be reduced (Walker & Clark, 1999)

Personality disorder continues to present considerable conceptual and therapeutic challenges. We still struggle with defining it, diagnosing it and dealing with its more destructive behavioural manifestations. As those behaviours become more dangerous and frightening to others, so we have seen that sections of the public, including government, hope that psychiatry can offer something that will make people not just feel better, but behave better. The clinician/researcher who could do such a thing might get a Nobel Prize (and make a lot of money). The more likely course for psychiatrists is that we will continue to have to manage very difficult people with scarce resources while somehow avoiding falling into either angry despair or mindless optimism. As Kipling suggests, 'triumph' and 'disaster' may both be psychological impostors.

Disclaimer

Although the facts are clinically accurate, Kieran's case is fictitious and does not represent any real patient, alive or dead. The views expressed here are those of the author alone, and do not represent the views of West London Mental Health Trust.

References

Adshead, G., Falkov, A. & Gopfert, M. (2004) Personality disorder in parents: developmental perspectives and interventions. In *Parental Psychiatric Disorders: Distressed Parents and Their Families* (eds M. Gopfert, J. Webster & M. V. Seeman), pp. 217–240. Cambridge University Press.

Agich, G. (1993) *Autonomy in Long-Term Care*. Oxford University Press.

Andrews, D. A. & Bonta, J. (2006) *The Psychology of Criminal Conduct* (4th edn). LexisNexis.

Barlow, K., Miller, S. & Norton, K. (2007) Working with people with personality disorder: utilising service users' views. *Psychiatric Bulletin*, **31**, 85–88.

Bass, C. & Murphy, M. (1995) Somatoform and personality disorders: syndromal comorbidity and overlapping developmental pathways. *Journal of Psychosomatic Research*, **39**, 403–427.

Bateman, A. W. & Fonagy, P. (2012a) Borderline personality disorder. In *Handbook of Mentalizing in Mental Health Practice* (eds A. W. Bateman & P. Fonagy), pp. 273–288. American Psychiatric Publishing.

Bateman, A. W. & Fonagy, P. (2012b) Antisocial personality disorder. In *Handbook of Mentalizing in Mental Health Practice* (eds A. W. Bateman & P. Fonagy), pp. 289–308. American Psychiatric Publishing.

Blackburn, R. (1998) Psychopathy and the contribution of personality to violence. In *Psychopathy: Antisocial, Criminal and Violent Behaviour* (eds T. Millon, E. Simonson, M. Birket-Smith, *et al*), pp. 50–68. Guilford Press.

Boorse, C. (1975) On the distinction between illness and disease. *Philosophy and Public Affairs*, **5**, 49–68. Reprinted (1999) in *Meaning and Medicine: A Reader in the Philosophy of Health Care* (eds J. Lindemann Nelson & H. Lindemann Nelson), pp. 16–27. Routledge.

Carlson, E., Egeland, B. & Sroufe, A. J. (2009) A prospective investigation of borderline personality symptoms. *Development and Psychopathology*, **21**, 1311–1334.

Castillo, H. (2000) *Personality Disorder: Temperament or Trauma?* Mind Advocacy Service, Colchester General Hospital.

Cawthra, R. (2000) Commentary on Recent developments in borderline personality disorder. *Advances in Psychiatric Treatment*, **6**, 217–218.

Craft, M., Stephenson, G. & Granger, C. (1964) The relationship between severity of personality disorder and certain adverse childhood influences. *British Journal of Psychiatry*, **110**, 392–396.

Department of Health (1996) *NHS Psychotherapy Services in England: Review of Strategic Policy (H56/001 0900 1P)*. Department of Health.

Dolan, B. M., Warren, F. M., Menzies, D., *et al* (1996) Cost-offset following specialist treatment of severe personality disorders. *Psychiatric Bulletin*, **20**, 413–417.

Dozier, M. & Tyrrell, C. (1998) The role of attachment in therapeutic relationships. In *Attachment Theory and Close Relationships* (eds J. A. Simpson & W. S. Rholes), pp. 221–248. Guilford Press.

Eldergill, A. (1999) Psychopathy, the law and individual rights. *Princeton University Law Journal*, **III**, 1–30.

Engelhardt, T. (1999) The disease of masturbation: value and the concept of disease. In *Meaning and Medicine: A Reader in the Philosophy of Health Care* (eds H. Lindemann Nelson & J. Lindemann Nelson), pp. 5–15. Routledge.

Ferguson, B. & Milton, J. (2000) Editorial. *Irish Journal of Psychological Medicine*, **17**, 3–4.

First, M. B., Cuthbert, B., Krystal, J., et al (2002) Personality disorders and relational disorders: a research agenda for addressing crucial gaps in DSM. In *A Research Agenda for DSM-V* (eds D. J. Kupfer, M. First & D. A. Regier). American Psychiatric Press.

Fulford, K. W. (1989) *Moral Theory and Medical Practice*. Cambridge University Press.

Fulford, K. W. (2000) Disordered minds, diseased brains and real people. In *Philosophy, Psychiatry and Psychopathy: Personal Identity in Mental Disorder* (ed. C. Heginbotham), pp. 47–75. Ashgate Publishing.

Gunn, J. (1992) Personality disorders and forensic psychiatry. *Criminal Behaviour and Mental Health*, **2**, 202–211.

Gunn, J. (1999) Written evidence of Professor John Gunn. In *Report of the Committee of Enquiry into the Personality Disorder Unit, Ashworth Special Hospital. Vol. II: Expert Evidence on Personality Disorder. Cm 4195* (ed. Department of Health), pp. 207–218. TSO (The Stationery Office).

Henderson, S. (1974) Care-eliciting behaviour in man. *Journal of Nervous and Mental Disease*, **159**, 172–181.

Johnson, J., Cohen, P., Brown, J., *et al* (1999) Childhood maltreatment increases risk for personality disorders during early adulthood. *Archives of General Psychiatry*, **56**, 600–606.

Kendell, R. E. (1975) The concept of disease and its implications for psychiatry. *British Journal of Psychiatry*, **127**, 305–315.

Krawitz, R. (2001) Borderline personality disorder: foundation training for public mental health clinicians. *Australasian Psychiatry*, **9**, 25–28.

Lewis, G. & Appleby, L. (1988) Personality disorder: the patients psychiatrists dislike. *British Journal of Psychiatry*, **153**, 44–49.

Mechanic, D. (1978) *Medical Sociology: A Selective View* (2nd edn). Free Press.

Modestin, J., Oberson, B. & Erni, T. (1998) Possible antecedents of DSM-III-R personality disorders. *Acta Psychiatric Scandinavia*, **97**, 260–266.

Morse, S. (2006) Moral and legal responsibility and the new neuroscience. In *Neuroethics: Defining the Issues in Theory, Practice and Policy* (ed. J. Illes), pp. 33–46. Oxford University Press.

National Collaborating Centre for Mental Health (2009a) *Borderline Personality Disorder: Treatment and Management (NICE Clinical Guideline 78)*. National Institute for Health and Clinical Excellence.

National Collaborating Centre for Mental Health (2009*b*) *Antisocial Personality Disorder: Treatment, Management and Prevention (NICE Clinical Guideline 77)*. National Institute for Health and Clinical Excellence.

National Institute for Mental Health in England (2003*a*) *Personality Disorder: No Longer a Diagnosis of Exclusion. Policy Implementation Guidance for the Development of Services for People with Personality Disorder*. Department of Health.

National Institute for Mental Health in England (2003*b*) *The Personality Disorder Capabilities Framework*. Department of Health.

Norton, K. (1996) Management of difficult personality disorder patients. *Advances in Psychiatric Treatment*, **2**, 202–210.

Paris, J. (2003) Personality disorders over time. *Journal of Personality Disorders*, **17**, 479–488.

Remington, M. & Tyrer, P. (1979) The social functioning schedule – a brief semi-structured interview. *Social Psychiatry*, **14**, 151–157.

Scadding, J. (1988) Health and disease: what can medicine do for philosophy? *Journal of Medical Ethics*, **14**, 118–124.

Silver, A. (1999) (In)equality, (ab)normality and the Americans with Disabilities Act. In *Meaning and Medicine: A Reader in the Philosophy of Health Care* (eds H. Lindemann Nelson & J. Lindemann Nelson), pp. 28–37. Routledge.

Swanson, J. (1994) Mental disorder, substance abuse, and community violence: an epidemiological approach. In *Mental Disorder and Violence* (eds J. Monahan & H. Steadman), pp. 101–136. Chicago: University of Chicago Press.

Taylor, P. J. (1999) Written evidence of Professor Pamela Taylor. In *Report of the Committee of Enquiry into the Personality Disorder Unit, Ashworth Special Hospital. Vol. II: Expert Evidence on personality disorder. Cm 4195* (ed. Department of Health), pp. 489–500. TSO (The Stationery Office).

Tyrer, P. & Johnson, T. (1996) Establishing the severity of personality disorder. *American Journal of Psychiatry*, **153**, 593–597.

Tyrer, P., Casey, P. & Ferguson, B. (1991) Personality disorder in perspective. *British Journal of Psychiatry*, **159**, 463–471.

Vaillant, G. (1994) Ego mechanisms of defence and personality psychopathology. *Journal of Abnormal psychology*, **103**, 44–50.

Wakefield, J. (1992) Disorder as harmful dysfunction: a conceptual critique of DSM-III-R's definition of mental disorder. *Psychological Review*, **99**, 232–247.

Walker, R. & Clark, J. (1999) Heading off boundary problems: clinical supervision as risk management. *Psychiatric Services*, **50**, 1435–1439.

World Health Organization (1992) *The ICD-10 Classification of Mental and Behavioural Disorders: Clinical Descriptions and Diagnostic Guidelines*. WHO.

CHAPTER 12

Personality disorder: its impact on staff and the role of supervision

Estelle Moore

Summary Over the past decade attention to the provision of healthcare for individuals with personality disorder, particularly those who pose a risk to others, has substantially increased. Keeping pace with such developments with a suitably trained, consistent and motivated workforce, interfacing health and criminal justice systems where necessary, presents an enormous challenge. Staff must be experts in managing conflict at every level, while sustaining an optimistic and therapeutic orientation. Boundaried relationships provide the context for recovery for patients. Key principles and practices likely to promote resilience in personality disorder services, with a focus on the role of supervision, are outlined in order to support staff in keeping themselves afloat, their patients safe and their services on target.

'Staff are asked to engage the unhoused and the dangerous with all the physical and psychological intimacies of a feared hand-to-hand combat whilst also supposedly retaining an attitude of care and concern for a potential enemy.'

(Scanlon & Adlam, 2009: p. 133)

Spending time in the company of people with personality disorder is emotionally demanding (Cox, 1996; Alwin *et al*, 2006; Kurtz & Turner, 2007; Aiyegbusi, 2009). This complex work hardly gets a mention when things are going well, and perhaps rightly so, as it is the service recipients who make the changes that in turn can re-establish the confidence of others in them. Conversely, when things go wrong, the effect for all can be devastating.

In an ideal world, professional carers are trained to approach their task in a systematic way, have the advantage of peer support from colleagues who understand the aims of the job, and use both educational and supervisory frameworks for guidance. Training provides an academic understanding of personality disorder and can make an important difference to the extent to which problematic behaviour can be tolerated. A capacity to understand traumatic interpersonal situations is likely to limit their impact, and to operate as a protective factor for vulnerable persons (Fonagy & Target,

1997). Staff working with patients with a high propensity to act dangerously cannot operate safely without the support of colleagues and within an informed system that is designed to allow space for reflection.

However, as inquiries into systems at risk have illustrated, it is often those with the least training and fewer forums for accessing knowledge who spend the longest periods of time in contact with detained patients (Melia *et al*, 1999; Storey & Minto, 2000). Associated as it is with unresolved distress, the task of creating a healthy environment for patients with personality disorder is difficult, particularly if there has been previous interpersonal violence.

This chapter addresses some key factors in the professional training and development of staff who work in personality disorder services. It is assumed that staff appreciate the value of and need for a robust and healthy working alliance with service users (Safran, 1993), which can confer a protective and healing advantage for recovery: 'the chance to build a life' (Haigh, 2002). The challenge is to bring about change by helping both service users and staff to develop the capacity to tolerate dissonance without precipitating crises that derail the process of intervention (Jones, 2007).

The interpersonal impact of personality disorder

Arising from a complex interplay of genetic and environmental influences, personality disorder is undoubtedly shaped by psychosocial adversity – usually physical, sexual and/or emotional abuse – which leads to chronic distress and interpersonal disadvantage (Box 12.1).

Box 12.1   Core problems associated with personality disorder

- Difficulties in asking for help, presenting in 'crisis mode'
- Ambivalence about and rejection of treatment
- Lack of trust in others; fear of intimacy
- Compulsion to re-enact damaging aspects of formative relationships
- Needing opportunities to discharge psychic tension

Additional issues that increase risk to self and others include:

- misinterpretation of the motives of others, particularly when emotionally aroused
- 'pseudo-attachment' to helpers, who become vehicles for their unbearable emotion
- use of controlling and manipulative strategies to restore coherence to their sense of self
- taking action before thinking (impulsivity)
- being in an unknown environment: 'The greater the alienation from a secure base the greater the tendency to avoidance and unprovoked violence' (Holmes, 1996)

If a person has a diagnosis of personality disorder, they are likely to suffer more, and for longer, with other illnesses (Duberstein & Conwell, 1997; Paris & Zweig-Frank, 2001; Taylor, 2006). Almost by definition, they are more likely to have been misunderstood and unfavourably judged against community standards. Offenders with personality disorder can present simultaneously as 'fearsome perpetrators and traumatised victims' (Adshead *et al*, 2008), their vulnerability masked by the threat they simultaneously pose (Schafer & Peternelj-Taylor, 2003).

The three clusters of personality disorder in DSM-IV (American Psychiatric Association, 1994) include criteria that are best understood as an expression of the range of distinguishable defences that patients employ in their reactions to distress (Box 12.2). Put another way, most symptoms and signs of personality disorder are a means of coping with reactions to unbearable people in the past or present (Vaillant, 1994), usually people in caring roles.

It is therefore not surprising that powerful feelings between patients and their professional carers are an inevitable aspect of therapeutic relationships;

Box 12.2   DSM-IV classification of personality disorder (Axis II)

Cluster A: odd or eccentric disorders

- Paranoid personality disorder: irrational suspicions and mistrust of others
- Schizoid personality disorder: lack of interest in social relationships, seeing no point in sharing time with others, anhedonia, introspection
- Schizotypal personality disorder: odd behaviour or thinking

Cluster B: dramatic, emotional or erratic disorders

- Antisocial personality disorder: pervasive disregard for the law and the rights of others
- Borderline personality disorder: extreme 'black and white' thinking, instability in relationships, self-image, identity and behaviour, often leading to self-harm and impulsivity
- Histrionic personality disorder: pervasive attention-seeking behaviour, including inappropriately seductive behaviour and shallow or exaggerated emotions
- Narcissistic personality disorder: pervasive pattern of grandiosity, need for admiration, and a lack of empathy

Cluster C: anxious or fearful disorders

- Avoidant personality disorder: social inhibition, feelings of inadequacy, extreme sensitivity to negative evaluation and avoidance of social interaction
- Dependent personality disorder: pervasive psychological dependence on other people
- Obsessive–compulsive personality disorder: rigid conformity to rules, moral codes and excessive orderliness

(American Psychiatric Association, 1994)

and are not always positive (Hayes, 2004). In an early description of 'hateful patients' in general practice, Groves (1978) articulated the 'physician's dread' at encountering: the 'clinger' (who evokes aversion), the 'demander' (who evokes the desire to counterattack), the 'help rejecters' (who evoke depression) and the 'self-destructive deniers' (who evoke malice and rejection).

Although such pejorative labels are rarely helpful in treatment, they resonate with clinicians because they give voice to real experiences. The feelings of patients towards clinicians (with origins in earlier experiences) constitute 'transference'; 'countertransference' includes the feelings stirred up in the clinician, and the clinician's projections onto the patient. When staff refer to a patient as 'difficult', they may not be describing just a set of clinical signs/symptoms, but rather their own state of being/mind in that person's presence over time (Hinshelwood, 1999).

The defences that arise in interaction with patients with personality disorder tend to generate distinguishable reactions from professionals. Patients with cluster A disorders often engender professional detachment and distance because of problems with engagement. Paranoid–schizoid functioning exposes staff on wards to high levels of projection, especially of intense persecutory anxieties, the processing of which is extremely emotionally taxing (Aiyegbusi, 2009). Alliances robust enough for the treatment of personality disorder can be destabilised by the presence of active and intrusive psychotic symptoms (Taylor, 2006). Patients with cluster C disorders may struggle to ask for help, or engage obsessionally with it.

There is some clinical consensus that cluster B personality disorders in particular (including psychopathy; Hare, 1998) have a substantial impact on carers (National Institute for Mental Health in England, 2003; Rigby & Langford, 2004; Bland & Rossen, 2005; Perseius et al, 2007). Staff can become the target of intolerable feelings (of guilt, anxiety, depression, jealousy, hostility, neediness). Clarke & Ndegwa (2006) observed patterns of emotional abuse of staff by patients in a forensic medium secure unit. Male staff were vulnerable to reacting punitively; female staff were confronted with both subtle and explicit sexual harassment, or invited to behave flirtatiously as a means of charming away hostility. Patients with cluster B disorders may elicit care in ambivalent or hostile ways, which unconsciously confront or confirm their core beliefs about themselves and the world. Services working with people with personality disorder must anticipate and have a framework for addressing such needs.

Different disciplinary experience

The intensity of the exposure to difficult emotions within mental health services varies by profession. Nurses are required to relate to patients for prolonged periods of time (e.g. 8-hour shifts) and are therefore less protected than those (e.g. psychiatrists and psychologists) who provide sessional input to teams. Theirs is a highly specialised task, which is being redefined in various settings as a 'behavioural technician' role (Clarke & Ndegwa, 2006) or a unit-based therapy assistant. Inevitable differences of views between disciplines, and by role, can generate conflict in teams. In this chapter, the generic term 'staff' will refer to all mental healthcare workers notwithstanding these differences.

Common issues for staff in personality disorder services

Primary tensions in services for individuals who are legally detained, either under the Mental Health Act or in prison, oscillate between care and control, voluntary consent to coercion and treatment (Meux & Taylor, 2006). Staff are likely to struggle with their experience of patients as 'good' v. 'bad', people whom it is possible to include/treat or whom it is preferable to exclude; (rescuable) victims or (to be avoided) perpetrators (Box 12.3).

Tensions between personal and professional identities

Staff in mental healthcare and forensic settings are advised to operate with neutrality, to dress and behave professionally, and not to 'bring themselves' to work. Nevertheless, the 'person' is the first thing patients notice about their therapists: appearance, general manner, age, gender, disability, weight, height, skin colour, dress and hairstyle are 'all mutually assessed at some level before any words are spoken' (Scaife & Walsh, 2001: p. 39).

Box 12.3 Potentially 'toxic transference' in personality disorder services: common tests of staff integrity

Service users may:

- compare various members of nursing and multidisciplinary teams and their decisions
- provide minimal information to a member of staff to see how they cope
- make high numbers of complaints
- question others with the same therapist/nurse about actions that person took previously
- refuse to follow recommendations, thereby emphasising the vulnerability of staff, not of themselves
- seek to relate to staff by adopting their language, style and affectations
- single staff out for special attention/comment, gifts or favours, criticism or assault
- play different professionals off against one another, exploiting normal inter-professional rivalries
- flirt with or reject staff

Professionalism is, of course, essential, but it can belie the impact of operating in settings where power and hierarchy are defining features of the organisation, and the working conditions can be traumatic:

'working only with violent persons in closed settings for sustained periods of time is too great a stress for staff members who seek to preserve a therapeutic orientation' (Roth, 1985: p. 228).

What can happen to staff exposed to such pressures? Significant emotional stress can overflow into their personal lives and can create fears even within their families (Bowers *et al*, 2000). Repeated encounters with disturbing material at work can have an impact on choices beyond work: how people dress, conduct themselves, the relationships they form or avoid, and how they raise their children. Collaboration in the workplace flounders where differences between staff members' responses exist and, crucially, are not safely explored. Some common patterns in the 'interpersonal dance' (Duggan, 2005) between patients with personality disorder and staff are outlined below.

The pull to punish

People-centred occupations are intrinsically stressful (Coffey, 1999). Staff working with patients who have been violent are likely to be concerned about being the recipient of attacks and of being identified as aggressors (Doctor, 2008). Some therapeutic practices, such as large community meetings, can be experienced by staff as 'too risky' (Moore & Freestone, 2006). Interactions that alter or flatten the balance of power between staff and patients can generate a tendency to overcontrol in staff who are anxious about losing power. Bullying, intimidation and assaults on patients by staff have been associated with circumstances in which there are no safeguards on imbalances of power, and the majority operate in collusion with a custodial regime (Blom-Cooper, 1992; Fallon *et al*, 1999).

Obviously, a workforce needs to feel confident and skilled in managing high-risk situations effectively. Staff who are well trained in the management of violence describe the experience of feeling physically safe, yet emotionally vulnerable in the presence of patients with personality disorder (Kurtz & Turner, 2007). Hence, physical security is only part of the task of the service overall: the emotional world of the unit cannot be ignored.

Displacement and 'acting out' of distress

'Acting out' is an analytic phrase which implies the non-conscious and unplanned behavioural 'acting out' of intolerable feelings, impulses and beliefs, without the capacity to contain or manage them in other ways. It should not be confused with the sort of performance that an actor consciously engages in as part of a pre-determined role.

In the 'culture' of personality disorder services, it may still covertly be deemed unprofessional to admit to having or expressing personal feelings or emotions about patients' actions and, perhaps even more so, about the response of colleagues to challenging behaviour. If this is the case, then emotions can be dislocated or transposed and reattached to another idea (Vaillant, 1994). Frontline staff in a range of settings who are interviewed about job-related stress more often implicate working conditions and organisational pressures as more problematic for them than contact with patients (Kurtz, 2005). It is possible that it is much easier to transfer (displaced) feelings of anxiety and frustration onto concrete external issues than give voice to emotions about patients.

Personal reactions may be masked as professional opinions. The term 'splitting' is common parlance within multidisciplinary teams struggling to contain divergent views about how best to respond to challenging behaviour. Mirroring the primitive defence mechanism, through which 'good' and 'bad' objects are set in opposition, a patient's behaviour can provoke different members of the team to ally to a greater or lesser extent with one another either in defence of or in opposition to the patient.

If there is a discrepancy between a personal reaction to behaviour (e.g. serious self-harm/shock and anger) and a professional intervention (calm and neutral), how does it get resolved? Norton & Dolan (1995) have illustrated the process by which 'many psychiatric hospitals are in effect, like acting out patients, in that they tend to display only a narrow repertoire of relatively inflexible responses [to distress]'. Acting out in the context of cluster B personality disorder is a process through which the direct behavioural expression of an unconscious wish/conflict allows the individual to remain unaware of the idea/emotion that the action accompanies.

Acting out serves two functions: expressive (communicating intense and urgent need) and defensive (preventing the destruction of integrity) (Campling, 1996). Staff who are experienced in working with people with personality disorder typically recognise the behavioural component of acting out as a surface marker of a concurrent emotional problem, but even so, such actions can impair collaboration.

Those not immediately involved with the patient (but perhaps with responsibilities such as supervisors and managers) can also evidence intense reactions. The more frustration staff that experience, the more the patient acts out and stalemate can ensue (Norton & Dolan, 1995). Regulation of affect, acknowledgement of the need for staff and patients to vent emotion, and adherence to relationship roles create the security that is essential for therapeutic responses when patients are both distressed and highly distressing in the actions they undertake (Adshead, 2002).

Complex and damaging repetitions

Individuals who were traumatised within their family environment are vulnerable in terms of the long-term maladaptive effect of their reaction to the trauma, and their reduced resilience in the face of it (Fonagy & Target,

1997). Lack of resolution of abusive experience, often via inhibition of reflective functioning, reduces the likelihood of forming meaningful and successful adult relationships (McGauley & Rubitel, 2006).

Unresolved distress is communicated via uncomfortable feelings that carers experience and through behavioural re-enactments of past traumatic experiences. Staff actions and interpersonal styles often trigger such conflict re-enactments through the process of 'projective identification' (whereby 'bad' feelings, impulses and beliefs are projected onto staff, who experience the patient's emotions as their own). For example, a frightened patient may consider his named nurse to be persecutory and be unusually hostile towards her (due to fear), while the named nurse experiences her patient as frightening. Staff may find themselves subjected to the hatred and rejection that patients were exposed to in earlier circumstances (Neeld & Clark, 2009). The challenge of distinguishing which feelings belong to whom, when and possibly why is essential to the building of psychotherapeutic alliances, especially in forensic settings (Aiyegbusi, 2004).

Boundary violations

The experience of a therapeutic alliance can trigger in patients an 'aching awareness' (Campling, 1996) of the extent of former neglect and loss, and frantic demands for staff time can be the consequence. This often materialises (and can become dangerous) at breaks or terminations in therapeutic contact. At such times patients may draw on contact-maintaining behaviour (e.g. threats of self-harm) and/or further seek 'concrete evidence' (e.g. a sign of commitment or a declaration of intimacy) of attachment from staff (Campling, 1996). This does not mean that therapy is necessarily contraindicated, but that attachment-related distress must be anticipated. If the capacity for mentalisation in close relationships (i.e. the understanding of behaviour in terms of the associated mental states in self and others) is not recovered in therapy, change is unlikely. Patients with borderline personality disorder are particularly vulnerable to the activation of their attachment systems in one-to-one sessions (Fonagy & Bateman, 2006).

Feeling attraction or love for a therapist can be a normal part of therapy that requires a 'working through' by the patient within a healthy alliance (Disch, 1993). Ideally, the therapist also works through their negative and positive emotions towards the patient. However, difficulties arise if any eroticism of the transference or countertransference becomes secret and acted upon. Although the most notorious boundary violations are sexual (and may initially be viewed as positive by both the member of staff and the patient), there are other types of boundary violation that are also harmful, such as breaches of confidentiality and scapegoating.

An established author in this field, Gutheil (2005) cautions as to the need for 'non-judgemental clarity' in the area of boundary problems, given the 'perils of confusion'. He distinguishes 'boundary crossing' (transient, non-exploitative deviations from 'classical'/general practice that do no harm, and may even facilitate alliance) from 'boundary violation' (essentially harmful deviations from the normal parameters of treatment). One essential test of this distinction is whether the events in question can be discussed during therapy or supervision. 'Explore before action' is a useful recommendation for staff responses when working with people with personality disorder.

No discipline is immune to perpetrating misuses of professional power; neither gender nor seniority are necessarily protective factors. Any actions that meet the needs of the staff member rather than those of the patient are ethically unjustifiable (Pope & Vetter, 1991; Peterson, 1992; Thomas-Peter & Garrett, 2000). This is because such violations exploit power disparities and imbalance relations in favour of the more powerful (Llewelyn & Gardner, 2009).

The damage to patients of breaches in the professional duty of care is phenomenal, exacerbating loss of trust in carers, and extensive distress and isolation that may endure for many years (Disch, 1993; Thomas-Peter & Garrett, 2000). Equally, the damage caused by boundary violations has an impact on the wider institution, undermining its capacity for effective treatment (Gutheil & Gabbard, 2003).

Specific impacts on staff range from the experience of constant anxiety in the workplace to suspension and dismissal (with concomitant loss of job, status and income). Those who are witness to colleagues 'crossing the line' are likely to experience feelings of uncertainty about previous evaluations of their colleagues' work, divided loyalties and moral distress (Peternelj-Taylor, 2003), such that the directive always to place the patient's welfare above all other considerations can become difficult to follow (Thomas-Peter & Garrett, 2000). All involved know that boundary violations are harmful, but they still occur.

Early detection of warning signs (the use of 'red flag' systems) is perhaps the best form of prevention: violations rarely happen 'out of the blue' (Gutheil, 2005). Self-assessment checklists are available that promote self-monitoring for 'blind spots' in relational security (e.g. Love, 2001). Slippages (behaviour that falls into the grey area between staying within or crossing boundaries) preceding violation are known to include over-familiarity, inappropriate favouritism and the exchange of promises/gifts (Webb, 1997; Walker & Clark, 1999). A lack of consequence for seemingly minor breaches decreases the likelihood of arresting toxicity in alliances before enduring harm has occurred (Box 12.4). The boundary seesaw model (Hamilton, 2010) supports a collective conceptualisation of boundaries in practice and generates clear guidelines for staff on how to relate in a balanced and professional way.

Summary

Defensive attitudes and practices are known to obstruct therapeutic opportunities at every level of the institution (Menzies Lyth, 1960; Norton

---

Box 12.4 Potentially unhelpful staff responses to 'toxic' challenges

Rejection/overcontrol

- Dismissive, belittling, pessimistic attitudes
- Use of physical restraint and obtrusive levels of observation
- Inappropriate prescribing or forcible use of medication
- Absence of interest in the causes of challenging behaviour and withdrawal of contact as a sanction; dehumanising or 'switching off'
- Criticism of expressed needs/actions (patients portrayed as attention-seekers, manipulative, trouble-makers, 'not mentally ill', bed-wasters)

Overinvolvement

- Detachment/separation from professional roles (e.g. keeping secrets)
- Disagreement within teams rehearsed in the company of the patient
- Criticism or belittling of other professionals' opinions
- Failure to put the patient's needs first; collusion with boundary violations
- Complying with patients' wishes for physical/sexual contact, special private time
- Personalising the therapeutic relationship or claiming special privacy
- Flirtation as a response to hostility

& Dolan, 1995). Conflict in professional relationships is inevitable, but the risk is higher in personality disorder services because, by definition, people with personality disorder have a compromised set of skills to enable them to handle distress safely. The context for the management of cluster B personality disorder is often controlling and hierarchical, which gives rise to another layer of manipulation (and iatrogenic outcomes; Fonagy & Bateman, 2006; Jones, 2007). When patients and staff rely on (maladaptive) survival skills, this maintains potentially unhealthy relationships in systems that have the power to detain (Box 12.3). Policies on conduct (and what will happen in the event of misconduct) should be accessible to all.

What can be done to create healthy and hopeful services for personality disorder?

The goal of the healthy personality disorder service is to promote safe containment or, in National Health Service terminology, security. What are some of the essential elements in such a system of care?

Mackie (2009) usefully describes three types of containment that reduce fear in staff and patients. 'Concrete' containment is embodied in the buildings, bricks and mortar, doors, walls and locks of the hospital or unit. 'Chemical' containment (medication) represses some disturbance and can provide respite from disabling (Axis I) symptoms. 'Emotional' containment is generated within safe, stable and supportive relationships with people in any setting, allowing people who are alienated and disturbed or aggressive to be re-introduced to 'doses of reality' and the company of others. A fourth form of containment is procedural, and it is provided in policies involving multiple checks and balances that institutions put in place to ensure safety. Since exposure to intense emotional experience associated with psychopathology is inevitable (Cox, 1996), the primary objectives for the clinical workforce become: selection, training, support and effective management.

Selection

Choosing staff who can 'contain'

Who might be best suited to working with people with personality disorder? Such a question is of interest to anyone seeking to recruit motivated, secure and reliable colleagues. People may be attracted to such posts for a whole range of reasons, most of which, it has been suggested, pale into insignificance in the face of the dynamic processes that they will encounter in the workplace. Scanlon & Adlam (2009) refer to the notion of 'psychic survival' as a key competence: conferring the ability to retain a clear sense of separateness, to be able to think your own thoughts while remaining functional and effective.

Similarly, Maden (2006) notes that different skills are required of staff working in personality disorder services than other mental healthcare services, and that the ability of staff to resolve conflict assertively might be a useful predictor of future resilience in the role. Thomas-Peter & Garrett (2000) recommend that staff who appear vulnerable to establishing unethical relations should not be selected for roles in forensic environments. This can be difficult to identify during a selection process, and may also change over the duration of a career. Relationship tensions outside the workplace can put staff at risk of emotional strain and potentially unhelpful self-disclosure, communicating mutuality rather than collaboration for treatment purposes (Walker & Clark, 1999). Procedures such as personal health checks, certainly pre-employment and regularly (annually) post-employment, have been proposed for staff in regular contact with patients with personality disorder (Lord, 2003; Sainsbury Centre for Mental Health, 2009).

A genuine interest in the work is likely to be a helpful starting place. The capacity to form secure attachments with others is also important, and has been associated with higher ratings of the therapeutic alliance by staff and patients in psychotherapy services (Eames & Roth, 2000).

Staff motivations and interests

Staff attitudes to their role as agents of help can make a difference to the nature and quality of the care patients receive. There is evidence that critical views about patients with enduring and complex disorders can change with psychoeducational training (Finnema *et al*, 1996; Willetts & Leff, 1997; Hazelton *et al*, 2006). Specifically, attributions about the causes of behavioural problems are important in determining the emotional and behavioural responses of staff.

Experience is another factor, with less-trained staff being more critical and emotionally cold, with higher levels of expressed emotion (Van Humbeeck & Van Audenhove, 2003). Dennis & Leach (2007) report high expressed emotion in male healthcare support staff who endorsed elements of burnout, including depersonalisation and low personal accomplishment. In forensic services, high expressed emotion is linked to less favourable outcomes for patients with complex needs, including personality disorder (Moore *et al*, 2002). Views can shift considerably following experiences of assault: in the immediate aftermath, staff victims are more likely to express criticism and to reject patients (Cottle *et al*, 1995).

Mothersole (2000) highlights voyeuristic motivations, particularly in forensic units, whereby staff may gain a vicarious excitement or notoriety from their connection to certain offender patients.

Training

Opportunities to learn about core competencies

'Relational security' is dependent on a multidisciplinary workforce that can enhance and develop therapeutic programmes (Exworthy & Gunn, 2003). Working as a newcomer in a personality disorder service is likely to be highly anxiety-provoking: the process of induction and the behaviour and attitudes of key mentors make an important contribution. From the outset, the tensions between security and care will be evident to inexperienced staff (who may find themselves swinging between inclinations to care v. reject, to protect v. punish, to operate with overconfidence v. hesitation) as they make sense of how to amalgamate complex information about the clinical task.

Longer-serving/senior staff are role models (Crichton, 1998), and much therefore depends on the psychological health of the unit. Whole teams and organisations can become dysfunctional, so that the external world reflects grave and disabling splits in the patients' internal world, in a 'some staff good, most staff bad' caricature (Tuck, 2009). Learning to operate with self-awareness might be considered a fundamental skill, a prerequisite for working with people with personality disorder.

What should a training package for staff on personality disorder units include?

Health, safety, violence and risk training are typically mandatory. Service users with personality disorder have recommended that training staff to develop empathy and understanding of the disorder would also help (Haigh,

199

2002). Skills in treating others respectfully while under pressure to do otherwise should probably be a fundamental training goal: understanding personality pathology and the nature of change provides an essential foundation (Livesley, 2005).

A formal introduction to what would constitute inappropriate interaction (Thomas-Peter & Garrett, 2000) and how to set and maintain boundaries are also core competencies. More complex interpersonal therapeutic skills, including appropriate emotional availability for patients in distress (Zeddies, 1999), typically demand longer post-qualification training. Knowledge of services is also important: what range of services is available to the patients? What is the contribution of (other) disciplines? What are the politics of the setting? (Scaife, 2001).

Training for staff must be well timed. For staff who appear 'burnt out' ('I've seen all this before – they'll never change. I'm basically here to pay the mortgage'), mistimed training may actually intensify such beliefs. Extended contact with very slow-to-change populations can cause staff to identify with the hopelessness that patients encounter, and the 'no-win' position of offender patients in relation to the society that has excluded them (Lowdell & Adshead, 2009). Conversely, a risk for well-intentioned staff is that they are seen as overattentive, perhaps too ready to do things for patients, rather than helping them to accomplish their own goals.

Creating a context for boundaried practice: the clinical importance of supervision

No one can fully process emotional reactions at the time of their occurrence, and people will vary in their preparedness and ability to acknowledge or express uncomfortable feelings. Sometimes services claim to promote safe expression of feeling, while in reality they stigmatise and discriminate against those who give voice to any struggles. The term supervision is often misused in this way: staff thought to be 'at risk' who are directed to attend 'more supervision' might see this as a form of discipline rather than as a resource for safe exploration and learning.

Clear therapeutic objectives and clinical supervision provide the framework within which alliances for change can be generated with patients. Supervisory relationships should either preclude the simultaneous existence of relationships or, where dual relationships pertain (e.g., with a line manager and a clinical supervisor), this should be acknowledged and the implications addressed (Scaife, 2001: p. 45).

In essence, supervision refers to a range of key ideas (Scaife, 2001) about how to provide support, reflective space, regulation of the supervisee and the establishment of the 'limit[s] that promote integrity' (Katherine, 1991). Empowerment of the supervisee is a key function of the supervisory alliance but is often poorly implemented in secure environments (Storey & Minto, 2000). To managers less exposed to clinical challenges, supervision might be viewed as irrelevant to the task, ineffective, expensive and ultimately unavailable owing to lack of good supervisors. Problems such as this must be addressed in any therapeutic service for patients with personality disorder. There are two primary aspects to supervision: (1) establishing and maintaining appropriate boundaries for professionals and services; and (2) attending to the needs (for safety, personal development, etc.) of the staff member.

The setting and maintenance of boundaries is therefore a key supervisory task, and one that official inquiries often highlight as having failed (Exworthy & Gunn, 2003). Boundaries must be regarded as flexible standards of good practice, the application of professional judgements, and not as rigidly adhered to lists of 'generically forbidden behaviour' (Hermansson, 1997; Gutheil & Gabbard, 2003). Boundaries define relationships and roles. A good definition of the nature of a 'boundary' in clinical practice is 'the edge of appropriate professional contact' (Gutheil, 2005). Accepting boundaries implies that we acknowledge that 'there are limits to what we can do, with whom and when, central to which are a commitment to non-exploitation of the other, and trust' (Llewelyn & Gardner, 2009).

Boundaries are maintained, and limits set, by staff working in multi-disciplinary teams via the communication of clear expectations about behaviour. Since exchanges between patients with personality disorder and staff can be 'covert' (Duggan, 2005), it is very important that staff have a safe place to describe and discuss how best to respond to such challenges. Certain useful strategies for maintaining boundaries are co-working, allocation of roles, and sharing the burden in demanding work (Melia et al, 1999).

Support

The role of supervision in maintaining 'optimal' working alliances

Supervision has a number of functions that are formative (lifelong learning and professional development), restorative (a space for support, shared understanding and acknowledgement of impacts) and normative (concerned with good practice standards). The supervisor's role is to attend both to the actions and reactions of the staff member and team, and to the knowledge, feelings and qualities that influence the alliance with the patient. The aim of the process is to ensure the best possible practice whatever the context, and to enhance the staff members' range and depth of clinical skills. Clinical supervision has been defined by Mothersole (2000) as a 'scheduled regular meeting in which a clinician meets with a fellow professional with the express purpose of examining their work'.

In the past, transfer to a colleague, team or service who could 'stand' the patient (Groves, 1978) was considered a solution to patients who engendered difficult feelings in professionals. Nowadays, treatment alliances in personality disorder services ideally involve a level of compassionate neutrality on the part of the professional. It is helpful (with the assistance of supervision) to process challenging events without aggression, outrage, withdrawal or compliance. An understanding of the unconscious message of challenging behaviour has the potential to arrest vicious cycles of rejecting re-enactments.

Some patients with personality disorder will be unaware of their impact on others, but are nevertheless held accountable for it, as if they could/ should do something about this. Rather, it must be the staff who provide the routes to repair ruptures in professional alliances as they develop. Staff should not expect to like or be liked by all patients (Moran & Mason, 1996). Nevertheless, they must always treat all services users with respect (Sainsbury Centre for Mental Health, 2009).

It is essential for patients with personality disorder to experience clinicians as personal, human and authentic (Safran, 1993). As Kraus & Reynolds (2001) put it, 'the person in the clinician must meet the person in the patient'. The adoption of an inquisitive (not expert) stance enables staff to retrace steps in an interaction or series of encounters that have 'gone wrong', and to take the initiative in building and rebuilding bridges (Fonagy & Bateman, 2006).

Drawing on research involving patients with serious and long-term mental health problems, Repper *et al* (1994) describe how successful staff realise the need to balance 'realism' (taking a long-term perspective) with optimistic hope of change and growth, appreciating that, given the nature of the patients' problems, recovery will be a fluctuating process.

Group approaches to supervision

Reflective practice

Reflective practice is a group technique that involves all professionals (regardless of experience or training) meeting together to talk about patients and their feelings towards them. This is recommended practice for all staff working with people with personality disorder as an essential part of the job (National Institute for Mental Health in England, 2003). As the term implies, reflection is the opposite of operating mindlessly in response to problem behaviour, and reflective practice should increase the capacity of the organisation to mentalise. Reflective practice also allows for an external perspective on a clinical treatment system, which protects against boundary violations and abusive practice.

Master classes

Other types of group supervision may be helpful (Proctor & Inskipp, 2001). Among the advantages of working with others is the mutual recognition of expertise (Scaife, 2001: p. 104). Some group supervision takes the form of a 'master class', with supervisees acting as an audience. A disadvantage of this model can be that staff may feel deskilled as a consequence. This is particularly likely to happen in multidisciplinary forums where wide power differentials between staff exist. In participative and cooperative groups, responsibility for the tasks of the group is shared with a supervisor who teaches, encourages and facilitates. Although time can become an issue if not fairly shared, these models generally encourage skill development.

Peer surpervision

Peer supervision, as the name implies, involves colleagues in shared responsibility for supervision, leadership roles and responsibilities. Well-functioning peer groups can provide safe and trustable working alliances. Bland & Rossen (2005) describe the role of clinical nurse specialists in the provision of group supervision for nursing teams working with people with borderline personality disorder, and the resultant enhancement of job satisfaction for all. A possible difficulty with peer supervision as the sole source of reflective practice is that it may exclude other professionals and increase the risk of splits in a multidisciplinary team.

Responsive management

Learning from incidents

During the early 1990s, the introduction of the serious incident review had the adverse effect of fostering a 'blame culture' in some quarters of the healthcare service (Blumenthal & Lavender, 2001; Rose, 2008). Analysis of errors (e.g. root cause analysis) generates knowledge, but sometimes at a cost: over the past decade, there has been an expansion in the formal management procedures for dealing with bad outcomes. If an incident has occurred, the inclusion of a range of staff, and the use of external facilitators, promotes the production of reports to operational boards, whose task is then to analyse the failure of the system as a whole.

Rose (2008) has argued that good patient care is best served by the use of an inclusive review process that combines peer group front-line expertise with management inquiry skills. Untoward incidents in large organisations often have complex interrelationships and need to be reviewed in this light (Vincent et al, 2000). Recent work on the dissemination of learning points from serious incident reviews has highlighted how critical the process of communicating the findings is (Thinn, 2010). Frequently, the learning cycle is incomplete because key points are not accessibly and specifically communicated to front-line staff.

Key events can have a profound impact on individual clinicians and their inclination or suitability to remain in post. Areas of concern noted by staff working with people with personality disorder include both the work itself (ranging from reading forensic case-note material to being subject to verbal abuse or complaint, or suffering/witnessing a violent attack) and the way in which managers handle these occurrences (Bowers et al, 2000).

Box 12.5 Management-led strategies to promote patients' health and recovery in personality disorder services

- Retain professional roles: always keep the duty of care in focus
- Select motivated staff
- Provide training on personality disorders, boundary setting and maintenance
- Attend to changes in staff attitude/interest/morale
- Promote an 'empathic balance' between trust and control: share decisions (rules agreed by peers are more likely to be accepted than those imposed by parental figures)
- Establish a culture of reflective enquiry: 'Can we safely explore together what might be happening here?'
- Include appropriate use of humour
- Respond swiftly but calmly to rule-breaking; operate with 'firmness without retribution'; do not retaliate; do not over-react
- Provide opportunities for detained persons (and staff) to 'let off steam'
- Communicate the learning points from serious incidents/set-backs specifically and directly to all staff

---

When incidents of crisis or acute distress in clinical work occur early in the person's career and are survived, this can enhance resilience. Senior managers have a responsibility to understand and anticipate the potential for these events, and to operate to minimise any 'casualties' of the process. All staff involved in any complaint or investigatory process should have access to (external) support (Bowers *et al*, 2000) (Box 12.5).

Evidence of the benefits of supervision: enhancing morale

As Scaife (2001) observes, supervision is not the 'panacea for dealing with [all] work-related issues'. The aims and purposes of supervision may not be realised, and typically especially not for those most at risk of defaulting from the professional task. Equally, many of the functions of supervision can be achieved in other ways via less 'formal' relationships (over a cup of coffee) in the workplace. However, in support of its role, vital in modern, effective healthcare systems, there is evidence that supervision is associated with positive outcomes (Milne, 2007).

The benefits of participation in clinical supervision can be highly significant: enhancing a sense of coherence and creativity, reducing job-related strain and increasing satisfaction (Berg & Hallberg, 1999). A number of factors contribute to rewarding, 'happy' work environments in mental healthcare (Bowers *et al*, 2009): services that are well organised, that have clearly defined and consistently implemented policies (e.g. relating to abuse directed at staff), that educate and rotate their staff, and that see retaining a sense of humour as valued and essential (Moran & Mason, 1996).

The positives of working with individuals with personality disorder are rarely explicitly articulated in practitioner literature, where the complexities of the task tend to be more fully addressed. However, the benefits of persisting with complexity can greatly enrich interpersonal flexibility and professional and personal communication skills, albeit alongside an ongoing acknowledgement of our limitations. As Layden and colleagues (1993) put it: being a therapist of a patient with borderline personality disorder 'is to be acutely reminded that one is a human being'. If staff feel secure in the support of colleagues, with a sense of purpose in their encounters, they stand some chance of accepting distress, sometimes responding with creativity, and structuring the relational environment such that those in their company might begin to do the same:

> 'It is always encouraging to see newer residents being encouraged, cajoled, soothed, challenged and constrained by residents further on in therapy, who a few months earlier, were exhibiting the same sorts of destructive ambivalence' (Campling, 1996: p. 544).

What could be more rewarding than that?

References

Adshead, G. (2002) Three degrees of security: attachment and forensic institutions. *Criminal Behaviour and Mental Health*, **12**, S31–45.

Adshead, G., Bose, S. & Cartwright, C. (2008) Life after death: working with men who have killed. In *Murder* (ed. R. Doctor), pp. 9–33. Karnac.

Aiyegbusi, A. (2004) Thinking under fire: the challenge for forensic mental health nurses working with women in secure care. In *Working Therapeutically with Women in Secure Mental Health Settings* (eds N. Jeffcote & N. Watson), 108–119. Jessica Kingsley Publishers.

Aiyegbusi, A. (2009) The dynamics of difference. In *Therapeutic Relationships with Offenders: An Introduction to the Psychodynamics of Forensic Mental Health Nursing* (eds A. Aiyegbusi & J. Clark-Moore), pp. 69–80. Jessica Kingsley Publishers.

Alwin, N., Blackburn, R., Davidson, K., *et al* (2006) *Understanding Personality Disorder: A Report by the British Psychological Society*. British Psychological Society.

American Psychiatric Association (1994) *Diagnostic and Statistical Manual of Mental Disorders (4th edn) (DSM-IV)*. APA.

Berg, A. & Hallberg, I. R. (1999) Effects of systematic clinical supervision on psychiatric nurses' sense of coherence, creativity, work-related strain, job satisfaction and view of the effects from clinical supervision: a pre-post test design. *Journal of Psychiatric and Mental Health Nursing*, **6**, 371–381.

Bland, A. R. & Rossen, E. (2005) Clinical supervision of nurses. *Working with patients with borderline personality disorder. Issues in Mental Health Nursing*, **26**, 507–517.

Blom-Cooper, L. (1992) *Report of the Committee of Inquiry into Complaints about Ashworth Hospital (Cm 2028)*. HMSO.

Blumenthal, S. & Lavender, T. (2001) *Violence and Mental Disorder: A Critical Aid to the Assessment and Management of Risk*. Jessica Kingsley Publishers.

Bowers, L., McFarlane, L., Kiyimba, F., *et al* (2000) *Factors Underlying and Maintaining Nurses' Attitudes to Patients with Severe Personality Disorder: Final Report to National Forensic Mental Health R&D*. Department of Mental Health Nursing, City University.

Bowers, L., Allan, T., Simpson, A., *et al* (2009) Morale is high in acute inpatient psychiatry. *Social Psychiatry Psychiatric Epidemiology*, **44**, 39–46.

Campling, P. (1996) Maintaining the therapeutic alliance with personality-disordered patients. *Journal of Forensic Psychiatry*, **77**, 535–550.

Clarke, A. & Ndegwa, D. (2006) Forensic personality disorder in an MSU: lessons learnt after two years. *British Journal of Forensic Practice*, **8** (suppl. 4), 29–33.

Coffey, M. (1999) Stress and burnout in forensic community mental health nurses: an investigation of its causes and effects. *Journal of Psychiatric and Mental Health Nursing*, **6**, 433–443.

Cottle, M., Kuipers, L., Murphy, G., *et al* (1995) Expressed emotion, attributions and coping in staff who have been victims of violent incidents. *Mental Handicap Research*, **8** (suppl. 3), 168–183.

Cox, M. (1996) Psychodynamics and the special hospital 'road blocks and thought blocks'. In *Forensic Psychotherapy: Psychodynamics and the Offender Patient* (eds C. Cordess & M. Cox), pp. 433–448. Jessica Kingsley Publishers.

Crichton, J. H. M. (1998) Psychodynamic perspectives on staff response to inpatient misdemeanour. *Criminal Behaviour and Mental Health*, **8**, 266–274.

Dennis, A. M. & Leach, C. (2007) Expressed emotion and burnout: the experience of staff caring for men with learning disability and psychosis in a medium secure setting. *Journal of Psychiatric and Mental Health Nursing*, **14**, 267–276.

Disch, E. (1993) When intimacy goes awry. *Dulwich Centre Newsletter*, **3&4**, 21–26.

Doctor, R. (ed.) (2008) Introduction. In *Murder*, pp. 1–7. Karnac.

Duberstein, P. R. & Conwell, Y. (1997) Personality disorders and completed suicide: a methodological and conceptual review. *Clinical Psychology: Science and Practice*, **4**, 359–376.

Duggan, C. (2005) Dynamic therapy for severe personality disorder. In *Personality Disorders and Serious Offending: Hospital Treatment Models* (eds C. Newrith, C. Meux & P. Taylor), 146–160. Hodder Arnold.

Eames, V. & Roth, A. (2000) Patient attachment orientation and the early working alliance: a study of patient and therapist reports of alliance quality and ruptures. *Psychotherapy Research*, **10** (suppl. 4), 421–434.

Exworthy, T. & Gunn, J. (2003) Taking another tilt at high secure hospitals: the Tilt Report and its consequences for secure psychiatric services. *British Journal of Psychiatry*, **182**, 469–471.

Fallon, P., Bluglass, R., Edwards, B., *et al* (1999) *Report of the Committee of Inquiry into the Personality Disorder Unit, Ashworth Special Hospital (Vol. 1) (Cm 4194, II)*. TSO (The Stationery Office).

Finnema, E. J., Louwerens, J. W., Slooff, C. J., *et al* (1996) Expressed emotion on long-stay wards. *Journal of Advanced Nursing*, **24**, 473–478.

Fonagy, P. & Bateman, A. (2006) Progress in the treatment of borderline personality disorder. *British Journal of Psychiatry*, **188**, 1–3.

Fonagy, P. & Target, M. (1997) Attachment and reflective function: their role in self-organization. *Development and Psychopathology*, **9**, 679–700.

Groves, J.. E. (1978) Taking care of the hateful patient. *New England Journal of Medicine*, **298**, 883–887.

Gutheil, T. G. (2005) Boundary issues and personality disorders. *Journal of Psychiatric Practice*, **11**, 421–429.

Gutheil, T. G. & Gabbard, G. O. (2003) Misuses and misunderstandings of boundary theory in clinical and regulatory settings. *Focus*, **1**, 415–421.

Haigh, R. (2002) *Services for People with Personality Disorder: The Thoughts of Service Users*. Department of Health (http://www.dh.gov.uk/prod_consum_dh/groups/dh_digitalassets/@dh/@en/documents/digitalasset/dh_4130844.pdf).

Hamilton, L. (2010) The boundary seesaw model: good fences make for good neighbours. In *Using Time, Not Doing Time: Practitioner Perspectives on Personality Disorder and Risk* (eds A. Tennant & K. Howells), pp. 81–94. John Wiley & Sons.

Hare, R. (1998) The Hare PCL-R: some issues concerning its use and misuse. *Legal and Criminological Psychology*, **3**, 99–119.

Hayes, J. A. (2004) The inner world of the psychotherapist: a program of research on countertransference. *Psychotherapy Research*, **14** (suppl. 1), 21–36.

Hazelton, M., Rossiter, R. & Milner, J. (2006) Managing the 'unmanageable': training staff in the use of dialectical behaviour therapy for borderline personality disorder. *Contemporary Nurse*, **21**, 120–130.

Hermansson, G. (1997) Boundaries and boundary management in counselling: the never-ending story. *British Journal of Guidance & Counselling*, **25**, 133–146.

Hinshelwood, R. D. (1999) The difficult patient: The role of 'scientific psychiatry' in understanding patients with chronic schizophrenia or severe personality disorder. *British Journal of Psychiatry*, **174**, 187–190.

Holmes, J. (1996) *Attachment, Intimacy, Autonomy: Using Attachment Theory in Adult Psychotherapy*. Jason Aronson.

Jones, L. (2007) Iatrogenic interventions with 'personality disordered' offenders. *Psychology, Crime & Law*, 13, 69–79.

Katherine, A. (1991) *Boundaries: Where You End and I Begin*. Simon & Schuster.

Kraus, G. & Reynolds, D. J. (2001) The 'ABC's' of the Cluster B's: identifying, under-standing, and treating Cluster B personality disorders. *Clinical Psychology Review*, **21**, 345–373.

Kurtz, A. (2005) The needs of staff who care for people with a diagnosis of personality disorder who are considered a risk to others. *Journal of Forensic Psychiatry and Psychology*, **16**, 399–422.

Kurtz, A. & Turner, K. (2007) An exploratory study of the needs of staff who care for offenders with a diagnosis of personality disorder. *Psychology and Psychotherapy*, **80**, 421–435.

Layden, M. A., Newman, C. F., Freeman, A., et al (1993) *Cognitive Therapy of Borderline Personality Disorder*. Allyn & Bacon.

Livesley, W. J. (2005) Principles and strategies for treating personality disorder. *Canadian Journal of Psychiatry*, **50**, 442–450.

Llewelyn, S. & Gardner, D. (2009) Boundary issues in clinical psychology. *Clinical Psychology Forum*, **193**, 5–9.

Lord, A. (2003) Working with personality-disordered offenders. *Forensic Update*, **73**, 31–39.

Love, C. C. (2001) Staff-patient erotic boundary violations. *Journal of Psychosocial Nursing*, **7**, 4–7.

Lowdell, A. & Adshead, G. (2009) The best defence: institutional defences against anxiety in forensic services. In *Therapeutic Relationships with Offenders: An Introduction to the Psychodynamics of Forensic Mental Health Nursing* (eds A. Aiyegbusi & J. Clark-Moore), pp. 53–67. Jessica Kingsley Publishers.

Mackie, S. (2009) Reflecting on murderousness: reflective practice in secure forensic settings. In *Therapeutic Relationships with Offenders: An Introduction to the Psychodynamics of Forensic Mental Health Nursing* (eds A. Aiyegbusi & J. Clark-Moore), pp. 93–104. Jessica Kingsley Publishers.

Maden, T. (2006) DSPD: origins and progress to date. *British Journal of Forensic Practice*, **8**, 24–28.

McGauley, G. & Rubitel, A. (2006) Attachment theory and personality disordered patients. In *Personality Disorder and Serious Offending: Hospital Treatment Models* (eds C. Newrith, C. Meux & P. Taylor), pp. 69–80. Hodder Arnold.

Melia, P., Moran, T. & Mason, T. (1999) Triumvirate nursing for personality disordered patients crossing the boundaries safely. *Journal of Psychiatric and Mental Health Nursing*, **6**, 15–20.

Menzies Lyth, I. (1960) *The Functioning of Social Systems as a Defence Against Anxiety – A Report*. Centre for Applied Social Research, Tavistock Institute of Human Relations.

Meux, C. & Taylor, P. (2006) Settings for the treatment of personality disorder. In *Personality Disorder and Serious Offending: Hospital Treatment Models* (eds C. Newrith, C. Meux & P. Taylor): 205–15. Hodder Arnold.

Milne, D. (2007) An empirical definition of clinical supervision. *British Journal of Clinical Psychology*, **46**, 437–447.

Moore, C. & Freestone, M. (2006) Traumas of forming: the introduction of community meetings in the Dangerous and Severe Personality Disorder (DSPD) environment. *Therapeutic Communities*, **27**, 193–209.

Moore, E., Yates, M., Mallindine, C., *et al* (2002) Expressed emotion between staff and patients in forensic services: changes in relationship status at 12 month follow up. *Legal and Criminological Psychology*, **7**, 203–218.

Moran, T. & Mason, T. (1996) Revisiting the nursing management of the psychopath. *Journal of Psychiatric and Mental Health Nursing*, **3**, 189–194.

Mothersole, G. (2000) Clinical supervision and forensic work. *Journal of Sexual Aggression*, **5** (suppl. 1), 45–58.

National Institute for Mental Health in England (2003) *Breaking the Cycle of Rejection: The Personality Disorder Capabilities Framework*. Department of Health.

Neeld, R. & Clark, T. (2009) The patient, her nurse and the therapeutic community. In *Therapeutic Relationships with Offenders: An Introduction to the Psychodynamics of Forensic Mental Health Nursing* (eds A. Aiyegbusi & J. Clark-Moore), pp. 157–170. Jessica Kingsley Publishers.

Norton, K. & Dolan, B. (1995) Acting out and the institutional response. *Journal of Forensic Psychiatry*, **6**, 317–332.

Paris, J. & Zweig-Frank, H. (2001) A 27 year follow-up of patients with borderline personality disorder. *Comprehensive Psychiatry*, **42**, 482–487.

Perseius, K. I., Kaver, A., Ekdahl, S., *et al* (2007) Stress and burnout in psychiatric professionals when starting to use dialectical behavioural therapy in the work with young self-harming women showing borderline personality symptoms. *Journal of Psychiatric and Mental Health Nursing*, **14**, 635–643.

Peternelj-Taylor, C. (2003) Whistleblowing and boundary violations: exposing a colleague in the forensic milieu. *Nursing Ethics*, **10**, 526–537.

Peterson, M. (1992) *At Personal Risk: Boundary Violations in Professional–Client Relationships*. Norton.

Pope, K. S. & Vetter, V. A. (1991) Prior therapist-patient sexual involvement among patients seen by psychologists. *Psychotherapy*, **28**, 429–438.

Proctor, B. & Inskipp, F. (2001) Group supervision. In *Supervision in the Mental Health Professions. A Practioner's Guide* (ed. J. Scaife), pp. 99–121. Brunner-Routledge.

Repper, J., Ford, R. & Crooke, A. (1994) How can nurses build trusting relationships with people who have severe and long-term mental health problems? Experiences of case managers and their clients. *Journal of Advanced Nursing*, **19**, 1096–1104.

Rigby, M. & Langford, J. (2004) Development of a multi-agency experiential training course on personality disorder. *Psychiatric Bulletin*, **28**, 337–341.

Rose, N. (2008) Oxford serious incident review: 7 years on. *Psychiatric Bulletin*, **32**, 307–309.

Roth, L. H. (ed.) (1985) *Clinical Treatment of the Violent Person*. Guilford Publications.

Safran, J. D. (1993) Breaches in the therapeutic alliance: an arena for negotiating authentic relatedness. *Psychotherapy*, **30**, 11–24.

Sainsbury Centre for Mental Health (2009) *Personality Disorder: A Briefing for People Working in the Criminal Justice System*. Sainsbury Centre for Mental Health (http://www.scmh.org.uk/pdfs/personality_disorder_briefing.pdf).

Scaife, J. (2001) *Supervision in the Mental Health Professions: A Practioner's Guide*. Brunner-Routledge.

Scaife, J. & Walsh, S. (2001) The emotional climate of work and the development of self. In *Supervision in the Mental Health Professions. A Practioner's Guide* (ed. J. Scaife), pp. 30–51. Bruner-Routledge.

Scanlon, C. & Adlam, J. (2009) Nursing dangerousness, dangerous nursing and the spaces in between: learning to live with uncertainties. In *Therapeutic Relationships with Offenders:*

An Introduction to the Psychodynamics of Forensic Mental Health Nursing (eds A. Aiyegbusi & J. Clark-Moore), pp. 127–142. Jessica Kingsley Publishers.

Schafer, P. & Peternelj-Taylor, C. (2003) Therapeutic relationships and boundary maintenance: the perspective of patients enrolled in a treatment program for violent offenders. *Issues in Mental Health Nursing*, **24**, 605–625.

Storey, L. & Minto, C. (2000) Mental health: the use of clinical supervision in secure environments. *British Journal of Nursing*, **9**, 2226–2231.

Taylor, P. J. (2006) Co-morbidity and personality disorder: the concept and implications for treatment of personality disorder co-morbid with psychosis. In *Personality Disorder and Serious Offending: Hospital Treatment Models* (eds C. Newrith, C. Meux & P. Taylor), pp. 170–182. Hodder Arnold.

Thinn, K. (2010) Reporting on incidents. *Health Service Journal*, 11 May (http://www.hsj.co.uk).

Thomas-Peter, B. & Garrett, T. (2000) Preventing sexual contact between professionals and patients in forensic environments. *Journal of Forensic Psychiatry*, **11**, 135–150.

Tuck, G. (2009) Forensic systems and organisational dynamics. In *Therapeutic Relationships with Offenders: An Introduction to the Psychodynamics of Forensic Mental Health Nursing* (eds A. Aiyegbusi & J. Clark-Moore), pp. 43–52. Jessica Kingsley Publishers.

Vaillant, G. E. (1994) Ego mechanisms of defence and personality psychopathology. *Journal of Abnormal Psychology*, **103** (suppl. 1), 44–50.

Van Humbeeck, G. & Van Audenhove, C. (2003) Expressed emotion of professionals towards mental health patients. *Social Psychiatry and Psychiatric Epidemiology*, **12**, 232–235.

Vincent, C., Stanhope, N. & Taylor-Adams, S. (2000) Developing a systematic method of analysing serious incidents in mental health. *Journal of Mental Health*, **9**, 89–103.

Walker, R. & Clark, J. J. (1999) Heading off boundary problems: clinical supervision as risk management. *Psychiatric Services*, **50**, 1435–1439.

Webb, S. R. (1997) Training for maintaining appropriate boundaries in counselling. *British Journal of Guidance & Counselling*, **25** (suppl. 2), 175–188.

Willetts, L..E. & Leff, J. (1997) Expressed emotion and schizophrenia: the efficacy of a staff training programme. *Journal of Advanced Nursing*, **26**, 1125–1133.

Zeddies, T. J. (1999) Becoming a psychotherapist: the personal nature of clinical work, emotional availability and personal allegiances. *Psychotherapy*, **36**, 229–235.

Part 3
Specific treatment approaches

CHAPTER 13

Treating personality disorder: methods and outcomes

Anthony W. Bateman and Peter Tyrer

Summary The growing demand for effective treatments for personality disorder has not been met adequately by the development of appropriate clinical services. However, there has been a significant shift from the view that personality disorder is untreatable; we do have treatments that have at least some efficacy and a number of countries have issued national guidance on the treatment of some personality disorders. This chapter summarises some of the current evidence regarding which psychological treatments are effective for personality disorder.

Although every known treatment is used at some time for conditions that are deemed untreatable, almost all of the treatments for personality disorder that carry some element of respectability are included under one of the headings in Table 13.1. In discussing the efficacy of treatments for personality disorders, we have to be aware of the special problems associated with assessment of these conditions:

(a) the high level of comorbidity with other disorders, of both personality and mental state (Tyrer *et al*, 1997);

Table 13.1 Summary of treatments used for personality disorder

Type of treatment	Main purpose of treatment
Behaviour therapy	To improve maladaptive behaviour
Cognitive analytic therapy	To achieve greater self-understanding
Cognitive–behavioural therapy	To alter dysfunctional core beliefs
Dialectical behaviour therapy	Initially to reduce self-harm; eventually to achieve transcendence
Nidotherapy	To achieve better environmental adjustment to minimise impact of disorder
Dynamic psychotherapy	To increase reflective capacity and emotional and interpersonal understanding
Therapeutic community	To effect attitudinal, social and behavioural change

(b) the fluctuating nature of personality status over time, mainly as a consequence of concomitant mood changes (Clark *et al*, 2003);

(c) the need for a long period of observation, preferably at least a year, before a treatment can be said to have been properly evaluated;

(d) the recognition that personality disorder is a multifaceted condition that can be influenced in many different ways and fully justifies the use of what are described as 'complex interventions' (Campbell *et al*, 2000) to treat it. Complex interventions lead to complex evaluations and consequent greater difficulty in interpreting results.

An important distinction in determining the value of an intervention is whether it has been demonstrated in standard practice or under strict experimental conditions. This was first highlighted by Schwarz & Lellouch (1967) in discussing randomised trials, and it is commonly described as the difference between an explanatory trial, i.e. a trial in which treatments are compared under ideal (experimentally manipulated) conditions, and a pragmatic trial, in which the study is carried out under the conditions normally appertaining to ordinary practice. In the latter type of trial, possible confounders to the intervention may be present, and although they could be removed, to do so would create an artificial environment that would not allow the results to be transferred to ordinary practice.

Schwarz & Lellouch showed that the results of these two types of trial can be very different, even though the treatments under test are the same. As personality disorders commonly occur in conjunction with other disorders, there is a place for both pragmatic and explanatory trials in their evaluation. In evidence-based psychiatry these are sometimes described as trials of efficacy (explanatory) and effectiveness (pragmatic). Each has its advantages and disadvantages, but in general it is common first to establish an intervention's efficacy under controlled conditions before testing it in ordinary practice. Owing to the formidable difficulties of meeting these requirements, summarised in Box 13.1, there has been a tendency for investigators to abandon them or at least to fulfil them only partially and the literature on treating personality disorder, particularly with psychotherapeutic interventions, is often difficult to interpret (Bateman & Fonagy, 2000).

Box 13.1 Requirements for establishing an effective treatment

- Efficacy over control treatments in randomised controlled trial of use for a pure form of the personality disorder
- Similar outcome in pragmatic randomised controlled trial
- Consistency across settings when used with appropriate treatment fidelity
- Maintenance of outcome over time (preferably more than 1 year) because of the long duration of personality disorder

Choice of outcome measures

Outcome measures have always been a problem in relation to psychiatric disorders, but these difficulties become even more pronounced in the case of personality disorders because there are no agreed common outcomes. The wide range of those that have been measured are summarised in Box 13.2. Personality disorders affect both the individual and society, and outcomes can be measured to cover all these possibilities.

The interaction between a personality disorder and a coexisting Axis I disorder could exaggerate or obscure a genuine treatment effect. Changes in symptoms may be a consequence of change in mental state disorders quite independent of personality. Treatment may improve the mental illness but not the personality dysfunction or *vice versa*, and improvement in one may follow improvement in the other. Conversely, it is well known that mental illness can create the impression of abnormal personality, but these characteristics change as the mental illness improves. Thus, any measured change in personality should be regarded in the first instance as an artefact related to improvement or deterioration in mental state.

Owing to these difficulties, there is a tendency to use single global outcome measures such as the Global Assessment Scale (Endicott *et al*, 1976) to determine the degree of improvement in personality disorders in long-term follow-up studies, although a battery of measurements, covering different domains, is normally used in short-term studies. Unfortunately, there is no standardised procedure for recording global outcome measures. However, it is reasonable to take into account any, several or all of the measures listed in Box 13.2, provided that there is a clear distinction between primary and secondary outcomes.

There are particular problems in assessing outcomes in the treatment of people with personality disorders who pose a risk to others. Most studies on psychological therapies with offenders (mainly in prison settings) have focused on reducing harm to others. Although the general public (and some forensic practitioners) may consider the reduction of risk to others to be the most important measure of treatment outcome, validly assessing this is complex. Frequency of re-offending is a comparatively easily measured statistic, although subject to recording and judicial variation over time,

---

Box 13.2 Outcome domains for personality disorder

- Symptomatic change
- Service usage and costs
- Social and interpersonal functioning, including harm to self
- Quality of life
- Incidents of societal conflict (e.g., contact with the police) and harm to others
- Reports from informants

---

which reduces its reliability. Rates of risk to others may be distorted by a range of factors, such as the long-term detention of high-risk patients and the non-detection of more competent offenders. Re-offending rates also do not address symptomatic or attitudinal personality change, which are equally important in relation to risk. Many measures of prosocial attitudes carry obvious social desirability, which may affect the validity of ratings, as will the context in which a rating is carried out.

Treatment options

Our interpretation of the treatment literature is subject to some degree of selection bias: one of us (A. B.) is interested in dynamic psychotherapy for the treatment of personality disorder and the other (P. T.) in the role of other approaches, particularly nidotherapy (Tyrer, 2009; see also Chapter 20, this volume). We will not discuss specific treatments for cluster A or cluster C disorders, because there is a lack of suitable evidence. We also will not discuss the treatment of antisocial personality disorder in detail, since this is considered in Chapter 3.

Many people with personality disorders have conditions with which they themselves are comfortable (i.e. that are ego-syntonic) and have no wish to change. However, there is considerable variation between personality disorders in this regard. Individuals who are unwilling to have treatment can be described as Type R (treatment-resisting), as opposed to Type S (treatment-seeking). Most of those with paranoid, antisocial and schizoid personality disorders come into the Type R category, whereas those with borderline, anxious and dependent personality disorders are more often Type S (Tyrer *et al*, 2003*a*). In addition, it is not known to what extent ongoing motivation for treatment engagement is a manifestation of dependency needs (e.g. dependent personality traits), or disengagement a manifestation of lack of responsiveness of service providers to a patient's idiosyncratic needs (e.g. in antisocial personality disorder). This classification is therefore of questionable utility and it is not necessarily lifelong. However, the distinction reminds clinicians to assess motivation to change and explains why most people who have a personality disorder (three out of four) do not attend for treatment as they are in the Type R group.

Meta-analyses of psychological treatments

There have been a number of meta-analyses of the effectiveness of dynamic psychotherapy and cognitive–behavioural therapy (CBT) in the treatment of personality disorders. In the earliest of these, Perry and colleagues (1999) found that all 15 studies of psychological treatments for personality disorders demonstrated improvement. The mean pre–post effect sizes within treatments were large: 1.11 for self-report measures and 1.29 for observational measures. In the three randomised controlled trials (RCTs), self-report measures showed that active psychotherapy was more effective than no treatment. In four studies, a mean of 52% of patients remaining in therapy recovered (defined as no longer meeting the full criteria for personality disorder) after a mean of 1.3 years of treatment. The authors concluded that psychotherapy was effective for personality disorders and calculated that it might give a significantly (up to a sevenfold) faster rate of recovery compared with the natural course of the disorders. But the paucity of randomised trials was notable.

A few years later things had improved, albeit by not much. Leichsenring & Leibing (2003) were able to include 14 studies of dynamic psychotherapy and 11 studies of CBT, although not all followed a randomised controlled design and meta-analysis should not normally be used with heterogeneous studies. In addition, the psychodynamic studies had a mean follow-up period of 1.5 years, compared with only 13 weeks for the CBT. Dynamic psychotherapy yielded a large overall effect size of 1.46, with effect sizes of 1.08 for self-report measures and 1.79 for observer-rated measures. The corresponding values for CBT were 1.00, 1.20 and 0.87.

The National Institute for Health and Clinical Excellence (NICE) also carried out meta-analyses of a wide range of studies of treatments for antisocial and borderline personality disorders, in preparation for their corresponding clinical guidelines (National Collaborating Centre for Mental Health, 2009a,b). The guideline development groups were unable to make a specific treatment recommendation for either disorder, concluding that the research literature was not extensive enough to allow firm conclusions to be reached from meta-analysis. Despite this, the two published guidelines do offer advice on the psychological treatment of both borderline personality disorder and antisocial personality disorder, together with areas for future research.

Psychological treatments

Dynamic psychotherapy (mainly individual)

Dynamic psychotherapy has long been recommended as a treatment for personality disorder. Most of the therapeutic interest in psychotherapy in this area has been for its use in borderline personality disorder (Higgitt & Fonagy, 1992).

There have been few published randomised trials of dynamic psychotherapy for personality disorders. Winston et al (1991) found no difference between short-term dynamic psychotherapy and brief adaptational psychotherapy, although both were superior to a waiting-list control. This study specifically excluded patients with borderline and narcissistic features, although a later study including some with cluster B disorders produced similar results (Winston et al, 1994). The most recent support for a psychoanalytically based approach has come from adaptations of dynamic therapy – mentalisation-based treatment and transference-focused psychotherapy.

In mentalisation-based treatment (MBT), interventions are organised to increase the reflective or mentalising capacity of the patient in the context of group and individual therapy. Mentalisation entails making sense of one's own actions and those of others on the basis of intentional mental states such as desires, feelings and beliefs. This capacity is enfeebled in people with borderline personality disorder, who are specifically prone to lose their ability to mentalise in interpersonal situations when they are anxious. So therapy actively focuses on developing their ability to maintain their understanding and recognition of the feelings they evoke in others and the feelings that others evoke in them during interpersonal interaction.

An initial randomised study comparing the effectiveness of a modified psychoanalytically oriented partial hospitalisation programme, later to be manualised as MBT in a partial hospital context, with standard psychiatric care for patients with borderline personality disorder (Bateman & Fonagy, 1999, 2001) suggested that MBT was superior to standard care. On all outcome measures there was significantly greater improvement in those allocated to psychotherapy. The improvement in symptoms and function were delayed by several months, but were greatest by the end of treatment at 18 months. In a follow-up study (Bateman & Fonagy, 2001), gains were maintained after a further 18 months, indicating that rehabilitative effects were stimulated during the treatment phase,. The treatment has also been found to be cost-effective (Bateman & Fonagy, 2003) but as yet its active components remain unclear, especially because it was not possible to show that mentalisation had increased in those patients who showed the most gains. A further follow-up of patients 8 years after the point of randomisation showed that differences between the two groups remained on a number of measures (Bateman & Fonagy, 2008).

A larger RCT, involving 134 patients randomised to out-patient MBT, demonstrated that this treatment was superior to structured clinical management on a number of measures (Bateman & Fonagy, 2009). Importantly, substantial improvements were observed in both treatment groups across all outcome variables, although patients randomly assigned to MBT showed a steeper decline in both self-reported and clinically significant problems, including suicide attempts and hospital admissions. Overall, the data suggest that structured treatments improve outcomes for individuals with borderline personality disorder, but a focus on specific psychological processes brings additional benefits to structured clinical support. Mentalisation-based treatment is relatively undemanding in terms of training, so it may be useful for implementation in general mental health services. Further evaluations by independent research groups are required. Promising data have recently become available on the effectiveness of a similar programme established in The Netherlands (Bales, 2012).

The other manualised dynamic therapy, transference-focused psycho-therapy (TFP), gives promising results in borderline personality disorder. In an RCT comparing TFP, dialectical behaviour therapy (DBT) and supportive psychotherapy (Clarkin *et al*, 2007), all three treatment groups showed significant positive change in depression, anxiety, global functioning and social adjustment over 1 year of treatment. Both TFP and DBT were significantly associated with improvement in suicidality. Only TFP and supportive psychotherapy were associated with improvement in anger. The authors concluded that people with borderline personality disorder respond to structured treatments in an out-patient setting with change in multiple domains of outcome. Transference-focused psychotherapy was associated with change in more domains than the other two treatments. Future research is needed to examine the specific mechanisms of change in these treatments beyond common structures, although some work has been done on this (Levy *et al*, 2006). Costs have not yet been examined.

A further study has compared TFP with a cognitive/dynamic therapy known as schema-focused psychotherapy (SFP) (Gieson-Bloo *et al*, 2006). Treatment was given over a period of 3 years to 88 individuals with borderline personality disorder. In an intent-to-treat analysis, patients who received TFP showed significantly less improvement than those who received schema-focused therapy over the 3 years, and TFP was more expensive. Both groups showed improvement, but changes in the group treated with SFP were greater and more prolonged than in the group treated with TFP. Economic analysis (Van Asselt *et al*, 2007) of the trial suggested that SFP was less costly than TFP.

The results of Gieson-Bloo *et al*'s study should be interpreted with caution. First, differences in outcome between the groups can be accounted for almost entirely by the higher drop-out early in treatment of patients in the TFP group: the study may really be about early management of borderline personality disorder. Differences in outcome disappear when 'completers' from each group are compared, and a more recent randomised trial showed that TFP was superior to community-based psychotherapy for borderline personality disorder (Doering *et al*, 2010). If there is indeed a higher drop-out rate during TFP, it is not a trivial finding. Engaging people with borderline personality disorder in long-term treatment is important. To further our understanding of the psychodynamic treatment of patients with this disorder, it would be helpful to know why more dropped out at an early stage from TFP than from SFP in the Gieson-Bloo *et al* study. Second, follow-up is required to determine whether treatment gains and group differences are maintained. Third, the results of such a long treatment need consideration in the context of follow-on research which suggests that over the same period around 40% of patients would have been expected to have improved (Zanarini *et al*, 2003). The question is why gains in treatment were not as large as expected in either or both treatments. Possible negative interaction between therapy and naturalistic outcome has been discussed by Fonagy & Bateman (2006). It remains possible that SFP simply had lesser iatrogenic effects than TFP. Schema-focused psychotherapy has not yet been compared with treatment as usual (TAU). Fourth, the SFP/TFP study (Gieson-Bloo *et al*, 2006) raises the issue of the transportability of a treatment (TFP) from a US home to a European context. Therapies in one cultural setting may need careful modification for another setting. Dialectical behaviour therapy, for example, seemingly transports to inner-city London only with considerable difficulty. When comparing therapies developed away from where they are trialled, therapists must be matched carefully for training, levels of training must be clarified, the previous experience of the therapists must be matched, and therapies must be appropriately modified for their new cultural and service context.

In a related RCT in which personality status was not recorded, although personality disorder is likely to have been present in a significant number of participants, Guthrie *et al* (2001) found that home-based dynamic/interpersonal psychotherapy was effective in reducing repetition of self-harm after 6 months.

Group psychotherapy

Non-controlled studies with day hospital stabilisation followed by out-patient dynamic group therapy indicate the utility of therapeutic groups in borderline personality disorder (Wilberg *et al*, 1998). Day hospital stabilisation included social interaction and milieu activities such as lunch together, cooking as a group and community support activities. In contrast, Marziali & Monroe-Blum (1995) found equivalent results in RCTS between group and individual therapy, concluding that on cost-effectiveness grounds group therapy is the treatment of choice. But further studies are needed to confirm their findings, especially since the treatment offered was less structured than most of the treatments discussed here and drop-out rates were high. There are no other studies of group psychotherapy as a specific treatment for personality disorder.

A review (Blackmore *et al*, 2009) found five RCTs of group psychotherapy, mostly using a mix of therapeutic techniques for a range of psychiatric disorders. The pattern of results in the studies suggested some effectiveness of group therapy for a range of clinical problems, but no evidence that benefits were specific to dynamic group psychotherapy or any other approach or that group therapy alone was particularly helpful in personality disorder. Nevertheless, there rightly remains considerable interest in group therapy as a useful and cost-effective intervention for patients with complex problems.

Cognitive analytic therapy

Cognitive analytic therapy (CAT) has been manualised for the treatment of borderline personality disorder and many are enthusiastic about its effectiveness. Initial indications that the method may be of help for some patients with the disorder (Ryle & Golynkina, 2000) led to a formal RCT involving adolescents (Chanen *et al*, 2008). Cognitive analytic therapy and good clinical care were compared in out-patients aged 15–18 years who fulfilled between two and nine of the DSM–IV criteria for borderline personality disorder. Of the 86 individuals initially randomised, 78 (CAT, $n = 41$; good clinical care, $n = 37$) were traced at follow-up. There was no significant difference between the outcomes of the treatment groups at 24 months on the pre-chosen measures but there was some evidence that patients allocated to CAT improved more rapidly. No adverse effect was shown with either treatment. The authors concluded that both interventions are effective in reducing externalising psychopathology in teenagers with subsyndromal or full-syndrome bipolar personality disorder but that larger studies are required to determine the specific value of CAT.

Cognitive analytic therapy is discussed in greater detail in Chapter 18.

Cognitive therapy

In cognitive therapy for personality disorders much greater emphasis is placed on changing core beliefs than dysfunctional thoughts and on maintaining a collaborative therapeutic alliance. Crisis intervention strategies are developed, training in self-help and self-monitoring skills is provided, and schema-focused conceptualisation is linked to behaviours (such as self-harm) that interfere with therapy.

Davidson & Tyrer (1996), in an open study, used cognitive therapy to treat two cluster B personality disorders: the antisocial and borderline types. Using single-case methodology, they evaluated a brief (10-session) cognitive therapy and reported improvement in target problems. Another small ($n = 34$) RCT has recently been carried out using brief cognitive therapy, linked to a manual incorporating elements of DBT, in the treatment of recurrent self-harm in those with cluster B personality difficulties and disorders (Evans *et al*, 1999). Self-harm repeaters with a parasuicide attempt in the preceding 12 months were randomly allocated to manual-assisted cognitive–behavioural therapy (MACT) or TAU. The rate of suicidal acts was lower with MACT and self-rated depressive symptoms also improved. Participants receiving MACT had a mean of 2.7 sessions, and the average cost of their care was 46% lower than for TAU.

These results led to a much larger study that we believe comes closest to the model of effectiveness and generalisability. This was an extension of the MACT study described above (Evans *et al*, 1999) with up to 7 sessions of treatment offered to those with recurrent self-harm, 42% of whom had a personality disorder. It differed from other studies in being larger ($n = 480$), being multicentered (five centres in Scotland and England), using ordinary therapists (trained in the approach) in the course of their normal work, and offering no special service for those in the trial. In particular, those who did not attend appointments were not visited at home, as this was not part of normal practice. The results were, in general, negative in terms of efficacy compared with treatment as usual (which included psychotherapy and problem-solving therapy). Only 60% of patients attended for face-to-face sessions of MACT. For the primary outcome (i.e., the proportion of patients who repeated self-harm after treatment), 39% of those allocated to MACT repeated compared with 46% allocated to TAU. Seven participants died by suicide, five of whom were in the TAU groups (Tyrer *et al*, 2003*b*). Frequency of self-harming behaviour was reduced by 50% in the MACT groups compared with TAU, but there was great variation in episodes of self-harm (Tyrer *et al*, 2004). There was no significant between-group difference in any of the secondary outcomes. However, analysis of taped interviews from the study revealed important differences between some of these outcomes in the MACT groups. These were associated with the competence of the therapists delivering MACT (Davidson *et al*, 2004). At 6 months, MACT had cost an average of £900 per patient less than TAU, but the cost saving did not remain significant at 12 months (Byford *et al*, 2003). Interestingly, in borderline personality disorder, MACT increased total costs and had less satisfactory results in reducing self-harm, in contrast to its lower cost and greater effect in other personality disorders (Tyrer *et al*, 2004).

More recent randomised trials have provided further data suggesting the utility of CBT in borderline personality disorder. In an RCT in which 104 individuals with the disorder received up to 30 sessions from therapists trained in advance, there was significant benefit on suicidal behaviour but a non-significant increase in emergency presentations in those allocated to CBT (Davidson *et al*, 2006*a,b*). The mean number of suicide attempts over the 2-year period of the study was lower for CBT than for TAU. Across both treatment arms there was gradual and sustained improvement in both primary and secondary outcomes, but the CBT arm used less resources, although no significant cost-effectiveness advantage was demonstrated. Those who received CBT carried out significantly fewer suicidal acts over the 2 years. They also reported fewer dysfunctional beliefs and had lower state anxiety scores and positive symptom distress.

The same research group used CBT to treat antisocial personality disorder (Davidson *et al*, 2008). Fifty-two men with a diagnosis of antisocial personality disorder, with acts of aggression in the 6 months prior to the study, were randomised to either TAU plus CBT to TAU alone. At 12-month follow-up, both groups reported a decrease in the occurrence of acts of verbal or physical aggression. Trends in the data in favour of CBT were noted for problematic drinking, social functioning and beliefs about others. But overall, CBT did not improve outcomes more than usual treatment.

There is an interesting contrast of extremes in terms of the duration and outcomes of treatments focusing on a cognitive therapeutic approach. While schema-focused therapy appears to be an effective long-term treatment (over 3 years), even the 30-session version of MACT is limited in its effectiveness. Both cognitive approaches are, however, promising and may occupy different niches in personality disorder services. The overall evidence in favour of CBT in treatment of personality disorder is relatively slim, with much of it coming from one research group.

Cognitive therapy is further discussed in Chapter 14.

Mixed therapeutic approaches

Black & Blum (2004) report on the development of 'systems training for emotional predictability and problem-solving' (STEPPS). This is a 20-week manualised programme that deploys psychoeducation, behavioural management and a focus on maladaptive schemas in a systemic context (including both professional and family carers). It is a group treatment offered as an adjunct to other treatment, rather than a sole intervention in its own right. Individuals enrolled in the STEPPS programme are encouraged to continue their usual care, including individual psychotherapy, medication and case management. All patients are required to designate a primary mental health professional who provides care on an ongoing basis and who can be reached in the event of a crisis.

In an RCT, 124 people with borderline personality disorder were randomly assigned to STEPPS plus TAU or TAU alone (Blum *et al*, 2008). Total score on the Zanarini Rating Scale for Borderline Personality Disorder was the primary outcome measure. Secondary outcomes included: measures of global functioning, depression, impulsivity and social functioning; suicide attempts and self-harm acts; and use of crisis services. Participants were followed up 1 year post-treatment. Those who had received STEPPS plus TAU showed greater improvement in the Zanarini scale total score and subscales assessing affective, cognitive, interpersonal and impulsive domains. STEPPS plus TAU also led to greater improvements in impulsivity, negative affect, mood and global functioning. These differences yielded moderate to large effect sizes. There were no differences between groups for suicide attempts, self-harm acts or hospital admissions. The study needs to be interpreted with caution because the discontinuation rate was high in both groups.

Dialectical behaviour therapy

Dialectical behaviour therapy (DBT) is a special adaptation of behaviour therapy. It was originally used to treat a group of repeatedly parasuicidal women with borderline personality disorder, where it led to a marked reduction in the frequency of self-harm episodes compared with TAU (Linehan *et al*, 1991). Although DBT reduces episodes of self-harm initially, it is less effective in the longer term. The therapy is manualised (Linehan, 1993) and it includes techniques at the level of behaviour (functional analysis), cognitions (e.g., skills training) and support (empathy, teaching management of trauma). The initial aim of DBT is to control self-harm, but its long-term purpose is to promote change in the emotion dysregulation that is judged to be at the core of borderline personality disorder (Robins, 2003), and this goes far beyond self-harm reduction.

The original trial of DBT (Linehan *et al*, 1991) involved 44 women who met DSM-III-R criteria for borderline personality disorder and had made at least two suicide attempts in the previous 5 years, with one in the preceding

8 weeks. Half of the group were assigned to DBT and the other half to the control condition (TAU in the community). Assessment was carried out during and at the end of therapy, and again after 1 year (Linehan *et al*, 1993). Individuals in the control group were significantly more likely to have made suicide attempts, spent significantly longer as in-patients over the year of treatment and were significantly more likely to have droped out of the therapies to which they were assigned. Follow-up was naturalistic, based on the proposition that the morbidity of the disorder being treated precluded termination of therapy at the end of the experimental period. At 6-month follow-up, those allocated to DBT continued to show less parasuicidal behaviour than controls, though at 1 year there were no between-group differences. At 1 year, individuals in the treatment group had had fewer days in hospital, but at the 6-month assessment there were no between-group differences on this measure. The authors concluded that DBT for 1 year, compared with TAU, led to a reduction in the number and severity of suicide attempts and decreased the frequency and length of in-patient admission. However, there were no between-group differences on measures of depression, hopelessness or reasons for living.

The widespread adoption of DBT for borderline personality disorder is a tribute to both the effectiveness of the treatment and its acceptability to patients and families. Turner (2000) observed a decrease in parasuicidal acts and self-harm at 6 and 12 months in 12 patients treated with DBT compared with 12 treated with client-centred therapy. Koons *et al* (2000) compared DBT with out-patient TAU in 28 participants and found a decrease in frequency of parasuicidal acts and self-injury at 3 and 6 months. Bohus *et al* (2004) explored an in-patient adaptation of DBT and found significant reduction in self-harm but a higher drop-out rate. Linehan and colleagues' replication of their original study with very similar findings gives further support to its effectiveness (Linehan *et al*, 2006). In this replication, TAU was performed by therapists chosen for their expertise in non-behavioural psychotherapies. Despite this, the results duplicate quite closely those of the 1991 study: the 52 patients randomised to DBT showed better outcomes in terms of suicide attempts and self-harm than the 49 randomised to treatment by the experts in other psychotherapies. It should be noted that the drop-out rate was only 30% in the DBT group but over 70% in the comparison group. However, the study compared a cohesive group of practitioners of DBT working as a team with a disparate group of therapists operating a variety of therapeutic models, most of whom were working independently. Thus, the comparison is not just between DBT and other approaches, but also between a team-based treatment approach and one using individual therapy provided by independent practitioners working alone.

With two notable exceptions, most studies of DBT have arisen from the original proponents of the treatment. The first independent randomised trial provided some support for the original Linehan *et al* study. Verheul and colleagues (2003) randomly allocated 58 Dutch women who met DSM-IV criteria for borderline personality disorder to 1 year of DBT or TAU, i.e., ongoing treatment in the community. Participants had been referred from addiction treatment or psychiatric services because the therapist and/ or patient felt that treatment was not working. Those not randomised to DBT were referred back to their original therapist, potentially creating a comparison group of disgruntled patients and therapists. Efficacy was measured in terms of treatment retention and course of high-risk suicidal, self-mutilating and otherwise self-damaging behaviours. Dialectical behaviour therapy resulted in better retention rates and significantly greater reductions of self-mutilating behaviours and self-damaging impulsive acts than TAU, especially among those with histories of frequent self-mutilation. The study suggests that DBT is superior to TAU in reducing self-harm in patients with borderline personality disorder; *post hoc* analyses suggested that those with more severe self-harming behaviour were helped most. This study was conducted in the Dutch healthcare system and it remains uncertain how well the treatment translates to different healthcare systems. Other studies have shown DBT to be no better than other active treatments such as the 12-step programme for opioid dependence (Linehan *et al*, 2002) or TAU in a UK context (Feigenbaum *et al*, 2011). Trials of DBT for people with borderline personality disorder and comorbid substance dependence continue to be undertaken.

A more recent study of DBT conducted independently of the developers of the treatment has produced interesting results. McMain and colleagues (2009) randomised 180 people with borderline personality disorder who had engaged in suicidal or non-suicidal self-harm in the previous 5 years to 1 year of DBT or general psychiatric management. At the end of the treatment period, both groups showed improvement on the majority of clinical outcome measures, including significant reductions in the frequency and severity of suicidal and non-suicidal episodes of self-harm. Both groups had a reduction in general healthcare utilisation, including emergency visits and psychiatric hospital days, as well as significant improvements in symptoms of borderline personality disorder, symptom distress, depression, anger and interpersonal functioning. No significant differences across any outcomes were found between groups.

Owing to its severity, symptomatology and high rates of co-occurring disorders, borderline personality disorder obviously affects family members, and interventions addressing their needs have been developed using the framework of DBT (Hoffmann *et al*, 2005). In a replication study of a 12-week community-based family education programme, Family Connections, 50 participants were assessed pre-, post-programme and at 6-month follow-up (Hoffman *et al*, 2005). Participating family members showed significant improvements on all well-being variables: burden, grief and empowerment, including a reduction in level of depression. Although psychoeducation and DBT-based techniques appear to reduce family stress, and interventions such as Family Connections show promise, the long-term effect of family interventions on patients' well-being remains to be demonstrated.

Returning to the effects of DBT on the symptoms of borderline personality disorder, research has yet to clarify what the active elements of DBT might be: individual psychotherapy, skills training, telephone consultation, therapist consultation team (Neacsiu *et al*, 2010). From the data of the McMain study discussed above (McMain *et al*, 2009) it would seem that change could still be due to non-specific factors related to the structure of treatment. Nevertheless, two studies have investigated the process of change by focusing on the possible influence of validation (Shearin & Linehan, 1992; Linehan *et al*, 2002) but their results are inconclusive.

What we know thus far is that adding a DBT skills training group to ongoing out-patient individual psychotherapies not using the DBT model does not seem to enhance treatment outcomes in borderline personality disorder. Given that DBT is described as primarily a skills training approach (Koerner & Linehan, 1992), this finding might indicate that its central skills training component may not be of primary importance. But individual DBT focuses on the strengthening of skills learned in the skills groups, and trying to combine a skills training group with an individual therapy that ignores or pays minimal attention to skills strengthening may invalidate what the patient has been taught in terms of utilising learned skills in an attempt to cope with everyday functioning. Some disagree with the policy of not admitting patients to hospital, except for a bare minimum period, since some studies show that the time and structure of an in-patient setting can be used to apparently good effect (Bohus *et al*, 2004).

Although there has been considerable interest in the use of DBT with other personality disorders in clusters A and C, as well as antisocial personality disorder, there is no current evidence that it is helpful in these groups.

For further discussion of DBT see Chapter 14.

Therapeutic community treatments

A therapeutic community may be defined as an intensive form of treatment in which the environmental setting (namely, a highly structured programme including group activities and interpersonal reflection) becomes the core therapeutic intervention. By a repeated process of group discussion, behaviour can be challenged and modified, and interpersonal understanding enhanced. The community process promotes democratic group living in a supportive but boundaried environment in which emotional issues are discussed openly and in which members use close adult relationships to learn from each other. Therapeutic communities have been set up worldwide; in Europe, they are found mainly in the UK, Holland, Germany and Greece.

The early therapeutic communities admitted people with a range of psychological and psychiatric disorders, and were not specifically for personality disorder. Later therapeutic communities focused on people with particular problems, such as addiction or criminal behaviour. Within the criminal justice systems of various countries, therapeutic communities have been set up to address violent offending behaviours (e.g. HM Prison Grendon in England and the van der Hoeven Clinic in Holland). Current therapeutic community services focus on personality disorder, and select and accept community members with all types of personality disorder (Davies *et al*, 1999).

Although therapeutic communities have been in existence for over 50 years, they have only recently been subjected to any type of systematic and controlled evaluation. The structure and content of therapeutic programmes are varied, and patient groups are largely self-selected, which makes comparison data difficult to interpret. Nevertheless, there is some consensus that outcomes are favourable for individuals who attend and complete the programme, and gains are maintained at follow-up (Dolan *et al*, 1997; Lees *et al*, 1999; Warren *et al*, 2004).

A systematic review of the literature and meta-analysis (Lees *et al*, 1999, 2004) concluded that therapeutic communities (particularly the so-called concept communities in the USA) were effective for those who attended them. However, positive effects were found primarily in secure treatment programmes for substance misusers, where there was a considerable degree of coercion and no emphasis was placed on the treatment of personality disorder. Even though the data so far meet level 1 criteria for National Health Service evidence (that is, a systematic review or meta-analysis of all relevant RCTs that show positive change; Howick *et al*, 2011), it is still not clear what therapeutic factors might be effective in therapeutic communities.

The systematic review of the efficacy of therapeutic communities carried out by NICE in its preparation of treatment guidelines for borderline personality disorder (National Collaborating Centre for Mental Health, 2009*b*) found 19 papers published in peer-reviewed journals between 1989 and 2007. Much of the work arose from the Henderson Hospital (now closed) and the Cassel Hospital, two residential therapeutic communities in the UK. The more common version in Europe is the democratic therapeutic community and no randomised trials have been carried out in this type of community. However, Dolan *et al* (1997) at the Henderson Hospital, which used a democratic therapeutic community approach, in a creative attempt to find an appropriate control group, used a non-admitted comparison sample to assess the effectiveness of treatment on core symptoms. Of the 137 patients in their study, 70 were admitted and 67 not admitted (for clinical or financial reasons). This is not a strict comparison group as less than 1 in 7 of those considered for the Henderson Hospital complete treatment (Rutter & Tyrer, 2003). There was significantly greater improvement in core features of personality disorder on the Borderline Syndrome Index in the admitted group than in the non-admitted group. Further work has suggested that therapeutic community treatment may show cost savings over treatment in general psychiatric services, primarily because of reducing the need for hospital admission (Davies *et al*, 1999).

Warren *et al* (2004) followed 135 patients referred to the Henderson Hospital between 1990 and 1994, 74 of whom were admitted. They measured a range of items indicating impulsivity 1 year after discharge for the admitted group and 1 year after assessment for the non-admitted group. Impulsivity had decreased significantly more in the admitted group, primarily on the variable of hitting others.

Three psychodynamically oriented treatment models delivered by the Cassel Hospital for a mixed group of personality disorders have been assessed for relative effectiveness:

(a) long-term residential treatment using a therapeutic community approach;
(b) briefer in-patient treatment followed by community-based dynamic psychotherapy (a step-down programme);
(c) general community psychiatric care.

Initial results suggested that the brief in-patient therapeutic community treatment followed by out-patient dynamic psychotherapy is more effective than both long-term residential therapeutic community treatment and general psychiatric care in the community on most measures, including self-harm, attempted suicide and readmission rates to general psychiatric admission wards; it is also more cost-effective (Chiesa *et al*, 2002). Follow-up at 36 months confirmed that patients in the step-down programme continued to show significantly greater improvement than the in-patient group on social adjustment and global assessment of mental health. In addition, they were found to self-mutilate, attempt suicide and be readmitted significantly less at 24- and 36-month follow-up (Chiesa & Fonagy, 2003). However, the study was not a randomised trial and the groups were not strictly comparable. Further follow-up at 72 months after intake indicated that patients treated in the step-down programme continued to show significantly greater improvement than those in long-term residential treatment or in community psychiatric care (Chiesa *et al*, 2006).

A further study of 73 patients admitted to the Cassel Hospital examined predictive factors of positive outcome (Chiesa & Fonagy, 2007). Among participants with cluster B personality disorders, younger age, higher general functioning at admission, longer duration of treatment, absence of self-harm, and having an avoidant personality disorder predicted better outcomes.

It has been hypothesised that extended hospital admission may engender pathological dependency and regression (Linehan, 1987). In a prospective study of 216 individuals with severe personality disorder treated at the Menninger Clinic for variable lengths of time in two psychoanalytically oriented in-patient units, researchers found positive change at discharge and 1-year follow-up, with no evidence of deleterious effects due to regression or dependency (Gabbard *et al*, 2000). Nevertheless, Main's (1957) classic paper should act as a reminder that regression and countertransference may pose considerable difficulties, mainly in the form of professional boundary violations, for teams treating patients intensively.

Other therapies that emphasise altering the environment to make a better fit to the patient include nidotherapy (see Chapter 20, this volume). Given the increasing range of treatments available for personality disorder, therapeutic communities need to come into the frame of comparison studies and further research should be undertaken (Haigh, 2002). There have been recent attempts to standardise and systematise therapeutic community programmes and structures through a standards-based quality network called the Community of Communities (Royal College of Psychiatrists, 2012). Such structuring may make research into the effectiveness of therapeutic communities easier. Advocates and researchers will need to work together to develop acceptable experimental designs so that therapeutic communities can be seriously evaluated alongside other treatments. A key methodological difficulty is that voluntariness may be a key factor in effectiveness, i.e. therapeutic communities are effective for those people with personality disorder who can engage with them. Another is that therapeutic communities may select services users with only mild to moderate disorders, who would respond to any intervention.

Therapeutic communities are discussed further in Chapter 19.

Conclusion

Despite our somewhat cautionary views, it is important to note that for the first time in the history of personality disorder, the condition is now regarded as potentially treatable. A number of treatments have been shown to be reasonably effective, particularly in borderline personality disorder, but how they effect change remains unknown. In particular, it is not clear whether any particular specific intervention is essential to improvement.

The research seems to indicate that sustained and consistent emphasis on a patient's way of thinking and/or behaving is therapeutic, irrespective of the specific theoretical model being followed. Hence, when specific treatments such as dialectical behaviour therapy, mentalisation-based treatment or transference-focused psychotherapy are compared with well-structured and thoughtful generic alternatives, the differences that emerge in outcomes are relatively small. Perhaps practitioners who treat patients with personality disorders need a primary theoretical model onto which they consistently map clinical and interactional data. Without this, therapy is in danger of becoming incoherent and therapists responsive rather than proactive, two features that are likely to make patients with personality disorders worse. It seems that a specific focus using a coherent theoretical model is the first step to improving outcomes for this disadvantaged group of patients.

References

Bales, D. (2012) Mentalization based treatment for borderline personality disorder: a Dutch replication study of MBT in a partial hospital setting. *Journal of Personality Disorders*, in press.

Bateman, A. & Fonagy, P. (1999) The effectiveness of partial hospitalization in the treatment of borderline personality disorder – a randomised controlled trial. *American Journal of Psychiatry*, **156**, 1563–1569.

Bateman, A. & Fonagy, P. (2000) Effectiveness of psychotherapeutic treatment of personality disorder. *British Journal of Psychiatry*, **177**, 138–143.

Bateman, A. & Fonagy, P. (2001) Treatment of borderline personality disorder with psychoanalytically oriented partial hospitalisation: an 18-month follow-up. *American Journal of Psychiatry*, **158**, 36–42.

Bateman, A. & Fonagy, P. (2003) Health service utilisation costs for borderline personality disorder patients treated with psychoanalytically oriented partial hospitalisation versus general psychiatric care. *American Journal of Psychiatry*, **160**, 169–171.

Bateman, A, & Fonagy, P. (2008) 8-year follow-up of patients treated for borderline personality disorder: mentalization-based treatment versus treatment as usual. *American Journal of Psychiatry*, **165**, 631–638.

Bateman, A. & Fonagy, P. (2009) Randomized controlled trial of outpatient mentalization-based treatment versus structured clinical management for borderline personality disorder. *American Journal of Psychiatry*, **166**, 1355–1364.

Black, D. W. & Blum, N. (2004) The STEPPS group treatment program for outpatients with borderline personality disorder. *Journal of Contemporary Psychotherapy*, **34**, 193–210.

Blackmore, C., Beecroft, C., Parry, G., *et al* (2009) *A Systematic Review of the Efficacy and Clinical Effectiveness of Group Analysis and Analytic/Dynamic Group Psychotherapy*. Centre for Psychological Services Research, School of Health and Related Research, University of Sheffield, UK (http://groupanalyticsociety.co.uk/wp-content/uploads/file/IGA_GAS_FINAL_REPORT.pdf).

Blum, N., St John, D., Pfohl, B., *et al* (2008) Systems Training for Emotional Predictability and Problem Solving (STEPPS) for outpatients with borderline personality disorder: a randomized controlled trial and 1-year follow-up. *American Journal of Psychiatry*, **165**, 468–478.

Bohus, M., Haaf, B., Simms, T., *et al* (2004) Effectiveness of inpatient dialectical behavioural therapy for borderline personality disorder: a controlled trial. *Behaviour Research and Therapy*, **42**, 487–499.

Byford, S., Knapp, M., Greenshields, J., *et al* (2003) Cost-effectiveness of brief cognitive behaviour therapy versus treatment as usual in recurrent deliberate self-harm: a decision-making approach. *Psychological Medicine*, **33**, 977–986.

Campbell, M., Fitzpatrick, R., Haines, A., *et al* (2000) A framework for the design and evaluation of complex interventions to improve health. *BMJ*, **321**, 694–696.

Chanen, A. M., Jackson, H. J., McCutcheon, L. K., *et al* (2008) Early intervention for adolescents with borderline personality disorder using cognitive analytic therapy: randomised controlled trial. *British Journal of Psychiatry*, **193**, 477–484.

Chiesa, M. & Fonagy, P. (2003) Psychosocial treatment for severe personality disorder: 36-month follow-up. *British Journal of Psychiatry*, **183**, 356–362.

Chiesa, M. & Fonagy, P. (2007) Prediction of medium-term outcome in Cluster B personality disorder following residential and outpatient psychosocial treatment. *Psychotherapy and Psychosomatics*, **76**, 347–353.

Chiesa, M., Fonagy, P., Holmes, J., *et al* (2002) Health Service use costs by personality disorder following specialist and non-specialist treatment: a comparative study. *Journal of Personality Disorders*, **16**, 160–173.

Chiesa, M., Fonagy, P. & Holmes, J. (2006) Six-year follow-up of three treatment programs to personality disorder. *Journal of Personality Disorders*, **20**, 493–509.

Clark, L. A., Vittengl, J., Kraft, D., *et al* (2003) Separating personality traits from states to predict depression. *Journal of Personality Disorders*, **17**, 152–172.

Clarkin, J. F., Levy, K. N., Lenzenweger, M. F., *et al* (2007) Evaluating three treatments for borderline personality disorder. *American Journal of Psychiatry*, **164**, 922–928.

Davidson, K. & Tyrer, P. (1996) Cognitive therapy for antisocial and borderline personality disorders: single case study series. *British Journal of Clinical Psychology*, **35**, 413–429.

Davidson, K., Scott, J., Schmidt, U., *et al* (2004) Therapist competence and clinical outcome in the prevention of parasuicide by manual assisted cognitive behaviour therapy trial: the POPMACT study. *Psychological Medicine*, **34**, 855–863.

Davidson, K., Norrie, J., Tyrer, P., *et al* (2006*a*) The effectiveness of cognitive behavior therapy for borderline personality disorder: results from the borderline personality disorder study of cognitive therapy (BOSCOT) trial. *Journal of Personality Disorders*, **20**, 450–465.

Davidson, K., Tyrer, P., Gumley, A., *et al* (2006*b*) A randomized controlled trial of cognitive behavior therapy for borderline personality disorder: rationale for trial, method, and description of sample. *Journal of Personality Disorders*, **20**, 431–449.

Davidson, K. M., Tyrer, P., Tata, P., *et al* (2008) Cognitive behaviour therapy for violent men with antisocial personality disorder in the community: an exploratory randomized controlled trial. *Psychological Medicine*, **39**, 569–577.

Davies, S., Campling, P. & Ryan, K. (1999) Therapeutic community provision at regional and district levels. *Psychiatric Bulletin*, **23**, 79–83.

Doering, S., Hörz, S., Rentrop, M., *et al* (2010) Transference-focused psychotherapy *v.* treatment by community psychotherapists for borderline personality disorder: randomised controlled trial. *British Journal of Psychiatry*, **196**, 389–395.

Dolan, B., Warren, F. & Norton, K. (1997) Change in borderline symptoms one year after therapeutic community treatment for severe personality disorder. *British Journal of Psychiatry*, **171**, 274–279.

Endicott, J., Spitzer, R. L., Fleiss, J. L., *et al* (1976) The Global Assessment Scale: a procedure for measuring overall severity of psychiatric disturbance. *Archives of General Psychiatry*, **33**, 766–771.

Evans, K., Tyrer, P., Catalan, J., *et al* (1999) Manual-assisted cognitive-behaviour therapy (MACT): a randomized controlled trial of a brief intervention with bibliotherapy in the treatment of recurrent deliberate self-harm. *Psychological Medicine*, **29**, 19–25.

Feigenbaum, J. D., Fonagy, P., Pilling, S., *et al* (2011) A real-world study of the effectiveness of DBT in the UK National Health Service. *British Journal of Clinical Psychology*, doi: 10.1111/j.2044-8260.2011.02017.x.

Fonagy, P. & Bateman, A. (2006) Progress in the treatment of borderline personality disorder. *British Journal of Psychiatry*, **188**, 1–3.

Gabbard, G., Coyne, L., Allen, J., *et al* (2000) Evaluation of intensive in-patient treatment of patients with severe personality disorders. *Psychiatric Services*, **51**, 893–898.

Gieson-Bloo, J., van Dyck, R., Spinhoven, P., *et al* (2006) Outpatient psychotherapy for borderline personality disorder: randomized trial of schema-focused therapy vs transference-focused therapy. *Archives of General Psychiatry*, **63**, 649–658.

Guthrie, E., Kapur, N., Mackway-Jones, K., *et al* (2001) Randomised controlled trial of brief psychological intervention after deliberate self-poisoning. *BMJ*, **323**, 135–137.

Haigh, R. (2002) Therapeutic community research: past, present and future. *Psychiatric Bulletin*, **26**, 65–68.

Higgitt, A. & Fonagy, P. (1992) Psychotherapy in borderline and narcissistic personality disorder. *British Journal of Psychiatry*, **161**, 23–24.

Hoffmann, P., Fruzzetti, A., Buteau, E., *et al* (2005) Family Connections: a program for relatives of persons with borderline personaltiy disorder. *Family Process*, **44**, 217–225.

Howick, J., Chalmers, I., Glasziou, P., *et al* (2011) The 2011 Oxford CEBM Levels of Evidence: Introduction. Oxford Centre for Evidence-Based Medicine (http://www.cebm.net/index.aspx?o=5653).

Koerner, K. & Linehan, M. M. (1992) Integrative therapy for borderline personality disorder: dialectical behaviour therapy. In *Handbook of Psychotherapy Integration* (ed J. C. G. Norcross): pp. 433–459. Basic Books.

Koons, C., Robins, C. & Tweed, J. (2000) Efficacy of dialectical behavior therapy in women veterans with borderline personality disorder. *Behavior Therapy*, **32**, 371–390.

Lees, J., Manning, N. & Rawlings, B. (1999) *Therapeutic Community Effectiveness: A Systematic International Review of Therapeutic Community Treatment for People with Personality Disorders and Mentally Disordered Offenders (Centre for Reviews and Dissemination Report 17).* University of York.

Lees, J., Manning, N. & Rawlings, B. (2004) A culture of enquiry: research evidence and the therapeuti community. *Psychiatric Quarterly*, **75**, 279–294.

Leichsenring, F. & Leibing, E. (2003) The effectiveness of psychodynamic therapy and cognitive behavior therapy in the treatment of personality disorders: a meta-analysis. *American Journal of Psychiatry*, **160**, 1223–1232.

Levy, K. N., Meehan, K. B., Kelly, K. M., *et al* (2006) Change in attachment patterns and reflective function in a randomized control trial of transference-focused psychotherapy for borderline personality disorder. *Journal of Consulting and Clinical Psychology*, **74**, 1027–1040.

Linehan, M. M. (1987) Dialectical behavioural therapy: a cognitive behavioural approach to parasuicide. *Journal of Personality Disorders*, **1**, 328–333.

Linehan, M. M. (1993) *The Skills Training Manual for Treating Borderline Personality Disorder.* Guilford Press.

Linehan, M. M., Armstrong, H., Suarez, A., *et al* (1991) Cognitive–behavioural treatment of chronically parasuicidal borderline patients. *Archives of General Psychiatry*, **48**, 1060–1064.

Linehan, M. M., Heard, H. L. & Armstrong, H. E. (1993) Naturalistic follow-up of a behavioral treatment for chronically parasuicidal borderline patients. *Archives of General Psychiatry*, **50**, 971–974.

Linehan, M., Dimeff, L., Reynolds, S., *et al* (2002) Dialectical behavior therapy versus comprehensive validation therapy plus 12-step for the treatment of opioid dependent women meeting criteria for borderline personality disorder. *Drug and Alcohol Dependence*, **67**, 13–26.

Linehan, M. M., Comtois, K. A., Murray, A. M., *et al* (2006) Two-year randomized controlled trial and follow-up of dialectical behavior therapy vs therapy by experts for suicidal behaviors and borderline personality disorder. *Archives of General Psychiatry*, **63**, 757–766.

Main, T. (1957) The ailment. *British Journal of Medical Psychology*, **30**, 129–145.

Marziali, E. & Monroe-Blum, H. (1995) An interpersonal approach to group psychotherapy with borderline personality disorder. *Journal of Personality Disorders*, **9**, 179–189.

McMain, S., Links, P., Gnam, W., *et al* (2009) A randomized controlled trial of dialectical behaviour therapy versus general psychiatric management for borderline personality disorder. *American Journal of Psychiatry*, **166**, 1365–1374.

National Collaborating Centre for Mental Health (2009*a*) *Antisocial Personality Disorder: Treatment, Management and Prevention (NICE Clinical Guideline 77).* National Institute for Health and Clinical Excellence.

National Collaborating Centre for Mental Health (2009*b*) *Borderline Personality Disorder: Treatment and Management (NICE Clinical Guideline 78).* National Institute for Health and Clinical Excellence.

Neacsiu, A. D., Rizvi, S. L. & Linehan, M. M. (2010) Dialectical behaviour therapy skills use as a mediator and outcome of treatment for borderline personality disorder. *Behaviour Research and Therapy*, **48**, 832–839.

Perry, J. C., Banon, E. & Ianni, F. (1999) Effectiveness of psychotherapy for personality disorder. *American Journal of Psychiatry*, **156**, 1312–1321.

Robins, C. (2003) Dialectical behavior therapy for borderline personality disorder. *Psychiatric Annals*, **32**, 608–616.

Royal College of Psychiatrists (2012) What is the Community of Communities? Royal College of Psychiatrists (http://www.rcpsych.ac.uk/quality/qualityandaccreditation/therapeuticcommunities/communityofcommunities1.aspx).

Rutter, D. & Tyrer, P. (2003) The value of therapeutic communities in the treatment of personality disorder: a suitable place for treatment? *Journal of Psychiatric Practice*, **9**, 291–302.

Ryle, A. & Golynkina, K. (2000) Effectiveness of time-limited cognitive analytic therapy of borderline personality disorder: factors associated with outcome. *British Journal of Medical Psychology*, **73**, 197–210.

Schwarz, D. & Lellouch, J. (1967) Explanatory and pragmatic attitudes in therapeutic trials. *Journal of Chronic Diseases*, **20**, 637–648.

Shearin, E. & Linehan, M. M. (1992) Patient–therapist ratings and relationship to progress in dialectical behaviour therapy for borderline personality disorder. *Behaviour Therapy*, **23**, 730–741.

Turner, R. (2000) Naturalistic evaluation of dialectical behaviour therapy-orientated treatment for borderline personality disorder. *Cognitive and Behavioural Practice*, **7**, 413–419.

Tyrer, P (2009) *Nidotherapy: Harmonising the Environment with the Patient*. RCPsych Press.

Tyrer, P., Gunderson, J., Lyons, M., *et al* (1997) Extent of comorbidity between mental state and personality disorders. *Journal of Personality Disorders*, **11**, 242–259.

Tyrer, P., Mitchard, S. & Methuen, C. (2003*a*) Treatment-rejecting and treatment-seeking personality disorders: Type R and Type S. *Journal of Personality Disorders*, **17**, 265–270.

Tyrer, P., Jones, V. & Thompson, S. (2003*b*) Service variation in baseline variables and prediction of risk in a randomised controlled trial of psychological treatment in repeated parasuicide: the POPMACT study. *International Journal of Social Psychiatry*, **49**, 58–69.

Tyrer, P., Tom, B., Byford, S., *et al* (2004) Differential effects of manual assisted cognitive behaviour therapy in the treatment of recurrent deliberate self-harm and personality disturbance: the POPMACT study. *Journal of Personality Disorders*, **18**, 102–116.

Van Asselt, A. D. I., Dirkson, C. D. & Arntz, A. (2007) The cost of borderline personality disorder: societal cost of illness in BPD-patients. *European Psychiatry*, **22**, 354–361.

Verheul, R., Van Den Bosch, L. M., Koeter, M. W., *et al* (2003) Dialectical behaviour therapy for women with borderline personality disorder: 12-month, randomised clinical trial in The Netherlands. *British Journal of Psychiatry*, **182**, 135–140.

Warren, F., Evans, C. & Dolan, B. (2004) Impulsivity and self-damaging behaviour in severe personality disorder: the impact of democratic community treatment. *Therapeutic Communites*, **25**, 55–71.

Wilberg, T., Friis, S., Karterud, S., *et al* (1998) Outpatient group psychotherapy: a valuable continuation treatment for patients with borderline personality disorder treated in a day hospital? A 3-year follow-up study. *Nordic Journal of Psychiatry*, **52**, 213–222.

Winston, A., Pollack, J., McCullough, L., *et al* (1991) Brief psychotherapy of personality disorders. *Journal of Nervous and Mental Disease*, **179**, 188–193.

Winston, A., Laikin, M., Pollack, J., *et al* (1994) Short-term dynamic psychotherapy of personality disorders. *American Journal of Psychiatry*, **15**, 190–194.

Zanarini, M. C., Frankenburg, F. R., Hennen, J., *et al* (2003) The longitudinal course of borderline psychopathology: 6-year prospective follow-up of the phenomenology of borderline personality disorder. *American Journal of Psychiatry*, **160**, 274–283.

CHAPTER 14

Skills-based therapies for personality disorder

Sue Evershed

Summary   Over recent years, a variety of therapies have been developed or adapted to treat personality disorder. This chapter reviews skills-based (as opposed to insight-based) treatments. Two approaches are outlined: cognitive–behavioural therapy and dialectical behaviour therapy. The chapter details the underpinning theory and models of personality disorder used by the two approaches, and describes how the therapy is applied. Evidence of therapeutic efficacy is presented, with information about accessing training and therapy materials.

Until recently, many practitioners regarded personality disorder as untreatable. Although initially seeming to be suitable for therapy, patients with personality disorder were often difficult to engage, attended therapy sporadically, and their self-damaging and violent behaviours interrupted treatment (Warren & Dolan, 1996). Many failed to improve with treatment, often engendering anger and hopelessness in therapists (Gunderson, 1984). Some clinicians thought not only that patients failed to respond to treatment, but that their problems were amplified by their involvement in therapy, simply because of the fundamental characteristics of their disorder (Harris *et al*, 1994; Reiss *et al*, 1996). As a consequence of such opinions, patients with personality disorder were commonly considered to be 'abusers' of mental health services (Warren & Dolan, 1996) and personality disorder became a 'diagnosis of exclusion' from services (National Institute for Mental Health in England, 2003).

Certainly, personality disorder was associated with longer, more costly treatment and higher attrition rates (Goldstein *et al*, 1998; Blackburn, 2000) and several studies indicated that its presence predicted poorer treatment outcome (Diguer *et al*, 1993; Hoglend, 1993; Reich & Vasile, 1993). However, this research mostly derived from studies examining standard treatments for emotional disorders, rather than treatments specifically designed for personality disorder. It could be argued that this is akin to offering aspirin to a person with a broken leg: the treatment addresses only one symptom rather than tackling the core problem.

Over the past 15 years, several new treatments have been designed to address personality disorder. There is a growing body of evidence suggesting that patients with personality disorder can respond to therapy. This is especially true for borderline personality disorder (Linehan *et al*, 1991; Shea, 1993; Davidson & Tyrer, 1996; Wilberg *et al*, 1999; Bateman & Fonagy, 2000; Ryle & Golynkina, 2000; Verheul *et al*, 2003; Fonagy & Bateman, 2006). Some treatments are beginning to show promise with other types of personality disorder, such as antisocial personality disorder, although more research is required to build a useful evidence base (Davidson, 2008; Duggan *et al*, 2008; Frisman *et al*, 2009). Overviews of treatments are now more positive about the possibility of treating personality disorders (Perry *et al*, 1999; Leichsenring & Leibing, 2003; see also Chapter 13, this volume).

These newer treatments range across the whole spectrum of theoretical models. Treatment approaches might be divided broadly into two subsets, on the basis of their conceptualisation and the process of therapeutic change: those that focus on the building of new skills and those that focus on the development of insight. (Of course, this is an artificial divide since most treatments incorporate the development of both skills and insight.) In this chapter, I will focus on therapies that use a skills-development approach. The goal of skills-based therapy is to increase the range of effective coping strategies to help patients identify and manage their cognitive, emotional and behavioural responses to events. Treatment aims to extinguish maladaptive thoughts and behaviours, and build new skills to help patients modulate underlying feelings and express them in a more adaptive manner. In particular, I will discuss cognitive approaches such as those proposed by Beck *et al* (2003) and Davidson (2007), which are based primarily on cognitive–behavioural therapy (CBT), and the more behaviourally oriented dialectical behaviour therapy (DBT; Linehan, 1993*a*).

Cognitive–behavioural therapy

A number of different cognitive and cognitive–behavioural therapies for the treatment of personality disorder have been developed in recent years. Although there are some conceptual differences between them, the various approaches have much in common and all have their roots in the early cognitive therapies. To minimise confusion, CBT here refers to the full range of cognitive and cognitive–behavioural approaches.

Cognitive–behavioural therapy was first developed more than two decades ago for the treatment of depression and other emotional disorders (Ellis, 1962; Beck, 1967). In its early years, CBT was largely insight-oriented, primarily using introspective techniques to effect change. However, Beck, Ellis and others began to incorporate a range of behavioural techniques to strengthen its effect on dysfunctional controlling belief systems (schemas). Over time, the model has been applied to the treatment of a variety of clinical disorders, including personality disorder. In the case of personality disorders, CBT therapists place a greater emphasis on developmental issues, the therapist–patient relationship and the need for a longer treatment.

Cognitive–behavioural therapy concentrates on problem behaviours rather than the criteria identifying personality disorders. In CBT, personality disorders are simply seen as patterns of dysfunctional beliefs and behaviours that are rigid, overgeneralised, compelling (hard to resist) and resistant to change. These beliefs and behaviours arise as a result of the operation of certain schemas or controlling beliefs that produce consistently biased judgements in the way individuals view the world, and that lead to a tendency to make cognitive errors in certain types of situations. Each type of personality disorder is characterised by a distinct cognitive profile (a mixture of beliefs, attitudes and affect organised around a broad overview of the nature of the self and the world).

Cognitive–behavioural therapy uses a biosocial model hypothesising that the origin of personality disorder lies in the interaction of the infant's inherent temperament and emotional experience of its caregivers. It takes an evolutionary perspective, suggesting that personality traits are 'strategies' favoured by natural selection that have evolved as a result of their ability to sustain life and promote reproduction. However, our environment has changed over time and although some strategies may still be functional, others may be a 'poor fit' with our current context. Cognitive–behavioural therapists see the strategies that are either underdeveloped or over-developed and those that are a poor fit as constituting personality disorder.

Environmental influences also play a part in the development of personality disorder by increasing or decreasing the expression of these innate tendencies. When repeatedly reinforced in childhood, the tendencies can lead to specific belief systems (schemas). Once a core schema is established, individuals will selectively attend to confirming evidence and will block any disconfirming evidence. Thus, core schemas will be continuously reinforced, becoming progressively more rigid and pervasive.

What happens in therapy?

Using structured, problem-focused individual (one-to-one) treatment, CBT aims to temper the cognitive profile and so modify dysfunctional emotional and social responses to events. The goal is not to replace the dysfunctional schemas, but to modify existing beliefs and develop new ones, providing the patient with more effective strategies for coping with problematic situations (Box 14.1).

One of the cardinal principles in CBT is the formation of a therapeutic alliance with the patient. This is done to keep the patient motivated and engaged throughout therapy, by instilling a sense of trust and collaboration. The process begins at the start of therapy through a collaborative formulation of the patient's problems. The formulation is a working hypothesis which links the long-standing problematic behaviours and interpersonal problems seen in personality disorder to a number of likely underlying core beliefs

---

Box 14.1 Key features of cognitive–behavioural therapy

Cognitive techniques are used to:
- identify and evaluate dysfunctional thoughts
- uncover core schema/beliefs
- restructure, modify and/or reinterpret core schema/beliefs

Behavioural techniques are used to:
- address self-defeating behaviours
- teach new adaptive skills
- promote skills rehearsal and generalisation by means of behavioural assignments

Imagery is used to help restructure past experiences

---

that have arisen as a result of childhood experiences. The formulation also assists in determining which strategies are likely to be the most effective in bringing about change.

Cognitive techniques

Cognitive techniques and strategies are used to alter maladaptive core beliefs about the self and the world. Various techniques are employed to help patients recognise maladaptive patterns of thinking and interpretation. The aim is to help them identify and evaluate dysfunctional automatic thoughts and to elicit the ultimate meaning of events: to uncover the core schema at work.

Once the core schemas are accessible, there are three key ways to confront them. Schema restructuring helps patients to transform a maladaptive schema to an adaptive one. Schema modification does not produce new adaptive schemas, but modifies dysfunctional schemas and so reduces their impact and their effect on patients' responses. Finally, schema reinterpretation makes minor changes to existing schema, helping patients to reinterpret them and adapt their lifestyles to manage dysfunctionality.

Behavioural techniques

Behavioural strategies are used to promote a reduction in self-harm and other maladaptive behaviours, as well as to help the patient develop better ways of coping with their difficulties. The goals of behavioural techniques are threefold. The therapist may need to address patients' self-defeating behaviours. They may also need to teach/coach patients in new adaptive skills. Finally, behavioural assignments can be used as homework to help test out dysfunctional or newer adaptive cognitions. Common behavioural techniques employed include activity monitoring and scheduling, skills training (including behavioural rehearsal, relaxation training and social skills training) and exposure techniques for anxiety-based difficulties.

Other techniques

Imagery techniques to enable the patient to 'relive' past traumatic events are also used. These help patients to restructure experiences and consequently modify associated attitudes and beliefs.

Length of treatment

Cognitive–behavioural approaches to personality disorder are less intensive in terms of time than most insight-based treatments or dialectical behaviour therapy, often lasting about 12 months, and thus are economical to implement (Byford *et al*, 2003).

Who does CBT work for?

Two randomised controlled trials have demonstrated that CBT is an effective treatment for patients with avoidant and cluster B personality disorder (Evans *et al*, 1999; Emmelkamp *et al*, 2006). Other trials have shown similar indications of promise in the treatment of borderline and mixed personality disorders but methodological difficulties and small treatment samples limit the validity of their findings (Tyrer *et al*, 2003; Davidson *et al*, 2006; Weinberg *et al*, 2006).

The results of a pilot trial suggest that CBT may also be a promising treatment for men with antisocial personality disorder, reducing some aspects of maladaptive functioning associated with the disorder (Davidson *et al*, 2009). However, more research needs to be undertaken to examine the value of CBT approaches with the different personality disorder types.

Training and implementation

Training is not yet available for CBT with personality disorder, but several training routes provide expertise in generic CBT. All doctoral clinical psychology courses in the UK now teach CBT methodology, so that clinical psychologists have a grounding in CBT techniques. Further training in CBT to certificate (10 days) and diploma level (18 days) is available from a variety of academic institutions, all of which are listed on the British Association for Behavioural and Cognitive Psychotherapies (BABCP) website (www.babcp.com). The BABCP has also published guidelines regarding the requisite training needed for a core professional to become an accredited CBT practitioner. This includes the completion of an accredited diploma-level course and a number of hours of supervised practice. Practitioners can continue their training to become eligible to supervise and train others.

Dialectical behaviour therapy

Developed in the USA by Marsha Linehan (1993*a,b*), dialectical behaviour therapy (DBT) was designed for women in the community who self-harm. It is a long-term, structured, cognitive–behavioural treatment intended to address the difficulties of borderline personality disorder.

Dialectical behaviour therapy is based on a biosocial theory of personality disorder in which biological factors and social learning interact reciprocally to bring about a dysfunction in the emotion regulation system. Biologically, patients are emotionally vulnerable. They are born with an autonomic nervous system that reacts excessively to relatively low levels of stress and takes longer than normal to return to baseline. Borderline personality disorder develops when such a child is brought up within an 'invalidating' environment, where the child's significant others negate and/or respond erratically (through denial, failure to respond or abuse) to the child's experiences and responses. This lack of consistent acknowledgement of emotions prevents the child from learning to understand their feelings, and promotes distrust in their own responses.

Dialectical behaviour therapy is based on cognitive–behavioural principles but instead of focusing merely on changing the patient, DBT also includes acceptance strategies, often referred to as validation techniques. These are intended to communicate to the patient that they are acceptable as they are and that many of their thoughts, feelings and behaviours, however dysfunctional, make sense in some way.

The balance between acceptance and change strategies in DBT forms the fundamental 'dialectic' from which DBT derives its name. The dialectical method described in Buddhist philosophy is a means of seeking truth through the integration or synthesis of contradictory facts. Thus in DBT, therapists attempt to balance the requirement to accept patients for themselves, while recognising the need for them to change.

In describing the characteristics of borderline personality disorder, Linehan refers to a set of 'dialectical dilemmas'. These dilemmas are experienced by patients as dimensions of response to stressful events. Since each pole on a dimension is experienced as distressing, patients oscillate between opposing poles. This helps to explain the emotional lability and rapid changes in opinion and perspective often observed in such individuals. The goal of therapy is to reduce this oscillation and help the patient manage their responses to events in a more integrated and adaptive way.

In terms of treatment, Linehan (1993a,b) focuses on personality disorder largely from a behavioural perspective: as a pattern of maladaptive behaviours. If the behaviours and underlying cognitions and emotions cease, so too does the diagnosis:

> 'In a nutshell, DBT is very simple. The therapist [...] blocks or extinguishes bad behaviors, drags good behaviors out of the patient, and figures out a way to make the good behaviors so reinforcing that the patient continues the good ones and stops the bad ones' (Linehan, 1993a: p. 97).

What happens in therapy?

Dialectical behaviour therapy integrates individual psychotherapy with concurrent skills training and skills generalisation strategies, usually through telephone consultation. Thus, patients are expected to attend

239

Box 14.2   Key features of dialectical behaviour therapy

Individual therapy
- Acceptance strategies (validation)
- Change strategies, including:
  - identification of a hierarchy of treatment targets
  - progress review on a daily diary card
  - behavioural chain analysis for each difficulty encountered
  - solution analysis to find more effective strategies

Group work
- Training new adaptive skills for:
  - interpersonal effectiveness
  - emotion regulation
  - distress tolerance
  - core mindfulness

Telephone consultation
- *'In vivo'* skills coaching to promote skills rehearsal and generalisation

---

one individual session, and one 2-hour group skills session every week (Box 14.2). In addition, they are encouraged to use a telephone consultation system, which allows them to access immediate (so-called *in vivo*) skills coaching when they are in crisis.

Individual therapy

Treatment begins with a motivational approach within individual therapy. In this phase, the therapist must gain the patient's commitment to the therapy and the therapeutic procedures (individual and group work, and skills coaching). This commitment includes an agreement to work on identified treatment targets. Patients are given a diary card listing their personal treatment targets on one side and the skills they will be learning on the other. Patients complete the diary every day, charting their progress on targets and listing the skills they have practised. The diary forms the basis of the individual sessions, with the therapist identifying the most serious problems encountered during the week to use as the focus for the session.

Treatment targets are organised into hierarchical stages and, with few exceptions, addressed in strict order. This organisation prevents therapists from being distracted into addressing the crisis of the moment. Individual therapy focuses initially on 'first-stage targets' of decreasing suicidal and life-threatening behaviour and reducing 'therapy-interfering behaviours' (particularly non-adherence and premature withdrawal from therapy). Put simply, this means that DBT's first set of targets ensure that the patient remains alive and in treatment. Behaviours that have a detrimental effect on quality of life form the remainder of the first-stage treatment targets.

Second- and third-stage targets include longer-term aspirations such as decreasing post-traumatic stress, increasing self-respect and achieving individual life goals.

Individual DBT uses a number of therapeutic strategies, but central to the treatment is the use of problem-solving strategies to elicit change. This entails the application of a behavioural chain analysis to each identified difficulty to determine what the problem is, what is causing it, what is interfering with its resolution and what aids are available to help solve it. A behavioural chain analysis is a detailed outline of the events and situational factors leading up to and following a particular problem. The analysis pays close attention to the reciprocal interaction between the environment and the patient's cognitive, emotional and behavioural responses.

Having determined the exact nature of the problem, a solution analysis (to identify alternative behavioural solutions) is undertaken to help the patient find more effective coping strategies. The patient is then instructed and coached in the new strategies. Behavioural chain analyses will indicate skills deficits, problematic reinforcement contingencies, inhibitions resulting from fear and guilt, and faulty beliefs and assumptions. Thus, the instructional/coaching phase integrates skills training, contingency management, exposure strategies and cognitive modification.

Dialectical behaviour therapy is unusual because it pays as much attention to helping patients understand and accept themselves and their situation as it does to helping them to change. Therefore, the use of problem-solving strategies is balanced by the use of validation strategies. There are two types of validation. In the first type the therapist highlights the wisdom in the patient's emotional, cognitive and behavioural responses. The second type of validation centres on the therapist's belief in the patient's ability to rebuild a life worth living, and building on the patient's strengths rather than weaknesses.

Essentially, individual therapy tailors the skills taught to the specific needs of the patient and assists in their application and generalisation to the patient's everyday life. However, it also provides the patient with a therapeutic attachment from which they can learn about attachments and relationships generally. For Linehan, the therapeutic alliance is the 'vehicle through which therapy occurs' as well as the therapy itself. A strong therapeutic relationship is also seen as essential because the relationship with the therapist is often the key reinforcer for the patient striving to change their behaviour: 'If all else fails, the strength of the relationship will keep a patient alive during a crisis' (Linehan, 1993a).

Group work

The group work component of DBT is the key method of increasing adaptive behavioural skills. Skills training comprises four modules, covering interpersonal effectiveness, emotion regulation, distress tolerance and core mindfulness.

Interpersonal effectiveness largely focuses on assertiveness skills. Patients are helped to understand their needs in relationships and to develop healthy and effective ways of dealing with others to get their needs met. This involves respecting themselves and others, communicating effectively, learning to say no, and repairing relationships. Skills in emotion regulation increase the individual's understanding of emotions. The group provides basic education about the nature and function of emotions, and how to not be overwhelmed by them. The module helps patients survive difficult times by teaching them to manage their lives even when they are feeling highly emotional. Patients are trained to soothe themselves in healthy ways and to manage their reactions to stressful events. Skills in core mindfulness are contemplative practices that originate in Zen Buddhism. The skills help patients control their concentration by directing attention on only one thing: the moment they are living in. Patients thus learn to control their minds, rather than letting their minds control them.

Telephone consultation

Unusually, patients in DBT are instructed to telephone their therapists for skills coaching if, outside of scheduled therapy time, they have urges to hurt themselves. The therapist does not undertake a full individual therapy session but simply talks the patient through the problem situation and coaches alternatives strategies to self-harm or suicidal behaviours. In this way, skills are strengthened and generalised and the patient is kept safe.

Length of treatment

Dialectical behaviour therapy is a long-term intervention (1–2 years or more). The group work component takes about 12 months to complete but patients are often recommended to repeat all or part of the programme. Individual therapy takes place before and during the skills component and often lasts long after the skills training has finished: until the diary card reflects an increased ability to manage the prescribed targets over a sustained period (3–6 months).

Who does DBT work for?

Two randomised controlled trials involving parasuicidal women with borderline personality disorder living in the community found that DBT was more effective than treatment as usual. Over a 12-month period, partici-pants receiving DBT were less likely to drop out of therapy and engaged in fewer and less severe parasuicidal acts compared with the treatment-as-usual group. They also had fewer in-patient days, reported less anger, and had fewer and less severe psychiatric symptoms. These improvements continued during the 1-year follow-up (Linehan *et al*, 1991, 1993, 1994).

Various adaptations have been made to DBT to treat different patient populations: adolescents, in-patients, British and Dutch patients, women with substance dependency, female war veterans, male and female forensic patients and women with eating disorders (Barley *et al*, 1993; Springer *et al*, 1996; Miller *et al*, 1997; Linehan *et al*, 1999; Swales *et al*, 2000; Koons *et al*, 2001; Low *et al*, 2001; Telch *et al*, 2001; Evershed *et al*, 2003; Verheul *et al*, 2003). Generally, results have been encouraging and support the value of DBT in treating people with borderline personality disorder.

Training and implementation

Two-week DBT intensive training courses enable teams to develop competence in this approach. Training can be undertaken by individuals but this is on the assumption that no therapist would attempt to treat patients without support and supervision from a DBT consultation team. Trainers assume that attendees are experienced clinicians. For training to competency level, there is only one training provider in the UK. Information about courses can be found online (www.dbt.uk.net for courses in the UK and www.behavioraltech.com for courses in the USA). Shorter, awareness training courses can be accessed through alternative training providers.

Critique of skills-based therapies

Skills-based therapies aim to extinguish problematic thoughts and behaviours, and to provide patients with a toolkit of adaptive skills to moderate and manage previously difficult situations. Primarily, therefore, skills-based therapies tend to focus on observable or accessible thoughts and behaviours as treatment targets and as outcome measures. These therapies pay far less attention to causal mechanisms and processes. The underlying reasons for these thoughts, beliefs and behaviours are not seen as a key emphasis for treatment. Some writers have argued that this could result in superficial change only: a focus on symptoms as opposed to the fundamental disorder (Roth & Fonagy, 2005). It is essential therefore, that evaluations of skills-based therapies include a means of monitoring levels of patient distress or well-being as well as behaviour change.

Further problems with skills-based treatments relate to the therapeutic processes which rely heavily on the use of self-report and self-monitoring techniques (e.g. diaries). There is an assumption that patients are able to access cognitions and emotions with minimal training, and that they can make changes to cognitions and behaviours with relative ease (Young *et al*, 2003). Even if one rejects the existence of an 'unconscious', it is clear that people can be blind to their thoughts and feelings, and that many behaviours and cognitions in individuals with personality disorder will be distorted, rigid and intractable, almost by definition.

A key criticism of CBT approaches in particular is that they emphasise techniques at the expense of the therapeutic relationship. In their defence, CBT practitioners are sensitive to the need to build an effective relationship, if only because patients are unlikely to complete homework tasks unless they trust and respect the therapist (Dallos *et al*, 2006).

243

Finally, further research is required into the efficacy of CBT for personality disorder (Young *et al*, 2001). A recent meta-analysis for CBT with major psychiatric disorders (Lynch *et al*, 2010) was pessimistic about its effects on disorders other than mood disorders. However, a review of the evidence for CBT and related therapies (including DBT) by Epp & Dobson (2010) was not so negative regarding its efficacy with borderline personality disorder.

One criticism of DBT is that the very structure that helps therapists maintain focus on key treatment targets (and avoid the distraction of the 'unrelenting crises' common in personality disorder) could in itself cause problems. Rigid adherence to the hierarchy of treatment targets could result in patients feeling 'unvalidated' by apparently uncaring therapists. Worse, it could lead therapists to ignore very real and dangerous crises, leaving patients to fend for themselves. Proponents of DBT would argue that such crises are likely to be seen as 'therapy interfering'. As such, they would rise up the hierarchy, allowing therapists to focus on them as a first-stage target.

Of perhaps more concern is the notion that patients will only be accepted into DBT once they have made a commitment to the treatment targets. Many prospective patients may find the idea of renouncing self-harm as a coping strategy (however maladaptive) to be unacceptable and will be unable to commit. They may then be prevented access to treatment while still engaging in potentially dangerous behaviour.

Both DBT and CBT have a limited but growing evidence base for use with personality disorder, but this does not mean that they are problem-free. All therapies have their weaknesses, and these two are no exception.

References

Barley, W. D., Buie, S. E., Peterson, E. W., *et al* (1993) Development of an inpatient cognitive-behavioural treatment programme for borderline personality disorder. *Journal of Personality Disorders*, **7**, 232–240.

Bateman, A. W. & Fonagy, P. (2000) Effectiveness of psychotherapeutic treatment of personality disorder. *British Journal of Psychiatry*, **177**, 138–143.

Beck, A. T. (1967) *Depression: Clinical, Experimental and Theoretical Aspects*. Harper & Row.

Beck, A. T. , Freeman, A., Davis, D. D., *et al* (2003) *Cognitive Therapy of Personality Disorders* (2nd edn). Guilford Press.

Blackburn, R. (2000) Treatment or incapacitation? Implications of research on personality disorders for the management of dangerous offenders. *Legal & Criminological Psychology*, **5**, 1–21.

Byford, S., Knapp, M., Greenshields, J., *et al* (2003) Cost-effectiveness of brief cognitive behaviour therapy versus treatment as usual in recurrent deliberate self-harm: a rational decision making approach. *Psychological Medicine*, **33**, 977–986.

Dallos, R., Wright, J., Stedmon, J., *et al* (2006) Integrative formulation. In *Formulation in Psychology and Psychotherapy: Making Sense of People's Problems* (eds L. Johnstone & R. Dallos), pp. 154–181. Routledge.

Davidson, K. (2007) *Cognitive Therapy for Personality Disorders: A Guide for Clinicians* (2nd edn). Routledge.

Davidson, K. (2008) Cognitive–behavioural therapy for personality disorders. *Psychiatry*, **7**, 117–120.

Davidson, K. M. & Tyrer, P. (1996) Cognitive therapy for antisocial and borderline personality disorders: single case study series. *British Journal of Clinical Psychology*, **35**, 413–429.

Davidson, K. M., Norrie, J., Tyrer, P., et al (2006) The effectiveness of cognitive behavior therapy for borderline personality disorder: results from the borderline personality disorder study of cognitive therapy (BOSCOT) trial. *Journal of Personality Disorder*, **20**, 450–465.

Davidson, K. M., Tyrer, P., Tata, P., et al (2009) Cognitive behaviour therapy for violent men with antisocial personality disorder in the community: an exploratory randomized controlled trial. *Psychological Medicine*, **39**, 567–577.

Diguer, L., Barber, J. P. & Luborsky, L. (1993) Three concomitants: personality disorders, psychiatric severity, and outcome of dynamic psychotherapy of major depression. *American Journal of Psychiatry*, **150**, 1246–1248.

Duggan, C., Huband, N., Smailagic, N., et al (2008) The use of psychological treatments for people with personality disorder: a systematic review of randomized controlled trials. *Personality and Mental Health*, **1**, 95–125.

Ellis, A. (1962) *Reason and Emotion in Psychotherapy*. Lyle Stuart.

Emmelkamp, P. M. G., Benner, A., Kuipers, A., et al (2006) Comparison of brief dynamic and cognitive–behavioural therapies in avoidant personality disorder. *British Journal of Psychiatry*, **189**, 60–64.

Epp, A. M. & Dobson, K. S. (2010) Evidence base for cognitive–behavioral therapy. In *Handbook of Cognitive Behavioral Therapies* (3rd edn) (ed. K. S. Dobson), pp. 39–73. Guilford Press.

Evans, K., Tyrer, P., Catalan, J., et al (1999) Manual-assisted cognitive-behavioural therapy (MACT): a randomized controlled trial of a brief intervention with bibliotherapy in the treatment of recurrent deliberate self-harm. *Psychological Medicine*, **29**, 19–25.

Evershed, S., Tennant, A., Boomer, D., et al (2003) Practice-based outcomes of dialectical behaviour therapy (DBT) targeting anger and violence, with male forensic patients: a pragmatic and non-contemporaneous comparison. *Criminal Behaviour and Mental Health*, **13**, 198–213.

Fonagy, P. & Bateman, A. (2006) Progress in the treatment of borderline personality disorder. *British Journal of Psychiatry*, **188**, 1–3.

Frisman, L. K., Mueser, K. T., Covell, N. H., et al (2009) Use of integrated dual disorder treatment via assertive community treatment versus clinical case management for persons with co-occurring disorders and antisocial personality disorder. *Journal of Nervous and Mental Disease*, **197**, 822–828.

Goldstein, R. B., Powers, S. I., McCusker, J., et al (1998) Antisocial behavioral syndromes among residential drug abuse treatment clients. *Drug and Alcohol Dependence*, **49**, 202–216.

Gunderson, J. G. (1984) *Borderline Personality Disorder*. American Psychiatric Association.

Harris, G., Rice, M. & Courmier, C. (1994) Psychopaths: is a therapeutic community therapeutic? *International Journal of Therapeutic Communities*, **15**, 283–299.

Hoglend, P. (1993) Personality disorders and long-term outcome after brief dynamic psychotherapy. *Journal of Personality Disorders*, **7**, 168–181.

Koons, C. R., Robins, C. J., Tweed, J. L., et al (2001) Efficacy of dialectical behavior therapy in women veterans with borderline personality disorder. *Behavior Therapy*, **32**, 371–390.

Leichsenring, F. & Leibing, E. (2003) The effectiveness of psychodynamic therapy and cognitive behavior therapy in the treatment of personality disorders: a meta-analysis. *American Journal of Psychiatry*, **160**, 1223–1232.

Linehan, M. M. (1993a) *Cognitive-Behavioural Treatment of Borderline Personality Disorder*. Guilford Press.

Linehan, M. M. (1993b) *Skills Training Manual for Treating Borderline Personality Disorder*. Guilford Press.

Linehan, M. M., Armstrong, H. E., Suarez, A., et al (1991) Cognitive-behavioral treatment of chronically parasuicidal borderline patients. *Archives of General Psychiatry*, **48**, 1060–1064.

Linehan, M. M., Heard, H. L. & Armstrong, H. E. (1993) Naturalistic follow-up of a behavioural treatment of chronically parasuicidal borderline patients. *Archives of General Psychiatry*, **50**, 971–974.

Linehan, M. M., Tutek, D. A., Heard, H. L., et al (1994) Interpersonal outcome of cognitive-behavioural treatment for chronically suicidal borderline patients. *American Journal of Psychiatry*, **151**, 1771–1776.

Linehan, M. M., Schmidt, H., Dimeff, L. A., *et al* (1999) Dialectical behavior therapy for patients with borderline personality disorder and drug dependence. *American Journal on Addictions*, **8**, 279–292.

Low, G., Jones, D., Duggan, C., *et al* (2001) The treatment of deliberate self-harm in borderline personality disorder using dialectical behaviour therapy: a pilot study in a high security hospital. *Behavioural and Cognitive Psychotherapy*, **29**, 85–92.

Lynch, D., Laws, K. R. & McKenna, P. J. (2010) Cognitive behavioural therapy for major psychiatric disorder: does it really work? A meta-analytical review of well-controlled trials. *Psychological Medicine*, **40**, 9–24.

Miller, A. L., Rathus, J. H., Linehan, M. M., *et al* (1997) Dialectical behaviour therapy adapted for suicidal adolescents. *Journal of Practical Psychiatry and Behavioural Health*, **3**, 78–86.

National Institute for Mental Health in England (2003) *Personality Disorder: No Longer a Diagnosis of Exclusion. Policy Implementation Guidance for the Development of Services for People with Personality Disorder*. Department of Health.

Perry, J. C., Banon, E. & Ianni, F. (1999) Effectiveness of psychotherapy for personality disorders. *American Journal of Psychiatry*, **156**, 1312–1321.

Reich, J. H. & Vasile, R. G . (1993) Effect of personality disorder on the treatment outcome of Axis I conditions: an update. *Journal of Nervous and Mental Disease*, **181**, 475–484.

Reiss, D., Grubin, D. & Meux, C. (1996) Young 'psychopaths' in special hospital: treatment and outcome. *British Journal of Psychiatry*, **168**, 99–104.

Roth, A. & Fonagy, P. (2005) *What Works for Whom? A Critical Review of Psychotherapy Research* (2nd edn). Guilford Press.

Ryle, A. & Golynkina, K. (2000) Effectiveness of time limited cognitive analytic therapy of borderline personality disorder: factors associated with outcome. *British Journal of Medical Psychology*, **73**, 197–210.

Shea, M. T. (1993) Psychosocial treatment of personality disorders. *Journal of Personality Disorders*, **7** (suppl), 167–180.

Springer, T., Lohr, N. E., Burchel, H. A., *et al* (1996) A preliminary report of short-term cognitive-behavioural group therapy for inpatients with personality disorders. *Journal of Psychotherapy Practice and Research*, **5**, 57–71.

Swales, M., Heard, H. L. & Williams, M. G. (2000) Linehan's dialectical behaviour therapy (DBT) for borderline personality disorder: overview and adaptation. *Journal of Mental Health*, **9**, 7–23.

Telch, C. F., Agras, W. S. & Linehan, M. M. (2001) Dialectical behavior therapy for binge eating disorder. *Journal of Consulting and Clinical Psychology*, **69**, 1061–1065.

Tyrer, P., Thompson, S., Schmidt, U., *et al* (2003) Randomized controlled trial of brief cognitive behaviour therapy versus treatment as usual in recurrent deliberate self-harm: the POPMACT study. *Psychological Medicine*, **33**, 969–976.

Verheul, R., Van Den Bosch, L. M. C., Koeter, M. W. J., *et al* (2003) Dialectical behaviour therapy for women with borderline personality disorder: 12-month, randomised clinical trial in The Netherlands. *British Journal of Psychiatry*, **182**, 135–140.

Warren, F. & Dolan, B. (1996) Treating the 'untreatable': a therapeutic community is the personality disorder. *International Journal of Therapeutic Communities*, **17**, 205–215.

Weinberg, I., Gunderson, J. G., Hennen, J., *et al* (2006) Manual assisted cognitive treatment for deliberate self-harm in borderline personality disorder patients. *Journal of Personality Disorder*, **20**, 482–492.

Wilberg, T., Urnes, O., Friis, S., *et al* (1999) One year follow up of day treatment for poorly functioning patients with personality disorders. *Psychiatric Services*, **50**, 1326–1330.

Young, J. E., Weinberger, A. D. & Beck, A. T. (2001) Cognitive therapy for depression. In *Clinical Handbook of Psychological Disorders* (3rd edn) (ed. D. Barlow), pp. 264–308. Guilford Press.

Young, J. E., Klosko, J. S. & Weishaar, M. E. (2003) *Schema Therapy: A Practitioner's Guide*. Guilford Press.

CHAPTER 15

Insight-oriented therapies for personality disorder

Kerry Beckley and Neil Gordon

Summary This chapter gives a brief overview of the insight-oriented psychological therapies that are commonly used to treat personality disorder. The approaches that have been selected represent contemporary psychotherapy treatments with an emerging evidence base. Each approach is explored briefly with reference to the underlying theory, what happens in therapy and who might be helped by the approach. The training involved and the way the intervention is implemented are also be discussed.

Psychological therapies for personality disorder have two broadly different conceptualisations of the way in which change can occur: through the development of insight or through the learning of new skills. Most utilise both, but some have a particular emphasis on enhancing insight. The main goal of insight-oriented therapies is to increase the client's awareness of their inner experience (i.e. of core needs, emotional experiences, beliefs and value bases). The therapist helps the person to make sense of their current problems in the context of their past experiences through the use of techniques aimed at accessing or intensifying inner experience.

The insight-oriented therapies that we focus on in this chapter are: psychodynamic/psychoanalytical approaches such as transference-focused psychotherapy (Kernberg, 2004); attachment-based approaches such as mentalisation-based treatment (Bateman & Fonagy, 2004); schema therapy (Young, 1990); and cognitive analytic therapy (Ryle, 1990).

Psychodynamic/psychoanalytical approaches

Psychodynamic/psychoanalytical therapies have developed from the work of Freud and those described as the psychoanalytical 'deviationists' (Gelso & Hayes, 1998), including Adler, Jung, Sullivan and Fromm. Practitioners of these therapies tend to view psychological distress as being related to unconscious mental processes (Jacobs, 1998). Freud's psychoanalytical approach has been developed by others, some following his basic assumptions, others taking more independent paths. The term psychodynamic describes a wider perspective that encompasses the various analytical approaches. Jacobs suggests that psychodynamic refers to the way in which the psyche (mind/emotions/spirit/self) is seen as active and not static. This activity is not confined to our interactions with other people: it is also suggestive of internal mental processes as dynamic forces that influence our relations to others.

Explanatory metaphors

Different theorists have relied on a variety of terms or metaphors to explain these mental processes. Freud (1949) referred to the id, ego and super-ego. Jung (1957) described the shadow, anima and animus. Winnicott (1958) discussed the true self and false self. These terms were attempts to describe the nature of these inner processes. It is important to understand that these processes are not necessarily connected with feelings towards anyone else; nor do they rely on an external person for their promptings (Jacobs, 1998). These internal aspects of the psyche are seen as developing and forming throughout childhood as counterparts to the external relationships that predominate at that time (with mother and father or parent substitutes). These factors are characterised metaphorically as dynamic forces within the psyche. The child's psychological development is therefore influenced not only by the nature of early relationships with parents, but also by the way the child perceives and fantasises about these relationships. Psychological development is seen as a process whereby the child's fantasy world is gradually modified by the experience of wider reality. An important notion in this approach is that the images formed in the mind of the child are never really lost but become internalised 'objects' with a life of their own. This internal world is perceived as a dynamic force that can re-emerge into conscious awareness, particularly at times of stress (Jacobs, 1998).

Mitchell & Black's (1995) accessible and erudite historical account of the many therapeutic approaches that have emerged from Freud and his followers in different parts of the world shows how the American and European psychoanalysts have followed different theoretical trajectories, often related to cultural differences and discontent with existing orthodoxy. More recently, Watchel (2008) has written about the movement towards what he refers to as the 'relational model of psychoanalysis', showing how it adopts a 'two-person' psychology that challenges the limitations of more traditional 'one-person' approaches. He argues that earlier conceptual models tend to overstress internal structures of the personality at the expense of attending to current experiences and the relational context of therapy. For readers interested in exploring the different contributions of theoretical perspectives that come under the umbrella term psychoanalytical, we recommend a book by Fonagy & Target (2003), which offers a critical reflection on the complex relationship between practice and theory in this field.

What happens in therapy?

In general terms, a psychodynamic therapist sees therapy as helping someone to explore their relationships with others. This is achieved by enabling the client to become more aware of internalised aspects of their personality. Since much of this mental activity is unconscious (outside of the person's awareness), the aim of therapy is to bring internalised conflict into conscious awareness and thus enable the person to deal more effectively with the demands of external reality. In discussing the significance of relationships, the therapist considers with the client not only links between the client's external and internal worlds, but also links between the past and the present. Through these temporal links, they explore whether the client is handling current relationships in a way that is influenced by past 'experience', both real and imagined. The client is then helped to explore how their experience of the therapy relationship reflects their relationships outside of therapy, as relationships in both arenas are intimately linked to early relationships with significant others (Casement, 1985).

The transference relationship, transference-focused psychotherapy and borderline personality disorder

The therapist encourages the client to 'transfer' into the therapy relationship feelings they experience in relationships with others, so that the client can explore the ways in which past relationships are being used inappropriately in understanding the present. This 'unreal' (Gelso & Hayes, 1998), or transference, relationship is central to psychodynamic approaches. It is used by the therapist to help the client gain insight into current distortions in their relationships caused by internalised experience of which they are not aware (Malan, 1979). It is the exploration of and working through the transference relationship that is central in helping the client to change.

Transference-focused psychotherapy (TFP), developed by Otto Kernberg and his colleagues to treat borderline personality disorder, is an example of how early psychoanalytical ideas, in this instance, object relations, have been successfully assimilated into contemporary psychotherapeutic approaches focused on personality disorder (Foelsch & Kernberg, 1998). The client's internal world is conceptualised as being made up of multiple sets of relationship dyads, comprising self–other representations with associated affects (Clarkin et al, 2007). Such dyads inform how we make sense of social encounters. In borderline personality disorder, these dyads are thought to be more polarised, exaggerated and often to contradict one another, leading to the commonly experienced identity confusion described by people with the disorder. In interpersonal contexts, the fragmented sense of self in borderline personality disorder can result in confusion and misperceptions, often accompanied by overwhelming emotional dysregulation. These polarised representations can lead the person to behave in self-destructive and self-defeating ways during social encounters.

For example, an individual whose object-relational internal world is commonly built around a fear that they will be rejected and abandoned may act in extremely jealous, angry and destructive ways when their partner shows any interest in other people.

The aim in TFP is to establish a safe and stable therapy relationship that provides a 'frame' within which the patient can experience, observe and reflect on their representations of others. Using the relationship with the therapist allows the patient safe exploration of painful feelings, ultimately leading to modification and integration of the internal representational world. The intimacy and power differentials in the therapist–patient relationship encourage an expression of core internal object relations associated with borderline pathology. Change is seen as emerging from the therapist's capacity to reactivate distorted internal object relations and then contain and process the associated emotional arousal, thus encouraging the patient's capacity for reflective functioning.

It could be argued that the other approaches discussed in this chapter could be traced to analytical routes and therefore fit under the inclusive label of psychodynamic approaches. Indeed, there appears be a process of intellectual rapprochement taking place in the field of personality disorder. This is evidenced by the fact that contemporary terms such as mentalisation and reflective functioning (see below), with their roots in developmental psychology and attachment theory, are being increasingly accepted within different therapeutic traditions. Essentially, this seems to reflect a realisation that these conceptual frameworks are assisting practitioners to make sense of the origins and impact of the pervasive perceptual distortions and painful affective states that underpin psychopathology.

Who does it work for?

Psychodynamic and transference-focused approaches are seen as having particular relevance to people with borderline or narcissistic personality organisation (Yeomans *et al*, 2002; Kernberg, 2004; Clarkin *et al*, 2007). In particular, these approaches can work to resolve the externalisation of unbearable self states (Fonagy *et al*, 2002). In this context, this relates to the tendency for those with attacking internal worlds to do what Spillius (1992: p. 62) describes as 'evocatory projective identification', where internalised and distressing self-perceptions are managed by generating feelings within others. For example, the victims of maltreatment and abuse often have, as a result of their attachment trauma, internalised unbearable and malevolent states of mind. To manage the emotional distress associated with this hostile and persecutory affect, they externalise these difficult emotions, often leading them to experience others as persecutory and abusing.

Tracing presenting problems to early developmental experiences and establishing ways of working with disabling affect also enables these models to be used effectively with anxiety and panic states (Milrod *et al*,

2007). Levy and his colleagues have also explored the potential of TFP to change attachment patterns and increase reflective function (Levy *et al*, 2006). These studies indicate the potential for using these approaches with a wide range of mental health problems emerging from developmental trauma associated with insecure and ambivalent attachment experiences.

Training and implementation

General psychoanalytical training in the UK continues to be offered by a range of key institutes with long traditions and particular cultures. Anthropologist James Davies, in his exploration of the socialisation processes involved in becoming a psychoanalyst, gives a useful overview of the major training organisations in this country, including the original Institute of Psychoanalysis in London, founded by Sigmund Freud (Davies, 2009). Numerous less established organisations offer a variety of psychodynamically informed training programmes, most of which emphasise the importance of personal therapy/analysis and case supervision as the cornerstones of professional development.

The latest version of the treatment manual describing TFP for borderline personality disorder was published in 2006 (Clarkin *et al*, 2006). Kernberg and his colleagues in the Personality Disorders Institute at Cornell University offer a range of specialist trainings and workshops, in the USA and throughout Europe, to enable experienced therapists to work with the structured frame of this manualised approach. These introduce the approach and focus on therapist countertransference and the importance of structure and containment within the therapeutic frame. The Cornell team also run case consultation groups for qualified mental health professionals. The objective of the group is not to provide individual case supervision, but rather to teach the basic principles of TFP through the presentation of clinical material by the participants.

Mentalisation-based treatment

Mentalisation-based treatment (MBT) is an innovative form of psychodynamic psychotherapy developed and manualised by Anthony Bateman and Peter Fonagy (Bateman & Fonagy, 2004). It is designed for individuals with borderline personality disorder, addressing their disorganised attachment and failure to develop mentalising capacities in the context of an early attachment relationship. The concept of mentalisation emerged from the psychodynamic literature of the 1960s and it is the process by which we implicitly and explicitly interpret our own actions and those of others as meaningful on the basis of intentional mental states (needs, feelings, beliefs and reasons). The ability to consider alternative possibilities can in itself lead to changes in our understanding of a situation. A mentalising stance allows us to be uncertain about the 'facts' of a situation through the consideration of the motivations of others. This process is disrupted in individuals with borderline and antisocial personality disorders, who struggle to remain attentive to other people's mental states and, as a consequence, misinterpret their motives.

The MBT model is underpinned by attachment theory (Bowlby, 1969). Social biofeedback in the form of mirroring parental affect is the principal means by which we acquire an understanding of our own internal states, which is an intermediate step in the acquisition of an understanding of others as separate and psychological entities. This process enables us to differentiate between the internal and external world. If it does not occur, personality disorder results and the individual experiences their internal reality in non-mentalising ways, such as psychic equivalence ('I think, therefore it is'), pretend mode (dissociation from real thoughts and feelings), telological thinking (an experience is valid only if there is tangible evidence of it) and the alien self (where the child does not develop a representation of self through mirroring and thus the image of the caregiver becomes part of the child's self-identity).

What happens in therapy?

The therapeutic aims of MBT are to promote mentalising about oneself, others and relationships. The mentalisation model offers a framework for treatment within which the practitioner integrates their existing skills. Three principal themes are kept in mind:

1   a constant attempt to establish and maintain an attachment relationship with the client;
2   the use of this relationship to create an interpersonal context in which understanding mental states is the focus;
3   the creation of situations in which understanding the client's self as intentional and real is prioritised and experienced as such by the client.

Emphasis is placed on the structure of therapy, the repairing of any ruptures in the therapeutic relationship, and the interpersonal and social domains of functioning. Limited self-disclosure by the therapist, with careful consideration of its usefulness, is essential in the promotion of mentalisation. Treatment is usually of 18 months duration and takes the form of 90-minute group sessions and 50-minute individual sessions held on alternate weeks in the context of a day hospital programme that incorporates other expressive therapies (such as art or drama). Staff are carefully selected and trained, and healthy functioning of the team is a priority.

The overall aim of treatment is to help the client establish a more robust sense of self so that they can develop more secure relationships. The combination of coordinated group and individual treatment is used to broaden the attachment relationships within which the individual can develop greater mentalising capacities. Treatment in both settings focuses on bringing clients' emotional expression within the normal range and developing a coherent self-narrative. The most important aim of therapy is the development of mentalising capacities to provide a buffer between feelings and action: clients learn to identify and manage their impulses and to consider and understand the perceived intentions of themselves and others.

Who does it work for?

Mentalisation-based treatment was originally developed for borderline personality disorder. It has been shown to be effective in a randomised controlled trial (RCT) in a partial hospitalisation programme (Bateman & Fonagy, 1999). Those receiving MBT demonstrated statistically significant decreases in depressive symptoms, suicidal and self-mutilatory acts and in-patient days, and improved social and interpersonal functioning in comparison with those receiving standard psychiatric care. They continued to make improvements in these areas over the following 18 months (Bateman & Fonagy, 2001) and these improvements were maintained 5 years after the point of discharge (Bateman & Fonagy, 2008). A further study showed MBT to be effective for borderline personality disorder in out-patients (Bateman & Fonagy, 2009). Participants were randomly allocated to MBT or structured clinical management considered to represent current best practice. Substantial improvements were found across all outcome measures in both groups, although MBT demonstrated greater benefits across a number of key variables, including suicide attempts and hospital admissions.

Training and implementation

As an approach, MBT is considered accessible to practitioners with existing therapeutic skills and experience in working with personality disorder. Bateman and Fonagy run four-day introductory and two-day advanced workshops, the latter aimed at those who wish to train others in using the approach. A 'do-it-yourself' guide to implementing the approach is included in their treatment manual (Bateman & Fonagy, 2004).

Schema therapy

Schema therapy (also known as schema-focused therapy) is an integrative model developed by Jeffrey Young. It extends standard cognitive–behavioural therapy by integrating concepts from psychodynamic approaches and gestalt therapy, placing a greater emphasis on the childhood origins of psychological problems. The model was initially developed for treating borderline and narcissistic personality disorders, but has since been applied to other types of personality disorder. Schema therapy is based on the premise that personality pathology develops from unmet core emotional needs in childhood that lead to the establishment of 'early maladaptive schemas'. These schemas, of which 18 have been identified, are understood as unconditional assumptions about the self and others that originate in childhood and become self-perpetuating over time. By definition, they are dysfunctional and result in psychological distress. They are thought to be the result of both the child's innate temperament and early experiences, and ongoing negative interactions with others. For example, Mistrust/ Abuse relates to the experience of others as intentionally hurtful and/or abusive, which leaves the individual with a heightened sensitivity to threat in relationships. The schema is based on real experiences, although the subsequent expectation that others will act in a harmful manner may not be real.

In adulthood, the individual engages in a variety of cognitive, affective and behavioural manoeuvres that enable them to maintain or adapt their schemas in order to avoid experiencing overwhelming psychological distress. These coping styles take the form of 'schema surrender' (giving in to the schema and accepting that the resulting negative consequences are unavoidable); 'schema avoidance' (avoiding internal and external triggers that may activate the schema); and 'schema overcompensation' (acting as though the opposite were true). Inherent in schema therapy is the assumption that everyone has maladaptive schemas and coping strategies, but that these are more rigid and extreme in individuals with personality disorders.

Early maladaptive schemas are trait-like entities, that is, enduring features of the personality, whereas 'schema modes' are the state-like, changeable manifestations of schemas. Schema modes are defined as 'self states' that temporarily come to the fore and dominate a person's presentation, and are made up of clusters of schemas and coping strategies. In people with severe personality disorders, whose personalities are poorly integrated, these states are relatively dissociated from one another. As a result, schema modes can shift rapidly from one state to another. The concept of schema modes enables therapists to work with these sudden and extreme emotional shifts more effectively. In the schema therapy model, the combination of early maladaptive schemas, coping responses and modes form the basis of personality disorders. Bernstein *et al* (2007) have extended the original model to incorporate schema modes that are more commonly seen in patients in forensic settings.

Schema therapy views the therapy relationship as being of central importance. Key relational strategies are empathic confrontation (validating the development and perpetuation of schemas while simultaneously confronting the necessity to change) and limited re-parenting (providing within the boundaries of the therapy relationship what an individual needed but did not get from their parents in childhood). Imagery work and gestalt techniques such as the empty chair are used extensively to access and work with emotional experiences.

What happens in therapy?

Schema therapy is a long-term intervention (2–3 years) that does not subscribe to a fixed protocol for session structure. However, there are seven distinguishable phases (Arntz & van Genderen, 2009) to providing therapy for borderline personality disorder:

1 assessment and formulation
2 treating Axis I symptoms
3 crisis management
4 therapeutic interventions with schema modes
5 treating childhood trauma
6 changing behavioural patterns
7 ending therapy.

In addition to a full diagnostic assessment (which is recommended), a number of questionnaires (inventories) are used in the assessment phase. The inventories, which can be found at www.schematherapy. com, are designed to elicit information about schemas and their origins, coping strategies and modes. At the start of treatment, the emphasis is on psychoeducation about personality disorder and the schema-focused model; chapters from a self-help book (Young & Kolsko, 1993) are used to help this process. If Axis I symptoms are present, these are prioritised for treatment where possible. Crises (such as self harm or suicide attempts) are attended to as and when this becomes necessary. The client is next helped to make cognitive and emotional changes regarding their current situation in order to bolster the 'healthy adult mode' before engaging in more in-depth work into the childhood origins of their current difficulties. Finally, the focus is shifted to further breaking of behavioural patterns and preparing for the ending of therapy. Unlike other approaches, there is a greater acceptance of some form of continued contact (albeit the occasional telephone call or card) as, in accordance with the concept of limited re-parenting, it is believed that the bond between therapist and client should remain until the client has developed other healthy relationships.

There are modifications to the phases of therapy for different personality disorder types, including narcissistic personality disorder (Young et al, 2003), antisocial personality disorder (Bernstein et al, 2007) and cluster C personality disorders (Arntz, 2012). The approach has also been adapted for group work (Farrell et al, 2009; Beckley & Gordon, 2010).

Who does it work for?

Most of the evidence thus far has been generated for borderline personality disorder. A multi-centre trial in The Netherlands reported that individual schema therapy led to recovery from borderline personality disorder in about half the sample, with two-thirds experiencing a clinically significant improvement (Giesen-Bloo et al, 2006). It was about twice as effective as transference-focused psychotherapy and, despite being a long-term, high-intensity intervention, it was less costly and had a much lower drop-out rate. Group-based schema therapy has also been found to be effective for borderline personality disorder, in a comparison with treatment as usual (Farrell *et al*, 2009). Bamelis *et al* (2012) provide a comprehensive review of the available evidence for schema therapy with other personality disorder diagnoses, Axis I disorders and in specific settings (forensic and substance misuse services).

Training and implementation

The International Society of Schema Therapy (ISST) has recently published guidelines regarding the training needed to become an accredited practitioner (International Society of Schema Therapy, 2011). Training is at three levels (basic, standard and advanced), which are determined by hours of workshop attendance and supervised practice. There are currently two training providers in the UK and others are expected to be established in due course. Practitioners who reach the advanced stage are eligible to train others.

Cognitive analytic therapy

Cognitive analytic therapy (CAT) was developed by Anthony Ryle in an attempt to provide effective and affordable psychological treatment of borderline personality disorder within the UK's National Health Service. It is an integration of object relations theory (Kernberg, 1975) and personal construct theory (Kelly, 1955), using more easily accessible cognitive language to explain psychoanalytic ideas. The model has continued to evolve, now incorporating Vygotskian theories regarding the social and cultural formation of mind (Leiman, 1994).

The basic assumption of CAT is that the child's early interpersonal experiences result in the development of processes and structures known as reciprocal role procedures, patterns of relating to the self and others. Reciprocal role procedures are linked sequences of mental and behavioural processes that serve as repeatedly used guidelines for purposive action. Three common patterns result in the continuation of harmful reciprocal role procedures: traps, snags and dilemmas. Traps relate to 'vicious circles' of repetitive ways of thinking, feeling and acting that the person struggles to escape. For example, Sam feels that others do not like her, so she avoids social situations, thus increasing her experience of isolation. Snags are the subtle negative aspects of goals that sabotage the efforts a person makes to achieve change: Sam is unwilling to modify her own social behaviour because she feels that other people should behave more sociably towards her. Dilemmas are the 'false choices' or narrow options that cause the individual to continue to act in unhelpful ways because they think that the consequences of their other options would be just as negative or even worse: Sam avoids social situations because she feels that her efforts to join in are often clumsy and they leave her feeling embarrassed, but this causes other people to think that she is rejecting them, so either way she ends up feeling anxious and isolated.

These three patterns form the 'procedural sequence model'. This takes the form of a series of mental processes: appraisal and planning of action based on an aim; enactment of the action or role; evaluation of the consequence of this action or role; and confirmation or revision of the attempt to meet the aim. There are clear similarities to concepts of cognitive–behavioural therapy, although in CAT they are explicitly linked to early attachment experiences through the implicit or explicit prediction that the person's actions will elicit the interacting other to reciprocate in the form of an anticipated role (such as abused–abuser). Problems caused by the persistent, unrevised use of ineffective reciprocal role procedures are called target problem procedures and therapy aims to identify and revise such procedures. These emotional roles are re-enacted within the therapeutic relationship (akin to the concept of transference) and the role of the therapist is to identify role procedures while not reciprocating them (akin to avoiding countertransference).

Sequential diagrammatic reformulation, the representation of the client's reciprocal role procedures in diagrammatic form, is a key feature of CAT that is developed collaboratively throughout therapy (see Figs. 18.1 and 18.2 in Chapter 18). The aim is to help the client to recognise their perception of self and others, make sense of how and why these positions developed, and to gain control of these interpersonal patterns though the development of self-knowledge. The reformulation creates within the client the capacity for continuous self-observation, and this is used in conjunction with the therapeutic alliance as the main agent of change.

What happens in therapy?

Typically, the therapy comprises 16 sessions, although further blocks of sessions are sometimes offered. The aim is to offer a relatively brief intervention without losing depth of psychological engagement and insight. The initial task is to complete a 'psychotherapy file', which asks about common problem procedures. The first three sessions are focused on assessment and initial formulation of the client's difficulties. The therapist then presents the patient with a written reformulation (Chapter 18, pp. 299–301). This includes a description of the client's life so far, the difficulties they have struggled with and how they have survived them, and a reformulation of their presenting complaints as target problem procedures to be worked on. This is also presented as a sequential diagrammatic reformulation. The client is asked to reflect on these and amend them if they want to, so that eventually a joint understanding is achieved.

Focus is then shifted to material that comes up in the course of the (largely unstructured) sessions, including current events, history and transference, all of which is discussed in terms of the target problem procedures. The aim is to develop the client's capacity to recognise faulty procedures, so that they can start to control and replace them. Homework assignments may be used to confront the client with their procedures and to reinforce the possibility of modification. Change is seldom complete by the end of therapy, but the client is left with the tools to continue working. The last three or four sessions focus on the ending of therapy and how this may affect the client, particularly if endings have been difficult in the past. A 'good-bye letter' is written by both therapist and client, to consider what has been achieved and what remains to be worked on. A follow-up appointment in two or three months is also usually offered.

Who does it work for?

A number of studies have indicated that CAT shows promise in treating personality disorder. An early comparison with Mann's time-limited psychotherapy (Mann & Goldman, 1982) indicated that CAT produced greater cognitive reorganisation, as measured by a repertory grid, than did the more purely analytic approach (Brockman *et al*, 1987). Single-case experimental design studies (Kellett, 2005, 2007) have demonstrated CAT's effectiveness with dissociative identity disorder and histrionic personality disorder. Although the evidence remains limited, applying mainly to borderline personality disorder, CAT is increasingly being used in forensic services for a wider range of personality disorders (Pollock, 2006).

Training and implementation

Practitioner training in CAT enables core professionals with previous therapy qualifications to develop competence in this approach. These courses usually last 2 years and lead to accreditation as a practitioner and eligibility for membership of the Association for Cognitive Analytic Therapy (www.acat.me.uk).

References

Arntz, A. (2012) Schema therapy for cluster C personality disorders. In *The Wiley-Blackwell Handbook of Schema Therapy: Theory, Research & Practice* (eds M. van Vreeswijk, J. Broersen & M. Nardort), pp. 397–414. Wiley:Blackwell.

Arntz, A. & van Genderen, H. (2009) *Schema Therapy for Borderline Personality Disorder*. Wiley-Blackwell.

Bamelis, L., Bloo, J., Bernstein, D., *et al* (2012) Effectiveness studies. In *The Wiley-Blackwell Handbook of Schema Therapy: Theory, Research and Practice* (eds M. van Vreeswijk, J. Broersen & M. Nardort), pp. 495–510. Wiley:Blackwell.

Bateman, A. & Fonagy, P. (1999) The effectiveness of partial hospitalisation in the treatment of borderline personality disorder: a randomised controlled trial. *American Journal of Psychiatry*, **156**, 1563–1569.

Bateman, A. & Fonagy, P. (2001) The treatment of borderline personality disorder with psychoanalytically orientated partial hospitalization: an 18 month follow-up. *American Journal of Psychiatry*, **158**, 36–42.

Bateman, A. & Fonagy, P. (2004) *Psychotherapy for Borderline Personality Disorder: Mentalization-Based Treatment*. Oxford University Press.

Bateman, A. & Fonagy, P. (2008) 8-Year follow-up of patients treated for borderline personality disorder: mentalization-based treatment versus treatment as usual. *American Journal of Psychiatry*, **165**, 631–638.

Bateman, A. & Fonagy, P. (2009) Randomized controlled trial of outpatient mentalization-based treatment versus structured clinical management for borderline personality disorder. *American Journal of Psychiatry*, **166**, 1355–1364.

Beckley, K. A. & Gordon, N. S. (2010) Schema therapy within a high secure setting. In *Using Time, Not Doing Time: Practitioner Perspectives on Personality Disorder and Risk* (eds A. Tennant & K Howells), pp. 95–110. Wiley-Blackwell.

Bernstein, D. P., Arntz, A. & de Vos, M. (2007) Schema focused therapy in forensic settings: theoretical model and recommendations for best clinical practice. *International Journal of Forensic Mental Health*, **6**, 169–183.

Bowlby, J. (1969) *Attachment and Loss: Vol. 1 Attachment*. Hogarth Press & Institute of Psychoanalysis.

Brockman, B., Poynton, A., Ryle, A., *et al* (1987) Effectiveness of time-limited psychotherapy carried out by trainees: comparison of two methods. *British Journal of Psychiatry*, **151**, 602–610.

Casement, P. (1985) *On Learning from the Patient*. Routledge.

Clarkin, J. F., Yeomans, F. & Kernberg, O. F. (2006) *Psychotherapy of Borderline Personality: Focusing on Object Relations*. American Psychiatric Publishing.

Clarkin, J. F., Levy, K. N., Lenzenwenger, M. F., *et al* (2007) Evaluating three treatments for borderline personality disorder: a multiwave study. *American Journal of Psychiatry*, **164**, 922–928.

Davies, J. (2009) *The Making of Psychotherapists: An Anthropological Analysis*. Karnac Books.

Farrell, J. M, Shaw, I. A. & Webber, M. A. (2009) A schema-focused approach to group psychotherapy for outpatients with borderline personality disorder: a randomized controlled trial. *Journal of Behaviour Therapy and Experimental Psychiatry*, **40**, 317–328.

Foelsch, P. A. & Kernberg, O. F. (1998) Transference-focused psychotherapy for borderline personality disorders. *Psychotherapy in Practice*, **4**, 67–90.

Fonagy, P. & Target, M. (2003) *Psychoanalytical Theories: Perspectives from Developmental Psychology*. Whurr.

Fonagy, P., Gergley, G., Jurist, E. L., *et al* (2002) *Affect Regulation, Mentalization and the Development of Self*. Other Press.

Freud, S. (1949) *An Outline of Psychoanalysis*. Hogarth Press.

Gelso, C. J., & Hayes, J. A. (1998) *The Psychotherapy Relationship: Theory Research and Practice*. John Wiley & Sons.

Giesen-Bloo, J., van Dyck, R., Spinhoven, P., *et al* (2006) Outpatient psychotherapy for borderline personality disorder: randomized trial of schema-focused therapy vs transference-focused psychotherapy. *Archives of General Psychiatry*, **63**, 649–658.

International Society of Schema Therapy (2011) Guidelines for certification. ISST (http://isst-online.com/node/234).

Jacobs, M. (1998) *The Presenting Past: The Core of Psychodynamic Counselling and Therapy*. Open University Press.

Jung, C. G. (1957) *The Undiscovered Self*. Penguin.

Kellett, S. (2005) The treatment of dissociative identity disorder with cognitive analytic therapy: experimental evidence of sudden gains. *Journal of Trauma & Dissociation*, **6**(3), 55–81.

Kellett, S. (2007) A time series evaluation of the treatment of histrionic personality disorder with cognitive analytic therapy. *Psychology and Psychotherapy*, **80**, 389–405.

Kelly, G. (1955) *The Psychology of Personal Constructs*. Norton.

Kernberg, O. (1975) *Borderline Conditions and Pathological Narcissism*. Jason Aronson.

Kernberg, O (2004) *Aggression, Narcissism, and Self-Destructiveness in the Psychotherapeutic Relationship: New Developments in the Psychopathology and Psychotherapy of Severe Personality Disorders*. Yale University Press.

Leiman, M. (1994) Projective identification as early joint action sequences: a Vygotskian addendum to the procedural sequence object relations model. *British Journal of Medical Psychology*, **67**, 97–106.

Levy, K. N., Meehan, K. B., Kelly, K. M., *et al* (2006) Change in attachment patterns and reflective functioning in a randomized controlled trial of transference focussed psychotherapy for borderline personality disorder. *Journal of Consulting and Clinical Psychology*, **74**, 1027–1040.

Malan, D. H. (1979) *Individual Psychotherapy and the Science of Psychodynamics*. Butterworths.

Mann, J. & Goldman, P. (1982) *A Case Book of Time Limited Psychotherapy*. McGraw-Hill.

Milrod, B., Leon, A., Busch, F. N., *et al* (2007) A randomized, controlled clinical trial of psychoanalytical psychotherapy for panic disorder. *American Journal of Psychiatry*, **164**, 265–272.

Mitchell, S. A. & Black, M. J. (1995) *Freud and Beyond: A History of Modern Psychoanalytic Thought*. Basic Books.

Pollock, P. H. (2006) Final thoughts: the way forward for cognitive analytic therapy in forensic settings. In *Cognitive Analytic Therapy for Offenders: A New Approach to Forensic Psychotherapy* (eds P. H. Pollock, M. Stowell-Smith & M. Gopfert), pp. 323–326. Routledge.

Ryle, A. (1990) *Cognitive-Analytic Therapy: Active Participation in Change. A New Integration in Brief Psychotherapy*. John Wiley & Sons.

Spillius, E. B. (1992) Clinical experiences of projective identification. In *Clinical Lectures on Klein and Bion* (ed. R Anderson), pp. 59–73)Routledge.

Watchel, P. L. (2008) Relational Theory and the Practice of Psychotherapy. Guildford Press.

Winnicott, D. W. (1958) *Through Paediatrics to Psychoanalysis*. Tavistock Publications.

Yeomans, F. E., Clarkin, J. C. & Kernberg, O. (2002) *A Primer on Transference Focussed Psychotherapy for Borderline Patients*. Jason Aronson.

Young, J. E. (1990) *Cognitive Therapy for Personality Disorders: A Schema-Focused Approach*. Professional Resource Exchange.

Young, J. E. & Klosko, J. S. (1993) *Reinventing your life*. Plume Books.

Young, J. E., Klosko, J. S. & Weishar, M. E. (2003) *Schema Therapy: A Practitioner's Guide*. Guilford Press.

CHAPTER 16

Treatment approaches for severe personality disorder

Mike Crawford

Summary This chapter describes general features of treatments for severe personality disorder that are believed to make them effective. The evidence base for the value of each of these aspects of the organisation and delivery of services has not been independently tested, but support for their value comes from the experiences of people who provide and use them and from the prominence given to them in treatment approaches that have been shown to be effective.

This chapter focuses on services for people who have 'severe' personality disorder, in which personality-related problems are complex and associated with grossly impaired social functioning and/or risk of severe harm to self or others (Tyrer & Johnson, 1996; Crawford *et al*, 2010). Although people with less severe forms of personality disorder can and often do benefit from interventions and treatments, those with severe personality disorder are more difficult to engage with services, more likely to drop out of contact and less likely to benefit from standard treatments (Crawford *et al*, 2009a). The nature of personality disorder and the challenges associated with providing services for people with such disorder have meant that standard approaches to delivering psychosocial treatments have had to be modified. For those with more severe problems, specialist treatment services are increasingly being provided. These aim to structure treatment to better help people who often have very complex needs. However, even these services do not engage many of those referred to them, and further work is needed to establish optimal methods for helping people with severe personality disorder.

Challenges to the development of therapeutic relationships

It is in the nature of personality disorder that those affected have difficulties in relationships with others and that these difficulties are generally manifested in relationships with healthcare professionals. Previous experiences of inconsistent or abusive care lead some people with severe personality disorder to experience the neutral actions of others as dismissive or threatening and to have concerns that professional carers may try to abandon or harm them. Such reactions can make it harder for professionals to form a therapeutic alliance with them. The tendency of individuals with severe personality disorder to separate out people and relationships into extreme forms of good or bad (Kernberg, 1984), and the ways that staff respond to this 'splitting', can make it difficult for teams to deliver a consistent and reliable service. Methods for assessing and responding to risk of harm to self and others that are based on the needs of people with other mental disorders that impair capacity may not provide a helpful framework for managing the chronic suicidal thoughts and recurrent acts of self-harm that are prominent among many people with severe personality disorder (Paris, 2002; Bateman & Fonagy, 2004).

Surveys of clinicians' attitudes towards people with personality disorder demonstrate that many hold ambivalent or negative views (Lewis & Appleby, 1988; Gallop *et al*, 1989). Given this, it is of little surprise that people with personality disorder are often dissatisfied with mental health services. In a survey of 50 people in the south of England, less than half said that they had been helped by mental health services and 80% believed that their care had deteriorated as a result of their being given a diagnosis of personality disorder (Ramon *et al*, 2001). Qualitative data collected by the National Institute for Mental Health in England provide graphic accounts of individuals' experiences of being refused treatment, being labelled 'attention-seeking' and referred to as 'bed-wasters' (Haigh, 2002).

Whatever treatment approach is taken, failure to recognise and attend to problems that can arise in relationships between staff and people with personality disorder is likely to limit any benefit individuals gain from their contact with services (Holmes, 1999).

Specific treatment approaches

During the past 20 years, a variety of psychological treatments have been developed that have been specifically designed for people with severe personality disorder. These have generally been based on existing forms of psychological treatment that have been modified to take account of the nature of personality disorder and the needs of people with these problems.

The form of treatment that has been most extensively researched in experimental studies, dialectical behaviour therapy, was developed in the USA by Marsha Linehan. The focus of most research in this area to date has been on women with borderline personality disorder who self-harm. Meta-analysis of randomised trials of dialectical behaviour therapy suggests that it leads to sustained reductions in the level of self-harming behaviour (Binks *et al*, 2006). Dialectical behaviour therapy is a modified form of cognitive–behavioural therapy delivered in individual and group sessions, together with additional telephone-based support. It uses established techniques for understanding the triggers and consequences of different behaviours, although changes were made in an attempt to increase commitment to treatment and reduce drop-out rates.

Foremost among these changes are an emphasis on 'dialectics' and 'validation', and the inclusion of skills training (Linehan, 1993). In this context, dialectics refers to the interrelated nature of actions and behaviour. In focusing on dialectics, the treatment draws attention to how hard it can be to change established patterns of behaviour. The therapy also aims to help people consider the impact that efforts to change may have on relationships with others. In dialectical behaviour therapy, 'validation' aims to help people make sense of the way in which temperament or past experiences may have led them to feel and react the way they did, while being clear about the way that current patterns of behaviour affect themselves and others.

Other attempts to modify existing psychological treatment approaches have also focused on the long-term nature of personality-related problems and the interpersonal nature of the problems that people with personality disorder experience. So, for instance, schema-focused therapy (Young, 1994) targets core pervasive beliefs that develop in early life, rather than the negative automatic thoughts and dysfunctional assumptions that tend to be the focus of cognitive therapy for mental disorders that develop in adulthood. Clinical trials of modified cognitive therapy for people with borderline personality disorder demonstrate reductions in suicidal behaviour (Davidson et al, 2006), reductions in psychopathology and improved quality of life (Giesen-Bloo et al, 2006).

Mentalisation-based treatment is a modified form of psychoanalytical therapy that aims to increase a person's capacity to 'interpret the actions of oneself and others as meaningful on the basis of intentional mental states' (Bateman & Fonagy, 2004). Like dialectical behaviour therapy, it combines individual and group-based treatment. The focus of therapy is on trying to help people develop a better understanding of the connections between their feelings, thoughts and actions, the actions of others and their relationships with other people. In a randomised trial of 44 people, mentalisation-based treatment delivered as part of a structured day-hospital programme was compared with fortnightly out-patient follow-up by a psychiatrist. Those receiving mentalisation-based treatment experienced marked reductions in use of in-patient mental health services, fewer episodes of self-harm and improved mental health (Bateman & Fonagy, 1999). These improvements were sustained 8 years later (Bateman & Fonagy, 2008).

Specialist treatment programmes

Bateman & Tyrer (2004) have described three different approaches to organising services for people with personality disorder: the sole practitioner; a 'divided functions' approach; and the specialist team. When delivering services to people with severe personality disorder, the sole practitioner and divided functions approaches may be difficult to sustain. For instance, if a person has high levels of contact with a number of different services, it can be difficult to ensure that care is coordinated and a consistent treatment plan is delivered. The divided functions approach, in which different healthcare professionals take responsibility for different aspects of treatment (such as medication review by a psychiatrist and psychological treatment from a psychotherapist), may make it difficult to tackle splitting if this arises. Although it may be possible to manage such problems through regular and effective communication, specialist personality disorder teams are specifically designed to deliver treatment in a coordinated way and ensure clear communication between team members.

Specialist treatment teams for people with personality disorder take many different forms and offer interventions of different intensities. An evaluation of 11 specialist community-based personality disorder services in England highlighted key features shared by the different services (Price *et al*, 2009) (Box 16.1). One of these features is the attention that specialist services for people with personality disorder pay to the recruitment, support and supervision of staff. The interpersonal nature of the problems of most people with severe personality disorder mean that staff working in personality disorder services are regularly exposed to negative transferences (see Chapters 6 and 12, this volume). Helping people manage their feelings

---

Box 16.1 Shared features of specialist personality disorder services in England

- They provide ongoing contact with service users over a relatively long periods, e.g. over a year
- They provide a range of interventions (e.g., care planning, crisis management, psychological interventions, peer support through a single team) and actively involve service users in choosing the service they receive
- They take steps to ensure comprehensive communication within the team
- Responsibility for client welfare is shared by members of a team, rather than by individual members of staff
- Limits on the availability of staff and other boundaries are made clear to service users at the start of treatment and stuck to throughout treatment
- They aim to demonstrate that the user is valued and valuable; the treatment approach aims to be validating rather than dismissive of the user's experience
- They negotiate short- and long-term treatment goals at an early stage
- They provide and promote choice, self-efficacy and personal responsibility and avoid trying to control or coerce service users
- They arrange more intensive services at times of crisis, including home treatment and/or residential care
- They try to obtain users' consent to contact, support and inform carers
- They should prepare service users for leaving and discuss discharge procedures well in advance

(Crawford *et al*, 2007)

Box 16.2 Characteristics that may help staff to work successfully with people with personality disorder

- The ability to be responsive and work flexibly with service users, but not at the expense of neglecting appropriate boundaries
- The ability to empower service users, even if this means letting them make some mistakes; staff who are controlling may be unsuited to working with people with personality disorder
- Emotional maturity and a high degree of personal resilience
- The ability to accept the limitations of what can be done
- A capacity to reflect on themselves and their work
- A willingness to discuss their own mistakes and uncertainties
- An ability to balance their work life with other aspects of their life
- A willingness to work as members of a team (to reach compromises and accept shared decision-making when this is possible, but to accept the decision of a clinical lead when agreement is not possible)

(Crawford *et al*, 2007)

---

towards the people they work with is an important part of delivering the service. Services therefore need to pay particular attention to recruiting staff who have the personal characteristics that may be needed to sustain work with this group (Box 16.2).

Services also provide opportunities for reflect practice and staff support. Available evidence suggests that where these reflective systems are operating effectively, staff working with personality disorder may be no more likely to experience dissatisfaction at work or burnout than those working with other forms of mental disorder (Crawford *et al*, 2011).

Importance of general aspects of treatment approach

National guidance on the treatment of borderline personality disorder in England endorses the importance of many of these shared features of specialist personality disorder services (National Collaborating Centre for Mental Health, 2009*a*). These guidelines state that people should be given information about a psychological treatment service before they are asked whether they want to use it. When providing psychological treatment for people with severe impairment, the guidelines also recommend that:

- treatment lasts for at least 3 months
- an integrated theoretical approach is used that is made explicit to the service user
- therapists receive regular supervision
- twice-weekly treatment sessions are considered
- treatment is delivered as part of a coordinated package of care
- effects of treatment are monitored across a broad range of outcomes.

These recommendations were based on the observation that outcomes from clinical trials of multicomponent interventions such as dialectical behaviour therapy and mentalisation-based treatment appear to be better than those based on 'stand-alone' psychotherapy. For women with borderline personality disorder who self-harm, the guidelines state that treatment within a comprehensive dialectical behaviour programme should be considered. These recommendations are based on current 'best-available' evidence. It is clear that for a range of other interventions that have been used to treat personality disorder, there is an absence of evidence from randomised trials, rather than evidence that they are not effective.

Support for these shared features of personality disorder treatment services also comes from a study that used the consensus-building Delphi technique to examine views of service users and providers about how personality disorder services should be organised and delivered (Crawford et al, 2008). Although there was agreement about several core features of such services, it was not possible to reach a consensus about other important aspects of service organisation, including the role of medication and use of compulsory treatment.

The finding that service users and providers agree about the key features of high-quality personality disorder services does not mean that services delivered in this way achieve better treatment outcomes, but studies comparing different models of service delivery have rarely been conducted. However, indirect evidence for the importance of the key features of services listed in Box 16.1 comes from those trials that have been completed. Early trials of interventions such as mentalisation-based treatment and dialectical behaviour therapy compared with treatment as usual demonstrated better treatment outcomes among those who received these therapies. Intriguingly, more recent studies comparing these interventions against 'enhanced' treatment as usual, in which greater effort is made to provide a control treatment that is consistent, emphasises active service user involvement and includes proper crisis planning and management, have demonstrated either fewer (Bateman & Fonagy, 2009) or no (McMain et al, 2009) additional benefits from these therapies. These findings further emphasise the importance of the way that treatment is organised and delivered rather than the particular therapeutic approach that is taken.

Antisocial personality disorder

Much of the impetus for developing better services for people with personality disorder in Britain has come from concerns about the way in which people with personality disorder who pose a risk to others have been treated. Official enquiries into homicides by people with severe personality disorder have pointed to problems with risk assessment and management and concluded that the individuals concerned were not provided with the services they needed (Francis *et al*, 2006). Among people with personality disorder, those with antisocial personality disorder pose the greatest risk to others. Antisocial personality traits include disregard for the rights of others and a lack of remorse when behaviour leads to harm to others. Levels of antisocial personality disorder are unsurprisingly higher among people in prison than in any other setting, with as many as 50% of all those in prison having the disorder (Singleton *et al*, 1998). It has been estimated that as many as 25% of all violent incidents are committed by people with antisocial personality disorder (Coid, 2003).

In recent years, specialist forensic services for people with severe personality disorder who are believed to be at high risk of further offending have been developed (Moran *et al*, 2008). However, such services are available for only a small minority of those with severe personality disorder who present a significant risk to others. Some general community-based services for people with personality disorder exclude those who are judged to pose a risk to others and few people with a history of offending access them (Crawford *et al*, 2007). Despite high levels of common mental disorders and substance misuse problems, available evidence suggests that most people with antisocial personality disorder are not in contact with mental health services (Ullrich & Coid, 2009) and that those who are receive little follow-up care (Crawford *et al*, 2009*b*).

One reason for this may be the lack of evidence for the effectiveness of treatment. A randomised trial of cognitive–behavioural therapy for 52 men with antisocial personality disorder was considered too small to be able to detect clinically significant changes in offending behaviour and mental health outcomes (Davidson *et al*, 2009). Among people with antisocial personality disorder who also have substance misuse problems, contingency management may provide a means of increasing engagement with services and reducing drug use (Messina *et al*, 2003).

No other clinical trials specifically for people who have antisocial personality disorder and are in contact with mental health services have been conducted. However, numerous randomised studies have been completed that aimed to reduce reoffending behaviour among people in contact with criminal justice services. Given the high levels of antisocial personality disorder among people in contact with such services, it has been argued that findings from these studies can be applied more generally to people with antisocial personality disorder. From studies involving people recruited in criminal justice services, the National Institute for Health and Clinical Excellence (NICE) used evidence of reduced reoffending following referral to group-based cognitive and cognitive–behavioural therapy as the basis for its advice that people with antisocial personality disorder should be offered such interventions (National Collaborating Centre for Mental Health, 2009*b*). The guidance also highlighted the importance of interventions that might prevent the development of antisocial personality disorder and of the training needs of staff working in health and social care.

Improving mental health service provision for offenders has become a priority in the UK (Ministry of Justice, 2009). However, providers of general mental health services appear to continue to be reluctant to treat people with antisocial personality disorder (Crawford *et al*, 2009b). Although further research into the feasibility and effects of interventions could inform the development of better services, persisting concerns about the nature of antisocial personality disorder and the appropriateness of offering 'treatment' to offenders with personality disorder (Chapter 11, this volume) seem likely to continue to act as barriers to treatment.

Gaps in knowledge and future service developments

Services for people with personality disorder remain at an early stage of development compared with those for individuals with mental disorders such as depression and psychoses. As a result, some fundamental aspects of the way that services are delivered are unclear and others are contentious. Chief among these are: service intensity, the approach taken to people who do not engage with services, the role of medication and the role of in-patient services.

Service intensity

At a time of global financial uncertainty, there is increasing pressure across health and social care services to cut treatment costs. Such pressures challenge perceived wisdom that services for people with personality disorder need to be delivered over long periods of time. Although very short interventions such as bibliotherapy for individuals with personality disorder who self-harm may not be effective (Tyrer *et al*, 2003a), other interventions, such as group-based problem-solving therapy, may be sufficient to enable people with personality disorder to make important changes in their lives after weeks rather than months of treatment (Huband *et al*, 2007; Blum *et al*, 2008). The potential value of peer support to help people with personality disorder has long been known, and new models for facilitating it may also provide less costly and more cost-effective ways of helping individuals who want help (Miller & Crawford, 2010).

Therapeutic communities (Chapter 19, this volume), which were originally designed as residential treatments, are now being delivered in community settings, and mentalisation-based treatment, which was initially developed as part of an intensive day treatment, is being evaluated as a twice-weekly intervention (UK trial ISRCTN57363317). Although clinical trials comparing intensive and less intensive models of treatment for personality disorders have rarely been conducted, controlled studies suggest that less intensive services may be equally or more effective than more intensive ones (Chiesa *et al*, 2004). Further work is needed to explore the cost-effectiveness of less intensive interventions.

Engagement with services

Despite considerable effort to engage people with personality disorder in specialist services, it is clear that many choose not to use them. For some, the way that services are organised, such as an emphasis on group-based treatment, provides a reason not to engage with them. Others do not see themselves as having a problem and are therefore unwilling to engage in a treatment directed at trying to help them make changes to their feelings, thoughts and behaviour (Tyrer *et al*, 2003*b*). An alternative approach to working with people with personality disorder is to help them identify and change aspects of their social environment in an attempt to ameliorate the impact of their personality (Tyrer *et al*, 2003*c*). Further information about this approach, which has been dubbed nidotherapy, can be found in Chapter 20.

Role of medication

People with personality disorder are at greater risk of other mental health problems such as anxiety and depression. Evidence from randomised trials of drug treatments for people with such conditions suggests that those with comorbid personality disorder are less likely to respond to pharmacotherapy than those without personality disorder (Newton-Howes *et al*, 2006; Gorwood *et al*, 2010).

The role of pharmacological interventions for individuals without comorbid psychiatric conditions is unclear. Although a number of clinical trials have suggested that, among select groups of people mainly with borderline personality disorder, antipsychotic drugs and mood stabilisers may be associated with changes in behaviour and mental health (Lieb *et al*, 2010), such studies tend to be small and have short follow-up periods. In clinical practice polypharmacy, poor adherence to treatment regimes and risk of self-poisoning mean that specialist services for people with personality disorder are more likely to be involved in helping people stop rather than start psychotropic medication (Crawford *et al*, 2007). The NICE guidelines on the treatment of borderline personality disorder conclude that medication should not be used in an attempt to treat borderline or antisocial personality disorders (National Collaborating Centre for Mental Health, 2009*a*). In the absence of compelling evidence for the effectiveness of drug treatments in those who do not have comorbid mental disorders, this conservative approach appears well judged.

Role of in-patient treatment

Some of the earliest attempts to design treatment programmes for people with severe personality disorder were based on treating people in residential settings. More recent evidence that community-based services are also able to help this group of people to attain better mental health has raised questions about the role of in-patient treatment. There is a consensus that some people with personality disorder may need to access in-patient care at times of severe crisis (see Chapter 6, this volume). However, concerns have been raised that repeated use of in-patient services can increase service dependency and reduce a person's capacity to develop and use effective coping strategies. Bateman & Fonagy (2004) suggest that in-patient treatment for individuals with borderline personality disorder should be:

- short term
- planned rather than emergency
- delivered on a voluntary rather than compulsory basis
- offered with the aim of achieving specific treatment goals.

In the absence of clear evidence on the impact of in-patient treatment for people with personality disorder, such advice seems well founded.

Conclusion

Available evidence suggests that people with severe personality disorder can attain improved health and social outcomes when they receive care that is well coordinated and delivered using a shared and consistent approach. Important questions about the most effective and cost-effective ways of helping individuals with personality disorder, especially antisocial personality disorder, remain. Meanwhile, when psychosocial treatments are offered, clear short- and long-term goals should be agreed before treatment starts and staff providing services should be adequately trained and supported.

References

Bateman, A. & Fonagy, P. (1999) Effectiveness of partial hospitalization in the treatment of borderline personality disorder: a randomized controlled trial. *American Journal of Psychiatry*, **156**, 1563–1569.

Bateman, A. & Fonagy, P. (2004) *Psychotherapy for Borderline Personality Disorder: Mentalization-Based Treatment*. Oxford University Press.

Bateman, A. & Fonagy, P. (2008) 8-year follow-up of patients treated for borderline personality disorder: mentalization-based treatment versus treatment as usual. *American Journal of Psychiatry*, **165**, 631–638.

Bateman, A. & Fonagy, P. (2009) Randomized controlled trial of outpatient mentalization-based treatment versus structured clinical management for borderline personality disorder. *American Journal of Psychiatry*, **166**, 1355–1364.

Bateman, A. & Tyrer, P. (2004) Services for personality disorder: organisation for inclusion. *Advances in Psychiatric Treatment*, **10**, 425–433.

Binks, C. A., Fenton, M., McCarthy, L., *et al* (2006) Psychological therapies for people with borderline personality disorder. *Cochrane Database of Systematic Reviews*, issue 1, CD005652.

Blum, N., St John, D., Pfohl, B., *et al* (2008) Systems Training for Emotional Predictability and Problem Solving (STEPPS) for outpatients with borderline personality disorder: a randomized controlled trial and 1-year follow-up. *American Journal of Psychiatry*, **165**, 468–478.

Chiesa, M., Fonagy, P., Holmes, J., *et al* (2004) Residential versus community treatment of personality disorders: a comparative study of three treatment programs. *American Journal of Psychiatry*, **161**, 1463–1470.

Coid, J. (2003) Epidemiology, public health and the problem of personality disorder. *British Journal of Psychiatry*, **182** (suppl. 44), s3–s10.

Crawford, M. J., Rutter, D., Price, K., *et al* (2007) *Learning the Lessons: A Multi-Method Evaluation of Dedicated Community-Based Services for People with Personality Disorder*. National Coordinating Centre for the Service Delivery and Organisation (NCCSDO) Research Programme.

Crawford, M. J., Price, K., Rutter, D., *et al* (2008) Dedicated community-based services for adults with personality disorder: Delphi study. *British Journal of Psychiatry*, **193**, 342–343.

Crawford, M. J., Price, K., Gordon, F., *et al* (2009*a*) Engagement and retention in specialist services for people with personality disorder. *Acta Psychiatrica Scandinavica*, **119**, 304–311.

Crawford, M. J., Sahib, L., Bratton, H., *et al* (2009*b*) Service provision for men with antisocial personality disorder who make contact with mental health services. *Personality and Mental Health*, **3**, 165–171.

Crawford, M. J., Koldobsky, N., Mulder, R., *et al* (2010) Classifying personality disorder according to severity. *Journal of Personality Disorder*, **25**, 321–330.

Crawford, M. J., Adedeji, T., Price, K., *et al* (2011) Job satisfaction and burnout among staff working in community-based personality disorder services. *International Journal of Social Psychiatry*, **56**, 196–206.

Davidson, K., Norrie, J., Tyrer, P., *et al* (2006) The effectiveness of cognitive behavior therapy for borderline personality disorder: results from the borderline personality disorder study of cognitive therapy (BOSCOT) trial. *Journal of Personality Disorder*, **20**, 450–465.

Davidson, K. M., Tyrer, P., Tata, P., *et al* (2009) Cognitive behaviour therapy for violent men with antisocial personality disorder in the community: an exploratory randomized controlled trial. *Psychological Medicine*, **39**, 569–577.

Francis, R., Higgins, J. & Cassam, E. (2006) *Report of the Independent Inquiry into the Care and Treatment of Michael Stone*. South East Coast Strategic Health Authority, Kent County Council & Kent Probation Area.

Gallop, R., Lancee, W. J. & Garfinkel, P. (1989) How nursing staff respond to the label "borderline personality disorder". *Hospital and Community Psychiatry*, **40**, 815–819.

Giesen-Bloo, J., van Dyck, R., Spinhoven, P., *et al* (2006) Outpatient psychotherapy for borderline personality disorder: randomized trial of schema-focused therapy vs transference-focused psychotherapy. *Archives of General Psychiatry*, **63**, 649–658.

Gorwood, P., Rouillon, F., Even, C., *et al* (2010) Treatment response in major depression: effects of personality dysfunction and prior depression. *British Journal of Psychiatry*, **196**, 139–142.

Haigh, R. (2002) *Services for People with Personality Disorder: The Thoughts of Service Users*. Department of Health.

Holmes, J. (1999) Psychotherapeutic approaches to the management of severe personality disorder in general psychiatric settings. *CPD Bulletin Psychiatry*, **1**, 35–41.

Huband, N., McMurran, M., Evans, C., *et al* (2007) Social problem-solving plus psychoeducation for adults with personality disorder: pragmatic randomised controlled trial. *British Journal of Psychiatry*, **190**, 307–313.

Kernberg, O. F. (1984) *Severe Personality Disorders: Psychotherapeutic Strategies*. Yale University Press.

Lewis, G. & Appleby, L. (1988) Personality disorder: the patients psychiatrists dislike. *British Journal of Psychiatry*, **153**, 44–49.

Lieb, K., Völlm, B., Rücker, G., *et al* (2010) Pharmacotherapy for borderline personality disorder: Cochrane systematic review of randomised trials. *British Journal of Psychiatry*, **196**, 4–12.

Linehan, M. M. (1993) *Cognitive Behavioural Treatment of Borderline Personality Disorder*. Guilford Press.

McMain, S. F., Links, P. S., Gnam, W. H., *et al* (2009) A randomized trial of dialectical behavior therapy versus general psychiatric management for borderline personality disorder. *American Journal of Psychiatry*, **166**, 1365–1374.

Messina, N., Farabee, D. & Rawson, R. (2003) Treatment responsivity of cocaine-dependent patients with antisocial personality disorder to cognitive-behavioral and contingency management interventions. *Journal of Consulting and Clinical Psychology*, **71**, 320–329.

Miller, S. & Crawford, M.J. (2010) Open access community support groups for people with personality disorder: attendance and impact on use of other services. *Psychiatrist*, **34**, 177–181.

Ministry of Justice (2009) *The Bradley Report: Lord Bradley's Review of People with Mental Health Problems or Learning Disabilities in the Criminal Justice System*. Ministry of Justice.

Moran, P., Fortune, Z., Barrett, B., *et al* (2008) *An Evaluation of Pilot Services for People with Personality Disorder in Adult Forensic Settings*. National Coordinating Centre for the Service Delivery and Organisation (NCCSDO) Research Programme.

National Collaborating Centre for Mental Health (2009a) *Borderline Personality Disorder: Treatment and Management (NICE Clinical Guideline 78)*. National Institute for Health and Clinical Excellence.

National Collaborating Centre for Mental Health (2009b) *Antisocial Personality Disorder: Treatment, Management and Prevention (NICE Clinical Guideline 77)*. National Institute for Health and Clinical Excellence.

Newton-Howes, G., Tyrer, P. & Johnson, T. (2006) Personality disorder and the outcome of depression: meta-analysis of published studies. *British Journal of Psychiatry*, **188**, 13–20.

Paris, J. (2002) Chronic suicidality among patients with borderline personality disorder. *Psychiatric Services*, **53**, 738–742.

Price, K., Gillespie, S., Rutter, D., *et al* (2009) Dedicated personality disorder services: a qualitative analysis of service structure and treatment process. *Journal of Mental Health*, **18**, 467–475.

Ramon, S., Castillo, H. & Morant, N. (2001) Experiencing personality disorder: a participative research. *International Journal of Social Psychiatry*, **47**, 1–15.

Singleton, N., Meltzer, H. & Gatward, R. (1998) *Psychiatric Morbidity among Prisoners in England and Wales*. TSO (The Stationery Office).

Tyrer, P. & Johnson, T. (1996) Establishing the severity of personality disorder. *American Journal of Psychiatry*, **153**, 1593–1597.

Tyrer, P., Jones, V., Thompson, S., *et al* (2003a) Service variation in baseline variables and prediction of risk in a randomised trial of psychological treatment in repeated parasuicide: the POPMACT Study. *International Journal of Social Psychiatry*, **49**, 258–269.

Tyrer, P., Mitchard, S., Methuen, C., *et al* (2003b) Treatment rejecting and treatment seeking personality disorders: Type R and Type S. *Journal of Personality Disorder*, **17**, 263–268.

Tyrer, P., Sensky, T. & Mitchard, S. (2003c) Principles of nidotherapy in the treatment of persistent mental and personality disorders. *Psychotherapy and Psychosomatics*, **72**, 350–356.

Ullrich, S. & Coid, J. (2009) Antisocial personality disorder: co-morbid Axis I mental disorders and health service use among a national household population. *Personality and Mental Health*, **3**, 151–164.

Young, J. E. (1994) *Cognitive Therapy for Personality Disorders: A Schema-Focused Approach*. Professional Resource Press.

CHAPTER 17

Mindfulness in the psychotherapy of personality disorder

Chris Mace

Summary Mindfulness has become a popular topic among psychological therapists. This chapter explains what mindfulness is and how it can be developed, before exploring how it has been incorporated within psychoanalytic and cognitive–behavioural psychotherapies that can be used with people with personality disorders. These reflect general as well as specific presumed therapeutic actions. At present, variations in the way mindfulness is understood, taught and applied mean that it is too early to fully assess its potential, but its capacity to potentiate other kinds of intervention and to reduce reactivity to several kinds of problematic experience recommend it in work with people with clinically complex needs.

'Mindfulness' is a common translation of a term from Buddhist psychology that means 'awareness' or 'bare attention'. It is frequently used to refer to a way of paying attention that is sensitive, accepting and independent of any thoughts that may be present. The definitions in Box 17.1 represent some different ways of expressing this. Although mindfulness can sound quite ordinary and spontaneous, it is the antithesis of mental habits in which the mind is on 'automatic pilot'. In this usual state, most experiences pass by completely unrecognised, and awareness is dominated by a stream of

---

Box 17.1 Some definitions of mindfulness

Mindfulness is:

'facing the bare facts of experience, seeing each event as though occurring for the first time' (Goleman, 1988: p. 20)

'keeping one's consciousness alive to the present reality' (Hanh, 1991: p. 11)

'paying attention in a particular way: on purpose, in the present moment, and nonjudgmentally' (Kabat-Zinn, 1994: p. 4)

'awareness of present experience with acceptance' (Germer, 2005: p. 7)

---

internal comment whose insensitivity to what is immediately present can seem mindless. Although most people knowingly experience mindfulness for very brief periods only, it can be developed with practice.

Differences can be discerned in how different practitioners use mindfulness. Some of these reflect the hazards of translation and others reflect long-standing ambiguities within Buddhist psychology (for an extended discussion see Mace, 2008, 2009). One nuance that should not be overlooked, because it has implications for therapeutic practice, is evident from the way 'mindfulness' can be used to denote self-awareness or self-consciousness as well as an awareness of what is immediately present. There is an important element of self-recollection in traditional Buddhist conceptions of mindfulness too, evident when the awareness of internal psychological events such as feelings and patterns of thought is promoted through deliberate verbal reflection, as in: 'Now I am doing x, now I am feeling y'. This aspect has been played down in the contemporary definitions quoted in Box 17.1, but it has been important in the therapeutic use of mindfulness, particularly within dialectical behaviour therapy (DBT).

Once mindfulness is identified with a kind of self-consciousness, it is likely to become confused with Fonagy et al's (2002) concept of 'mentalisation'. As a reflective capacity that was neatly summarised by Elizabeth Meins as 'mind-mindedness', or the capacity to discern whole mental states in the self and others, mentalisation is distinct from mindfulness. Mindfulness remains a quality of awareness that is pre-reflective and independent of an ability to verbalise (Brown & Ryan, 2004). The capacities to be mindful and to mentalise are not exclusive and can complement one another in clinical practice (Wallin, 2007).

Interest in the potential health benefits of mindfulness has fuelled attempts to define its components more clearly through empirical research. These are in their infancy, but indicate that two components could be primary: the capacities to direct and maintain receptive awareness, and to sustain an accepting attitude towards all experience (Bishop et al, 2004). Studies of relatively inexperienced practitioners of mindfulness show such a high correlation between these aspects that it has been suggested the first alone might be taken as a marker of its depth (Brown & Ryan, 2004). However, more recent findings suggest that accumulating experience leads to a continuing deepening of non-reactivity once the capacity to maintain an open awareness develops to a consistent level (Lykins & Baer, 2009). Research continues to confirm that some facets of mindfulness emerge only with experience (Mace, 2006), making it essential that length of practice is taken into account in experimental assessments.

Given that not all commentators agree on what is specific to mindfulness, and its capacity to vary according to individuals' experience, generalisation about neurobiological correlates must be treated with caution. It does seem that development of the capacity to maintain a continuing non-verbal awareness of being aware is associated with increased coherence

---

Box 17.2 Techniques for experiencing mindfulness

Formal practices

- Sitting meditations (attending to breathing, body sensations, sounds, thoughts, etc.)
- Movement meditations (walking meditation, mindful yoga stretches)
- Group exchange (led exercises, guided discussion of experience)

Informal practices

- Mindful activity (mindful eating, cleaning, driving, etc.)
- Structured exercises (self-monitoring, problem-solving, etc.)
- Mindful reading (especially poetry)
- Mini-meditations (e.g. the '3 minute breathing space')

---

of electroencephalograph (EEG) activity, and that bilateral slowing is commonly found during mindful meditation (Austin, 2006).

More speculative findings concerning asymmetric prefrontal activation in new students of mindfulness remain to be confirmed (Treadway & Lazar, 2009), but have interesting implications as they have also been associated with positive changes in affect.

Techniques for developing mindfulness

Some people develop mindfulness because pursuits such as regularly playing a musical instrument can foster it. However, it is usually learned through a mixture of guided instruction and personal practice. The techniques that are generally used (Boxes 17.2 and 17.3) can be divided into those that require periods of withdrawal from other activities to practise extended exercises (formal practices) and those that can be undertaken throughout the day, amid other activities (informal practices).

Mindfulness and psychotherapy

Mindfulness places attention at the heart of psychotherapy. Given that psychotherapy depends so heavily on the interaction between therapist and patient, it is remarkable how little prominence attention has received. Notable exceptions have included Freud, who believed psychoanalysts' attention to be essential to their practice. The psychoanalyst should maintain:

'evenly hovering attention [...] all conscious exertion is to be withheld from the capacity for attention, and one's "unconscious memory" is to be given full play; or to express it in terms of technique, pure and simple: one has simply to listen and not to trouble to keep in mind anything in particular'. Failure to do this risks "never finding anything but what he already knows"' (Freud, 1912: pp. 111–112).

> **Box 17.3** Sample instructions for mindful breathing
>
> 1 Settle into a comfortable, balanced sitting position on a chair or floor in a quiet room.
> 2 Keep your spine erect. Allow your eyes to close.
> 3 Bring your awareness to the sensations of contact wherever your body is being supported. Gently explore how this really feels.
> 4 Become aware of your body's movements during breathing, at the chest, at the abdomen.
> 5 As the breath passes in and out of the body, bring your awareness to the changing sensations at the abdominal wall. Maintain this awareness throughout each breath and from one breath to the next.
> 6 Allow the breath simply to breathe, without trying to change or control it. Just noticing the sensations that go with every movement.
> 7 As soon as you notice your mind wandering, bring your awareness gently back to the movement of the abdomen. Do this over and over again. Every time, it is fine. It helps the awareness to grow.
> 8 Be patient with yourself.
> 9 After 15 minutes or so, bring the awareness gently back to your whole body, sitting in the room.
> 10 Open your eyes. Be ready for whatever's next.

An equally significant injunction of this kind can be found, appropriately, in the English psychoanalyst Wilfred Bion's *Attention and Interpretation*:

> 'the capacity to forget, the ability to eschew desire and understanding, must be regarded as essential discipline for the psycho-analyst. Failure to practise this discipline will lead to a steady deterioration in the powers of observation whose maintenance is essential. The vigilant submission to such discipline will by degrees strengthen the analyst's mental powers just in proportion as lapses in this discipline will debilitate them' (Bion, 1970: pp. 51–52).

The strictures of Freud and Bion are intended to sharpen the analyst's receptivity and acuity of observation, including the uncomprehending apprehension of features that would otherwise be obliterated by the usual habits of the analyst's mind. Attention becomes important because training it helps the analyst to observe and to analyse more effectively.

While Bion was still formulating his views on psychoanalytic procedure, Karen Horney had made attention the cornerstone of the analyst's technique. She insisted that effective work reflects the quality of the analyst's attention, which should be whole-hearted, comprehensive and productive. The first two of these characteristics stand for the functions of self-forgetting and openness that are effectively prefigured in Freud and Bion. The third introduces an additional element – how attention can 'set something going' for the patient in terms of their self-awareness and self-realisation (Horney, 1951: p. 189).

It may be no accident that Horney had some contact with Buddhism at the time of formulating how, in addition to helping the analyst function as a trained observer, the extension of attention towards the patient can be therapeutic in itself. Two other analytic writers who successfully integrated Buddhist understanding into their work have provided clarifications about 'bare attention'. Mark Epstein writes 'It is the fundamental tenet of Buddhist psychology that this kind of attention is, in itself, healing' (Epstein, 1996: p. 110). And Nina Coltart applies this directly to psychoanalysis:

> 'the teaching of Buddhism is what is called *bhavana* or the cultivation of the mind with the direct aim of the relief of suffering in all its forms, however small; the method and the aim are regarded as indissolubly interconnected; so it seems to me logical that neutral attention to the immediate present, which includes first and foremost the study of our own minds, should turn out to be our sharpest and most reliable therapeutic tool in psychoanalytic technique since there, too, we aim to study the workings of the mind, our own and others, with a view to relieving suffering' (Coltart, 1993: p. 183).

Epstein and Coltart also illustrate quite different ways of introducing mindful awareness to psychoanalytic psychotherapy. Coltart did nothing overtly to change the rules of analytic procedure with her patients. She recognised that the quality of her own close attention affected the atmosphere and activity of her sessions, commenting on how they acquired the quality of a meditation as she worked intuitively in a way she likens to Bion's ideal (Molino, 1998: p. 177). Epstein has long put analytic thinking, particularly that of Winnicott, in the service of what he refers to as Buddhist psychotherapy. This is reflected in his attitude to technique. He likens his role to that of a coach who teaches people how to venture into their unexperienced feelings. The methods he uses differ from patient to patient, and can include instruction in meditation.

Quite distinct ways of incorporating mindfulness into psychotherapy have arisen within the cognitive–behavioural tradition over the past 20 years. Cognitive psychology and Buddhist psychology are in broad agreement about the dependence of emotional disturbance on pervasive patterns of thinking and perception. In contrast to most psychodynamic therapies, recent cognitive–behavioural treatments tend to be designed as interventions for people with a specific set of clinical needs or disorder, rather than as a broad-range therapy. These aims have informed the design of a flood of new 'mindfulness-based' interventions, a sample of which are listed in Box 17.4.

Mindfulness-based stress reduction

Although Kabat-Zinn has always stated that mindfulness-based stress reduction (MBSR) is not a therapy (he feels that patients should assume continuing responsibility for their own health), its influence on overtly therapeutic interventions has been profound. Mindfulness-based stress reduction was developed for use in general hospitals with patients suffering

> **Box 17.4** Mindfulness in the cognitive–behavioural tradition
>
> - Mindfulness-based relapse prevention (Witkiewitz *et al*, 2005)
> - Mindfulness-based cognitive therapy (Segal *et al*, 2002)
> - Mindfulness-based eating awareness training (Kristeller & Hallett, 1999)
> - Dialectical behaviour therapy (Linehan, 1993)
> - Acceptance and commitment therapy (Hayes *et al*, 1999)

from painful, chronic, disabling or terminal conditions. Over the course of eight weekly sessions, alongside psychoeducation about the nature of stress and its amplification through habitual reactions, patients receive instruction and practice in the 'body scan' and sitting and movement meditations. The group format of therapy (up to 30 patients concurrently) encourages discussion. Individuals are expected to continue practising each exercise as it is introduced. Instructors are required to have extended personal experience of the techniques concerned, which they call upon in guiding patients through them. A trial of MBSR in a general hospital reported reductions in patients' levels of anxiety and depression (Reibel *et al*, 2001).

Mindfulness-based cognitive therapy

Mindfulness-based cognitive therapy (MBCT; Segal *et al*, 2002) adds training in specific cognitive skills to the framework of mindfulness-based stress reduction (MBSR; Kabat-Zinn, 1990). Very similar in content to MBSR, it is usually taught to patients in smaller groups. The training in mindfulness places marginally less emphasis on bodily movement and incorporates a '3 minute breathing space' – a very brief, transportable routine for rapidly restoring a mindful attitude that effectively bridges formal and informal practices. Instead of stress education, exercises for the monitoring and analysis of dysfunctional thinking and its specific relationship to mood are included. Although it is being increasingly used as a treatment, MBCT was originally developed as a preventive intervention for use with people with an established history of relapsing depression. Its demonstrable effectiveness in reducing the frequency of relapse in people who have had three or more depressive episodes has been attributed to its capacity to prevent chronic depressive ruminations from maintaining this vulnerability.

Mindfulness-based eating awareness training

Mindfulness-based eating awareness training (MB-EAT) is an extension of MBSR and MBCT designed for people with binge eating disorder. The programme, which usually continues for longer than 8 weeks, is based on the premised that mindfulness can reverse the lack of awareness of bodily and internal states that has been commonly observed among people with eating disorders. In practice, Kristeller & Hallett (1999) have found restoration of sensitivity to feelings of satiety to be therapeutically essential. A complementary goal with this population has been to provide a way of living with prominent guilt feelings. Meditations designed to foster feelings of forgiveness are a key component of the programme for this reason. (Here, modern practice is replicating traditional Buddhist training, where meditations to develop concentration and mindfulness are often interspersed with others that develop positive social emotions such as loving kindness or compassion.)

Dialectical behaviour therapy

Dialectical behaviour therapy (DBT) takes a didactic approach to 'mindfulness skills training', using both group and individual therapy. Compared to MBSR and MBCT, the teaching of mindfulness in DBT is more remedial in character and is arguably suited for people with more evident difficulties in maintaining attention. It is fitting that DBT is used primarily with people diagnosed with borderline personality disorder, who are frequently deficient in this respect. The mindfulness skills that are taught divide into two sets: the 'what' skills of observing, describing and participating, and the 'how' skills of being non-judgemental and compassionate. A variety of exercises are used and patients are encouraged to try them as they go about their usual business rather than in extended formal practices such as meditation. Unlike MBSR instructors and MBCT therapists, DBT therapists are not expected to have or to maintain personal practice of mindfulness, although many do. The understanding and quality of 'mindfulness' that is offered through this approach can vary significantly in practice. Although mindfulness occupied a pivotal position in the original formulation of the model, this appears to be reducing as it becomes more widely used.

Acceptance and commitment therapy

Acceptance and commitment therapy (ACT) is based on a radical behavioural analysis of patients' difficulties. From this, a selection of appropriate therapeutic strategems is made from a full and varied menu. They fall under six main headings, four of which are 'mindfulness functions': 'contact with the present moment', 'acceptance', 'cognitive defusion' and 'self as context'. The first two correspond to the receptive awareness and suspension of judgement that have been key to modern conceptions of mindfulness. The third, cognitive defusion, a deliberate dis-identification from thoughts, is the expected outcome of a series of exercises that focus directly on clients' relationship to their thoughts. Box 17.5 gives an example of a practical exercise that a therapist might introduce for this. In practice, it would be followed by detailed examination of the client's experience by the therapist to underline the intended lesson. The fourth function, self as context, is

---

Box 17.5 Exercise to help cognitive defusion

This exercise is to help you see the difference between looking at your thoughts and looking from your thoughts. Imagine you are on the bank of a steadily flowing stream, looking down at the water. Upstream some trees are dropping leaves, which are floating past you on the surface of the water. Just watch them passing by, without interrupting the flow. Whenever you are aware of a thought, let the words be written on one of the leaves as it floats by. Allow the leaf to carry the thought away. If a thought is more of a picture thought, let a leaf take on the image as it moves along. If you get thoughts about the exercise, see these too on a leaf. Let them be carried away like any other thought, as you carry on watching.

At some point, the flow will seem to stop. You are no longer on the bank seeing the thoughts on the leaves. As soon as you notice this, see if you can catch what was happening just before the flow stopped. There will be a thought that you have 'bought'. See how it took over. Notice the difference between thoughts passing by and thoughts thinking for you. Do this whenever you notice the flow has stopped. Then return to the bank, letting every thought find its leaf as it floats steadily past.

---

characteristic of ACT, referring to a shift of perspective in which the client is encouraged to check and reject assumptions about the substantiality and continuity of the experienced self.

The therapy is designed to be flexibly adapted to a wide range of clinical problems (and therapist preferences). As its exercises are often elaborate yet intended to be used across various situations, they do not always fit easily into the formal/informal framework of Box 17.2. If the repertoire of existing exercises does not match a particular clinical need, or a client's preferences, the therapist is encouraged to devise an alternative. Throughout, means are adjusted to goals. There is no requirement for therapist or patient to undergo formal meditation as a way to any of the mindfulness functions, although they are free to do so.

Although ACT has been used across a broad spectrum of conditions, it is finding increasing application in work with people with personality disorders. The freedom it offers to swing between its 'acceptance' and 'commitment' components parallels the switches between acceptance and change that are what makes the practice of DBT 'dialectical'.

Mindfulness and psychological distress

It is clear from the above that different mindfulness-based psychotherapies have different aims. Traditional mindfulness practice was expected to lead to differences at the level of being, in a way that is compatible with the optimistic formulations found in psychoanalytic conceptions of a 'true self'. The tendency of cognitive–behavioural practice has been to formulate goals that are more specific, problem oriented and measurable. This specificity is

> **Box 17.6**   Specific applications of mindfulness-based interventions
>
> Mood (anxiety, depression)
>
> Intrusions (ruminations, hallucinations, memories)
>
> Behaviours (bingeing, addiction, self-harm, violence)
>
> Problems of relating (attitudes, empathy)
>
> Problems of self (self-consciousness, self-hatred)

useful in summarising some of the phenomena to which mindfulness-based therapies have been applied (Box 17.6).

People who have circumscribed difficulties in one or two of these categories are likely to receive a traditional diagnosis from DSM-IV's Axis I (American Psychiatric Association, 1994). Mindfulness training is likely to help them through actions that differ depending on the problem concerned. The use of mindfulness to reduce subjective anxiety appears to be an example of facilitated exposure that aims to reverse affective avoidance by strengthening the capacity to face and investigate warded-off fears while maintaining an open and accepting attitude (Roemer & Orsillo, 2002). The application of MBCT in relation to depressive ruminations is hypothesised to bring about a general switch in 'mental mode'. Accordingly, mindfulness brings about a 'decentring' of each successive experience that is incompatible with the chain reactions characteristic of the ordinary mental mode. If depressive ruminations no longer receive the kind of reactive attention that allows them to amplify, the negative mood changes that are usually consequent on this will be prevented (Segal *et al*, 2002: p. 75). The expectation that MB-EAT relies on an increased capacity to recognise internal bodily cues has been mentioned already. Like the hypothesis of Segal and colleagues, it has received some support from process measures during clinical trials.

People whose difficulties encompass most or even all of the features listed in Box 17.6 are the most likely to be considered to have personality disorders. Acquisition of mindfulness skills seems an efficient method of simultaneously addressing several areas of problematic experience (Wupperman *et al*, 2009). In assessing the current state of mindfulness-based therapies for people with personality disorder, several observations should be made. First, other problematic feelings can be prominent in the experience of people diagnosed with borderline personality disorder – feelings of emptiness or abandonment, for instance. These are likely to benefit from additional therapeutic actions, including the demonstration of warmth and mentalisation as well as encouraging the development of a capacity for compassionate self-soothing (Gilbert, 2007). Second, the pre-eminent mindfulness-based treatment, DBT, continues to have demonstrably greater impact on self-harming than on other aspects of borderline personality disorder (Linehan *et al*, 2006). Third, despite the fact that the intervention has other components in addition to training in mindfulness skills, evaluations have not attempted to independently assess recipients' mindfulness in the course of treatment. Its contribution as a mediator therefore remains unclear. Fourth, much of the rationale for the apparent effects of mindfulness must remain speculative at this stage and alternative explanations can be found. For instance, when mindfulness within DBT has been associated with a reduction in impulsive behaviour, this has been attributed both to an improved awareness of all the processes that lead up to an action (e.g. Linehan, 1993: p. 63) and to greater acceptance of the painful negative emotions that otherwise trigger impulsive actions (e.g. Welch *et al*, 2006: p. 122).

It should not be assumed that all of the clinical consequences of mindfulness practice are necessarily always positive or therapeutic. Attrition during trials of mindfulness-based interventions is rarely explored and the whole question of side-effects is underresearched. Possible unintended effects that are known to be exacerbated during intensive training retreats include restlessness, anxiety, depression, guilt and hallucinosis (Albeniz & Holmes, 2000; Mace, 2006).

The therapeutic future of mindfulness

Recognising the importance of how attention is used in psychotherapy cuts across divisions between the cognitive–behavioural and psychodynamic approaches such as those considered here. The challenges it poses are both theoretical and practical. We have seen how a mindful therapy can have distinctive goals, as well as novel ways of conceptualising what therapeutic success depends upon. Informing these is a psychological understanding based on a view of individualism, and of how people affect one another, that is different from those underpinning most established therapeutic models.

The practical challenges differ according to therapists' practices and attitudes in ways that have also been illustrated. Some psychodynamic psychotherapists have changed the way they advise and instruct patients in order to help them develop mindfulness, but others have not. Some cognitive–behavioural psychotherapists have changed the way they attend to their own inner feelings so that they can work mindfully with patients, but others have not. In general, some therapists will relish such challenges and others will not, ensuring that enthusiasm for mindfulness-based interventions is likely to be balanced by considerable scepticism. While much remains to be worked out at theoretical and practical levels, the future of mindfulness-based therapies is likely to depend on demonstrations of their distinct, effective and lasting contributions that other clinicians cannot ignore.

- It will be evident there are many possible ways of incorporating mindfulness into psychotherapeutic practice. This diversity, coupled with the important fact that a state of consciousness such as mindfulness is both silent and invisible, is likely to complicate attempts to demonstrate independent clinical effects that can confidently be attributed to mindfulness and nothing else. Without objective corroboration of when a therapist or a patient is mindfully aware, it is difficult for comparative studies of treatment effects to be persuasive that mindfulness is a discriminating variable between groups and/or that it mediates any observed changes. Although worthwhile attempts are continuing to refine measures of mindfulness, these are limited by the lack of a consistent yet comprehensive operational definition. Ideally, this would be sensitive to differing degrees of attainment and supported by reliable neurophysiological markers.

In the meantime, studies of the outcome and process of mindful psychotherapies are necessarily limited in their scope and interpretation. It may be important to remember too that none of the therapeutic applications of mindfulness that have been investigated to date has a unique claim on its potential, in the way that a new drug treatment might be designed to fulfil a particular requirement. Even when drugs are created for specific purposes, they have a habit of revealing other, unexpected and sometimes more beneficial uses than those for which they were developed – as well as new and unsuspected side-effects. The present situation, in which the rapid growth of new, often manualised, mindfulness-based therapies is being accompanied by controlled studies that are restricted to consideration of a very narrow range of quantified outcomes, presents a contradiction. It lies in the contrast between the restrictiveness of this methodology and what mindfulness is already taken to be – a receptive state of awareness in which any and all experiences are accepted without automatic judgement.

Realisation of the potential range and modes of action of mindfulness in therapeutic settings may therefore need currently favoured methods of investigation to be complemented by others. These would pay far more detailed and inclusive attention to what happens within and between therapists and patients in terms of awareness during therapeutic sessions. Continuing attempts to establish the role of mindfulness in interventions for people with personality disorders, as elsewhere, seem likely to benefit from a more patient and phenomenologically alert approach to its description.

References

Albeniz, A. & Holmes, J. (2000) Meditation: concepts, effects and uses in therapy. *International Journal of Psychotherapy*, **5**, 49–58.

American Psychiatric Association (1994) *Diagnostic and Statistical Manual of Mental Disorders (4th edn) (DSM-IV)*. APA.

Austin, J. H. (2006) *Zen-Brain Reflections*. MIT Press.

Bion, W. (1970) *Attention and Interpretation*. Karnac.

Bishop, S. R., Lau, M., Shapiro, S., *et al* (2004) Mindfulness: a proposed operational definition. *Clinical Psychology: Science and Practice*, **11**, 230–241.

Brown, K. W. & Ryan, R. M. (2004) Perils and promise in defining and measuring mindfulness. *Clinical Psychology: Science and Practice*, **11**, 242–248.

Coltart, N. (1993) *Slouching towards Bethlehem... And Further Psychoanalytic Explorations*. Free Association Books.

Epstein, M. (1996) *Thoughts without a Thinker*. Duckworth.

Epstein, M. (1998) *Going to Pieces without Falling Apart*. Thorsons.

Fonagy, P., Gergely, G., Jurist, E., *et al* (2002) *Affect Regulation, Mentalization and the Development of the Self*. Other Press.

Freud, S. (1912) Recommendations for physicians on the psychoanalytic method of treatment. Reprinted (1953–1974) in the *Standard Edition of the Complete Psychological Works of Sigmund Freud* (trans. and ed. J. Strachey), vol. 12. Hogarth Press.

Germer, C. K. (2005) What is mindfulness? In *Mindfulness and Psychotherapy* (eds C. K. Germer, R. D. Siegel & P. R. Fulton), pp. 1–27. Guilford Press.

Gilbert, P. (2007) Evolved minds and compassion in the therapeutic relationship. In *The Therapeutic Relationship in the Cognitive Behavioral Psychotherapies* (eds P. Gilbert & R. L. Leahy), pp. 106–142. Routledge.

Goleman, D. (1988) *The Meditative Mind*. Putnam.

Hanh, T. N. (1991) *The Miracle of Mindfulness*. Rider.

Hayes, S. C., Strosahl, K. D. & Wilson, K. D. (1999) *Acceptance and Commitment Therapy: An Experiential Approach to Behavior Change*. Guilford Press.

Horney, K. (1951) The quality of the analyst's attention. Reprinted (1999) in *Karen Horney: The Therapeutic Process* (ed. B. J. Paris), pp. 186–190. Yale University Press.

Kabat-Zinn, J. (1990) *Full Catastrophe Living: Using the Wisdom of Your Body and Mind to Face Stress, Pain, and Illness*. Delacorte Press.

Kabat-Zinn, J. (1994) *Mindfulness Meditation for Everyday Life*. Piatkus Books.

Kristeller, J. L. & Hallett, C. B. (1999) An exploratory study of a meditation-based intervention for binge eating disorder. *Journal of Health Psychology*, **4**, 357–363.

Linehan, M. (1993) *Skills Training Manual for Treating Borderline Personality Disorder*. Guilford Press.

Linehan, M. M., Comtois, K. A., Murray, A. M., *et al* (2006) Two-year randomized controlled trial and follow-up of dialectical behaviour therapy versus therapy by experts for suicidal behaviors and borderline personality disorder. *Archives of General Psychiatry*, **48**, 1060–1064.

Lykins, E. L. B. & Baer, R. A. (2009) Psychological functioning in a sample of long-term practitioners of mindfulness meditation. *Journal of Cognitive Psychotherapy*, **23**, 226–241.

Mace, C. (2006) Long-term impacts of mindfulness practice on wellbeing: new findings from qualitative research. In *Dimensions of Well-being. Research and Intervention* (ed. A. Delle Fave), pp. 455–469. Franco Angeli.

Mace, C. (2008) *Mindfulness and Mental Health*. Routledge.

Mace, C. (2009) Mindfulness and technologies of healing: lessons from Western practice. In *Self and No-Self: Continuing the Dialogue Between Buddhism and Psychotherapy* (eds D. Mathers, M. E. Miller & O. Ando), pp. 132–143. Brunner-Routledge.

Molino, A. (1998) Slouching towards Buddhism: a conversation with Nina Coltart. In *The Couch and the Tree: Dialogues in Psychoanalysis and Buddhism* (ed. A. Molino), pp. 170–182. North Point Press.

Reibel, D. K., Greeson, J. M., Brainard, G. C., *et al* (2001) Mindfulness-based stress reduction and health-related quality of life in a heterogeneous patient population. *General Hospital Psychiatry*, **23**, 183–192.

Roemer, L. & Orsillo, S. M. (2002) Expanding our conceptualisation of and treatment for generalised anxiety disorder: integrating mindfulness/acceptance-based approaches with existing cognitive–behavioural models. *Clinical Psychology: Science and Practice*, **9**, 54–68.

Segal, Z., Williams, J. M. G. & Teasdale, J. (2002) *Mindfulness-Based Cognitive Therapy for Depression*. John Wiley & Sons.

Treadway, M. T. & Lazar, S. W. (2009) The neurobiology of mindfulness. In *Clinical Handbook of Mindfulness* (ed. F. Didonna), pp. 45–58. Springer.

Wallin, D. (2007) *Attachment in Psychotherapy*. Guilford Press.

Welch, S. S., Rizvi, S. & Dimidjian, S. (2006) Mindfulness in dialectical behavior therapy (DBT) for borderline personality disorder. In *Mindfulness-based Treatment Approaches: Clinician's Guide to Evidence Base and Applications* (ed. R. A. Baer), pp. 117–139. Academic Press.

Witkiewitz, K., Marlatt, G. A. & Walker, D. (2005) Mindfulness-based relapse prevention for alcohol and substance use disorders. *Journal of Cognitive Psychotherapy*, **19**, 211–228.

Wupperman, P., Neumann, C. S., Whitman, J., *et al* (2009) The role of mindfulness in borderline personality disorder features. *Journal of Nervous and Mental Disease*, **197**, 766–771.

CHAPTER 18

Cognitive analytic therapy for borderline personality disorder

Ian B. Kerr, Dawn Bennett and Carlos Mirapeix

Summary Cognitive analytic therapy (CAT) is a still-evolving integrative and relational model that conceptualises borderline personality disorder as a pervasive and complex dissociative disorder of the self arising largely as a consequence of long-term, developmental psychological trauma in the context of dysfunctional formative relationships and neurobiological vulnerability. Therapy aims initially at the collaborative creation, through a benign and non-collusive relationship, of empathic and validating descriptions and understandings of current difficulties and of their background through written (narrative) and diagrammatic reformulation. These aid self-reflective capacity and integration of the self. They also serve as 'route maps' for the work of therapy and contribute to the therapeutic alliance and to the negotiation of often 'difficult' transference–countertransference enactments. Many of the contributory and perpetuating factors of problems in borderline personality disorder are social and relational and these may be addressed using systemic 'contextual reformulation' in multidisciplinary team-based approaches. Cognitive analytic therapy offers a robust and coherent conceptual framework within which a range of further interventions can be undertaken for various problems and symptomatic behaviours.

In this chapter we describe the conceptual framework and key features of the cognitive analytic therapy (CAT) approach to borderline-type personality disorders (Ryle, 1997, 2004; Ryle & Kerr, 2002; Kerr & Ryle, 2005). We also consider how effective these may be for different patients in different settings and implications of this for further (comparative) research and evaluation. We note some current problems with the concept of borderline personality disorder. These include, in particular, ongoing uncertainty regarding its nosological status, its heterogeneity in terms of both apparent aetiology and clinical presentation, and the range of apparently different 'brand name' models that have addressed it, each with its own emphases and specialist terminology. It will be a major challenge for the future to clarify which approaches do in fact effect lasting change and how they do so, and to elucidate the undoubted considerable commonalities between differing models (Roth & Fonagy, 2004; National Collaborating Centre for Mental Health, 2009).

CAT as a model of development and psychopathology

A still-evolving integrative model of psychological development and therapy, CAT stresses the social and relational formation of the self and its 'psychopathology' (Box 18.1). It was first formulated by Anthony Ryle over a period of several decades, and has been extended both theoretically and clinically by a number of other workers, notably Mikael Leiman in Finland (Ryle & Kerr, 2002; Kerr & Ryle, 2005). Although initially representing an attempt to integrate the valid and effective elements of psychoanalytic object relations theory and the then evolving discipline of cognitive therapy (including, notably, Kelly's personal construct theory), CAT has subsequently been further transformed by consideration of Vygotsky's activity theory (Leiman, 1992; Ryle & Kerr, 2002), notions of a dialogical self deriving from Bakhtin (Leiman, 1992, 2004) and important developments in infant psychology (Stern, 2000; Trevarthen & Aitken, 2001; Reddy, 2008). The latter include findings stressing the actively intersubjective nature of developing infants and their predisposition and need for active, playful collaboration and 'companionship' (Trevarthen & Aitken, 2001). These findings have

---

Box 18.1 Key features of the cognitive analytic therapy model of development and psychopathology

The model is predicated on a fundamentally relational and social concept of self; this implies that individual psychopathology cannot be considered apart from the sociocultural context in which it arose and within which it is currently located.

In the context of individual genetic and temperamental variation, early socially meaningful experience is internalised as a repertoire of reciprocal roles.

A reciprocal role is a complex of implicit relational memory that includes affect and perception and is characterised by both child-derived and parent/culture-derived poles; a role may be associated with a clear dialogical 'voice'.

Enactment of a reciprocal role always anticipates or attempts to elicit a reciprocal reaction from a historic or current other.

Reciprocal roles and their recurrent procedural enactments determine both subsequent interpersonal interactions and also internal dialogue and self-management.

All mental activity, whether conscious or unconscious, is rooted in and highly determined by our repertoire of reciprocal roles.

Human psychopathology is rooted in and highly determined by a repertoire of maladaptive or unhealthy reciprocal roles.

More severe and complex damage to the self may occur as a result of chronic developmental trauma/deprivation, resulting in dissociation and disruption of the repertoire of reciprocal roles and consequent impairment of self-reflective and executive function. These phenomena are accounted for in the 'multiple self states model' of borderline personality disorder.

---

important implications for the aims and style of psychotherapy. In CAT, they have influenced the concept of the formation of the (highly social) self and, correspondingly, of its deformation or psychopathology. Cognitive analytic therapy describes early internalised, formative relational experience in terms of a repertoire of 'reciprocal roles', and describes the subsequent habitual coping or responsive (Leiman, 2004) behavioural patterns as 'reciprocal role procedures' (RRPs). These are understood to be partly determined by inherited temperamental variation and the neurobiological consequences of early (e.g. traumatic) experience. Common reciprocal roles range from, for example, 'properly cared for–properly caring for' at one extreme to 'neglected and abused–neglecting and abusing' at the other. Maladaptive reciprocal role procedures are important therapeutic targets.

Cognitive analytic therapy adopts a fundamentally relational focus, and stresses the importance of the transformative and mutative psychological internalisation within a developing 'individual' of surrounding social structures and conditions, and of semiotically mediated interpersonal experience. The outcome of this process is an 'individual' who cannot ever be simply individual, but who is socially formed and constituted by developmental interpersonal experience and cultural values and whose very sense of subjective self, relations with others, behaviour and values are socially determined and relative and, for the most, part unconscious. This viewpoint is further supported empirically by observational and experimental studies (Cox & Lightfoot, 1997; Reddy, 2008). An important corollary of the process of internalisation, understood in this Vygotskian sense, is that although it is an individual who experiences and presents with distress and disability, there is in an important sense no such thing as individual psychopathology – only sociopsychopathology (Kerr *et al*, 2007; Kerr, 2009). The implications of this statement, which may sound to most contemporary, post-Cartesian, Western sensibilities largely counterintuitive, will be elaborated below.

A further implication of the model, and of these understandings, is that ultimately therapy may only, or best, be achieved by engaging the ownership, support and participation of a broader community, notwithstanding that specialist understandings and expertise may be required to underpin or support mental health and well-being initiatives overall. But to move towards this, a major paradigm shift is required that our services and our society as a whole will need to address, implement and evaluate (James, 2007; Kerr & Leighton, 2008; Wilkinson & Pickett, 2009). At the least, in routine day-to-day work a coherent model of the socially constituted self can enable better communication and lessen professional stress.

The CAT model of borderline personality disorder

In common with approaches such as psychodynamic therapy, CAT adopts a dimensional approach to the conceptualisation of degrees of damage to and dysfunction of the self. This cuts across current conventional 'shopping list' diagnostic approaches that describe mental disorders as discrete and separate entities of comparable status. Borderline personality disorder is seen from a CAT perspective as a severe and complex disorder frequently characterised by considerable comorbidity. The self is understood as operating in states ranging from normal multiplicity through to those of overt dissociation (Ryle & Kerr, 2002; Ryle & Fawkes, 2007; Mirapeix, 2008). Lesser degrees of damage to the self are characterised by the presence of mildly dysfunctional or maladaptive reciprocal role procedures (Box 18.1) for coping, located within a more integrated self capable of self-reflection, empathic interactions with others and an advanced capacity for executive function. However, more severe degrees of damage are characterised by failure of integration of structures of the self (notably, its repertoire of reciprocal roles and reciprocal role procedures), and by lack of self-reflective capacity and problems associated with a coherent and continuous sense of identity (Ryle, 1997, 2004; Kerr & Ryle, 2005). Such disorder is also typically characterised by extreme psychological distress that may manifest as stress-related dissociation into different self states. Dissociation is also conceived of as the principle mechanism through which developmentally abusive, traumatic and depriving interpersonal experiences have a deleterious effect on the developing self. The damage is considered to occur in the context of likely neurobiological vulnerability through, for example, possibly impaired impulse control and/or proclivity to dissociation as a defensive mechanism in the face of (psychological) trauma (Ryle & Kerr, 2002).

This conceptualisation addresses and largely accounts for the range of psychopathology encountered in borderline personality disorder, in particular the tendency under pressure to switch suddenly and apparently unpredictably between different self states, with their associated differing reciprocal roles and reciprocal role procedures (Pollock *et al*, 2001). These switches between self states represent some of the most problematic and challenging enactments encountered in working in any capacity with people with borderline personality disorder, often causing such patients to be seen as 'difficult' or 'hard to help' – at least in the absence of a coherent model accounting for these interactions.

Self states and their identification

The presence of different self states has been empirically demonstrated and validated in several clinically based studies using the Personality Structure Questionnaire (PSQ) and the States Description Procedure (SDP). These instruments were developed from within CAT, but have come to have broader applicability (Bedford *et al*, 2009).

The PSQ consists of eight pairs of contrasting descriptions of the self, each item scored between 1 (stable) and 5 (changeable). The mean scores of samples of healthy people range from 19.7 to 23.3, whereas those of people with borderline personality disorder range from 30.4 to 31.3 (Pollock *et al*,

2001). Scores on the PSQ correlated with a number of other measures of identity disturbance and personality fragmentation, establishing the PSQ as a valid, psychometrically sound measure. The broader validity and utility of this measure has been subsequently demonstrated in this and other patient populations (Bedford *et al*, 2009).

The SDP (Bennett *et al*, 2005) involves patients in a process of guided introspection, generating detailed and clinically useful understandings of their states and state switches. The first part of the instrument consists of names and descriptions of 10 commonly encountered states, drawn from clinical experience and from Golynkina & Ryle's (1999) study of partially dissociated states in borderline personality disorder. Respondents are invited to identify any states that they experience, to modify the name of the state if they wish, and to select from or add to the listed descriptions. The second part of the SDP is completed for each of the identified states. It consists of detailed enquiries about the frequency, duration, mode and provocation of entry into and exit from the state, and the accompanying emotional and physical symptoms.

Bennett & Ryle (2005) report a series of 12 patients, all of whom had been diagnosed with borderline personality disorder and/or had scored 28 or over on the PSQ. All 10 states on the SDP were recognised by at least half the sample. The most common were the 'victim' and 'bully' states (all participants), the 'zombie' state (11 participants) and the 'high' state (10 participants). The fact that every patient identified with the 'bully' and 'victim' states supports the assumption that experiences of abuse are very frequently a forerunner of borderline personality disorder and demonstrates how patients may identify with both poles of the abusing–abused reciprocal role pattern. The 'victim', 'soldiering on' and 'zombie' states are also similar, in that all are associated with slowness and exhaustion. The 'soldiering on' and 'victim' states are more associated with anxiety and anger than is the 'zombie' state, which is more often associated with dissociative symptoms. The study confirmed that the description of borderline personality disorder in terms of alternating states is meaningful to patients, and the model of the self as made up of distinct, identifiable states was supported, as it had been by Golynkina & Ryle (1999).

In clinical practice, Hubbuck (2008) reported that, of 32 patients with borderline personality disorder who had completed the SDP, 29 (90.6%) thought that it was 'of value' or of 'considerable value' to their therapy. The SDP helps people with borderline personality disorder to change the way they think about their states of mind. Referring to discussions about their states, Hubbuck reported that 'most of these patients probably finished therapy viewing their states of mind as carriers of highly condensed, highly systemic, and highly important information about their life histories and life plans', able to ask themselves 'What named state of mind am I in at this moment; and what is the reason for it?'. This adds to the likelihood that conscious, positive 'exits' will be sought.

An individual case formulation in terms of partially dissociated states, to which the SPD can contribute, can supplement current formal diagnostic procedures and provide valuable understanding to therapists and others concerned with the treatment and management of borderline personality disorder. More generally, the multiple self-states model and the SPD make it clear that integration must be a central aim in the treatment of borderline personality disorder. It also explains how treatment procedures and clinicians' activities may represent inadvertent collusion with the dysfunctional reciprocal role patterns associated with borderline states, thus undermining that aim.

This conceptualisation of a range of different reciprocal roles and reciprocal role procedures predicts and accounts for the range of comorbid conditions encountered in borderline personality disorder, such as substance misuse, self-harm, anxiety and depression. Given that reciprocal roles associated with self states are characterised by internalised 'inner voices' and beliefs, these may constitute important therapeutic targets. These voices and beliefs may be enacted through coping or responsive reciprocal role procedures in relation to the 'real' outside world, but also, critically, through self-to-self and self-management reciprocal role procedures.

The multiple self-states model, as noted previously by Ryle & Kerr (2002), provides in addition a clinically important understanding of the instability and discontinuities noted, but not explained, in six of the nine features contributing to the diagnosis of borderline personality disorder in DSM-IV (American Psychiatric Association, 1994), namely: unstable intense interpersonal relationships, identity disturbance, impulsivity, affective instability, inappropriate intense anger, and transient paranoid and dissociative symptoms. It has been suggested that 'instability' usually means having fallen below the diagnostic threshold after a considerable length of time (Gunderson, 2003). However, this definition does not address the clinically challenging instabilities due to sudden self-state switches that are evident over short periods and characteristic of these disorders.

It is fundamental to the CAT conceptualisation of borderline personality disorder that widely different, often very extreme reciprocal role enactments may be encountered in work with a patient and that they are likely to elicit corresponding reciprocal role enactments (or reactions) from professionals. These may in turn be mirrored and amplified throughout a healthcare (or other) system. This can have a major effect on the outcome of therapy and of overall clinical management. It is also understood that, as a result of stress-related extreme dissociation, different self states will be encountered, each characterised by essentially very different reciprocal roles and procedures. These reactions may include, for example, 'desperate ideal care-seeking' or 'zombie' states, or enactments of abusive rage towards the self or others. A major interest of workers within the CAT tradition has been the systemic 'knock-on' effect of these enactments (Fig. 18.1) and the ways in

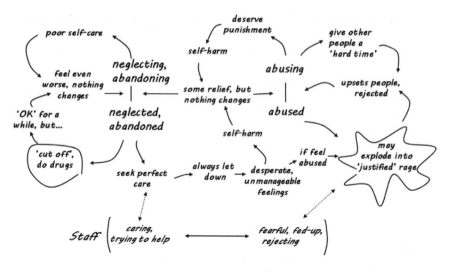

Fig. 18.1 Rudimentary contextual reformulation of a fictional patient with borderline personality disorder, showing basic reciprocal reactions and splitting in the staff team.

which they may provoke stress, disagreements, burnout and splits within services (Kerr, 1999; Ryle & Kerr, 2002). Although these differing role enactments are seen as problematic within CAT, the tools of reformulation and of extended contextual reformulation offer powerful means of both understanding and working with them (Kerr, 1999; Thompson *et al*, 2008). A further consequence for individual patients of dissociation into differing self states is a resultant difficulty in self-reflection, executive function or what might be called mentalisation (Bateman & Fonagy, 2004) or metacognition (Dimaggio *et al*, 2006).

A major aim of CAT is to enable a containing and collaborative understanding and insight into patients' dissociative states and switches. This helps them to reduce and contain intense and unmanageable emotional states that might otherwise lead to desperate coping behaviours (procedures) such as substance misuse or self-harm. It is implicit in the approach that patients may need active supportive assistance to deal with problems associated with these coping behaviours. However, CAT practitioners would not concur with the view asserted by, for example, practitioners of dialectical behaviour therapy, that these behaviours in themselves should always be addressed and contained first, without reference to their underlying recent or historic causes. It has been argued from a CAT perspective (Kerr & Ryle, 2005) that to do so may be an unwitting collusion with underlying historic reciprocal roles and that focus on behaviours such as self-harm or substance misuse can actually reinforce and represent a 're-run' of historic experiences such as being emotionally neglected, conditionally loved or not listened to.

CAT as treatment for borderline personality disorder

Cognitive analytic therapy has been employed for the most part as an individual therapy offered on a time-limited basis (Box 18.2). A time limit and 'ending well' are of fundamental importance in CAT. A typical initial contract would be for 24 weekly sessions. However, CAT is increasingly used as a common language to inform more intensive and/or team-based approaches (Sheard *et al*, 2000; Ryle & Kerr, 2002). One interest within CAT has been the use of shared contextual reformulation, either implicitly or explicitly, within treating teams. This use has been explored in a variety of settings, including intensive treatment programmes, therapeutic

---

Box 18.2 Key features of the cognitive analytic model of therapy for borderline personality disorder

Proactive and collaborative ('doing with') style, stressing the active participation of the patient/client.

Aims at non-judgemental description of, and insight into origins and nature of, psychopathology conceived as procedural enactments of reciprocal roles and associated dialogical voices, and of a tendency under stress to dissociate into different self states.

Aims to offer a new form of non-collusive relationship with a benign, thoughtful other that the patient/client can internalise in the form of new reciprocal roles and that enables the exploration of new perceptions of self and new ways of interacting with others; this is conceived of in terms of recognition and revision of maladaptive reciprocal role procedures.

Therapy is aided by the early collaborative construction of written and diagrammatic reformulations (conceived of as psychological tools) by the end of the initial phase of therapy. These serve as 'route maps' for therapy and also as explicit narrative and validating testimonies.

Therapy subsequently focuses on revision of maladaptive reciprocal role procedures and associated perceptions, affects and voices as they are evident in internal self-to-self dialogue and self-management, through enactments in the outside world, and also as manifest in the therapy relationship (as transference and countertransference).

Further techniques may facilitate this ranging from challenging of dialogical voices to behavioural experiments, mindfulness exercises, 'empty chair' work or active processing of traumatic memories.

The focus from the beginning is on a time limit (whether in individual therapy or CAT-informed approaches in other settings); 'ending well' is seen as an important part of therapy (experience of new reciprocal roles), and as a means of addressing issues surrounding loss and of avoiding protracted and collusive relationships.

Social rehabilitation is an important although often neglected aspect of therapy.

communities and day hospital services. The cognitive analytic approach is also increasingly used to inform broader consultancy work that does not necessarily involve individual therapy as such.

The therapeutic style of CAT is consistent with more recent findings on the nature of normal human growth and development, as mentioned above, and with emerging evidence on the features of successful psychotherapies. That is to say, it is proactive, collaborative, it stresses an active therapeutic alliance, and is clear and coherent to both professionals and patients. These characteristics are stressed in treatment guidelines such as that for borderline personality disorder published by the National Institute for Health and Clinical Excellence in England (National Collaborating Centre for Mental Health, 2009). Cognitive analytic therapy focuses on the internalised social and relational origins of a patient's difficulties and problems (in terms of their repertoire of reciprocal roles and reciprocal role procedures) and offers a means of addressing these both in general and as they are enacted within the therapeutic relationship. Thus, a major focus in therapy is work on what might be called transference and countertransference, although these are thought of and described rather more specifically in terms of named reciprocal role enactments. This work is aided by the use of summary reformulation letters and maps. These are conceived of in the language of Vygotsky as psychological tools. Joint construction of these can be seen as a form of narrative therapy (Dimaggio et al, 2005, 2006) or of testimony and also as an exercise in validation as stressed in dialectical behaviour therapy (Linehan, 1993). They also effectively serve as jointly agreed 'route maps' for the subsequent course of therapy.

Therapy in CAT focuses initially, therefore, on the collaborative exploration and making sense of the patient's formative interpersonal and social experiences in terms of reciprocal roles, the coping patterns (reciprocal role procedures) emanating from them and, importantly, their consequences. The latter usually reinforce initial formative experiences in 'vicious cycles'. Many of these procedures and self states may be identified from the psychotherapy file (discussed in 'Use of adjuvant paperwork' below). Therapy focuses on helping patients to reflect and 'try things differently' in the context of a more benign and facilitating relationship. Ideally, the patient will internalise this relationship as an important aspect of therapy, although this is rarely in itself enough to effect significant change. However, the relationship might also constitute collusion with the patient, in a 'needy victim–sympathetic carer' reciprocal role, to the neglect of other, more difficult reciprocal role enactments. It is important to be aware of such collusion in professional work – especially since it may unwittingly perpetuate or exacerbate the difficulties with which the patient presents (see the case study of Anna below).

A further aim in work with individuals who have extreme damage to the self is the clear depiction of the various self states that they experience, of what provokes their switches and of the consequences of coping procedures (reciprocal role procedures) emanating from them. This offers a coherent overview of often very confusing and distressing subjective states that is frequently very containing for the patient and, through its collaborative construction, strengthens the therapeutic alliance. Although with less unwell patients this mapping is normally attempted only after several sessions, paradoxically with very disturbed patients it is often helpful to attempt even a rudimentary version as quickly as possible – perhaps in the first meeting. In CAT both the written narrative reformulation and the diagram (or map) imply also the need to articulate 'exits' or 'aims' to help the patient move on and attempt things differently. Later phases of therapy offer an opportunity to process and 'work through' often painful formative experience and, possibly, major losses. Aims might include, for example, not repeating familiar coping reciprocal role procedures, or noting and challenging a critical inner voice.

Any more practical or behavioural work in CAT is always under-taken in the context of a shared reformulation, i.e. an understanding and appreciation of the interpersonal origins and nature of dysfunctional coping strategies (reciprocal role procedures) and their consequences. In our experience, not only may more relational therapeutic approaches be engaged in alongside more behavioural interventions – in practice, they may be necessary to enable such interventions, notwithstanding the need at times for emergency interventions for difficult behaviours such as self-harm, perhaps with brief hospital admission. These considerations would also apply to complementary approaches sometimes used within a CAT framework, such as creative therapies or 'empty chair' work attempting to access and process difficult memories (see the case study below). At times, interventions such as somatosensory approaches (Ogden *et al*, 2006) or a more active cognitive–behavioural desensitisation may be necessary, and the help of colleagues might be sought to undertake them. Some patients might receive eye movement desensitisation and reprocessing (EMDR) nested within a traditional CAT therapy (see Ryle & Kerr, 2002).

In common with most, particularly Western-based, therapies focusing on the individual (with the possible partial exception of some therapeutic community approaches (Kennard, 1999; National Collaborating Centre for Mental Health, 2009), the challenge of social reintegration and rehabilitation is frequently not addressed in CAT, although for many (see the case study below) this is a massive and debilitating problem.

Later phases of therapy and ending

Beyond the reformulation phase, work on maintaining a focus on recognising and revising maladaptive reciprocal role procedures (through clearly stated aims and exits) continues, aided by the tools of reformulation. Other important work, such as working through or grieving for previous losses or traumatic events, may also be undertaken (sometimes using complementary techniques). Existential issues relating to the meaning and purpose of life might be acknowledged, although focus will also be maintained on current life experience, for example in the family, at work or, importantly, within therapy. All of these will be respected and validated, but also recurrently challenged (non-judgementally) through the use of the previously jointly agreed reformulations. The latter also help to defuse the intensity and perceived personalisation of transference or countertransference enactments.

For good theoretical and clinical reasons, as already mentioned, all CAT-based approaches maintain firm focus on time limitation and ending well (Box 18.2). This maintains impetus, activity and, arguably, hope within therapy. It also minimises the temptation to drift into interminable, potentially collusive, relationships that may generate both dependency and demoralisation in the patient and, possibly, also in the therapist. Reciprocal roles enacted in such relationships include the 'superior empowered therapist–hopeless needy patient' or, more insidious, the mutually narcissistic 'special, admired, indispensable therapist–special, needy, admiring patient'. Ending well is seen as a therapeutic aim in itself, and is characterised ideally by enactment of new or modified reciprocal roles and reciprocal role procedures. These would include roles characterised by open dialogue and sharing of powerful and possibly angry or distressed feelings about ending and loss – as opposed to having to resort to more familiar historic defensive, avoidant or symptomatic reciprocal role procedures such as 'soldiering on', 'placating' or 'illness behaviours'. By this stage, it is hoped that, to some extent, a new, benign reciprocal role based on the experience of therapy will have been internalised. It should be stressed that time limitation and focus on ending well in CAT are not a response to economic pressure or the restricted delivery of an intervention that should ideally be much longer – notwithstanding the fact that an important part of Ryle's initial aim was to offer a good-enough therapy to as many patients as possible in a public health service.

Having said all this, it is recognised that individuals presenting with borderline personality disorders frequently remain fragile and vulnerable and may merit multidisciplinary and longer packages than less disturbed or damaged individuals with simpler conditions (for example, depressive disorders). More extended follow-up and support (ideally psychologically informed) may be required, including social rehabilitation and 'remoralisation', both of which are, in our experience, frequently underemphasised and underdeployed in these contexts. Reformulation frequently reveals particular formative (and current) sociocultural contexts that are beyond the remit or power of mental health professionals to address or modify. Nonetheless, sociocultural micromapping may be important in identifying and acknowledging the impact of such influences and how they might affect attempts to offer therapy or social assistance.

This process has obvious parallels and overlaps with the 'social-power mapping' (the structuring of who or what holds the power in an individual's social environment) described by Hagan & Smail (1997). However, the CAT approach offers a clearer and more effective means of conceptualising and dealing with the risk of collusion either directly with a patient or with a professional care group by means of techniques such as contextual ('systemic') reformulation or mapping (Fig. 18.1) (Ryle & Kerr, 2002). Indeed, cognitive analytic principles are being increasingly used to inform systemic consultancy work, both clinical and organisational. We have argued that sociocultural micromapping is always applicable, even if not very obviously, with every 'individual' treated or cared for by mental health services (Kerr, 1999; Ryle & Kerr, 2002). An important consequence of these considerations has been the recognised need to develop more complex models of treatment for borderline personality disorder. These could be based on CAT, but they could equally make use of other paradigms, such as Livesely's eclectic approach (Mirapeix *et al*, 2006). In CAT-based models, efforts at rehabilitation would be particularly emphasised, given their theoretical and practical importance and their striking absence in, for example, the North American literature.

Use of adjuvant paperwork

Various paper-based tools are routinely employed in CAT. In addition to the SDP, PSQ and contextual reformulation, patients routinely fill in a questionnaire called a psychotherapy file. A purpose of the file is to identify dysfunctional reciprocal roles and reciprocal role procedures (described by Ryle in terms of traps, snags and dilemmas; Ryle & Kerr, 2002). They might also complete a broad assessment measure such as the Clinical Outcomes in Routine Evaluation – Outcome Measure (CORE–OM; Evans *et al*, 2002) (including its distinct risk subscale). Such instruments are of considerable benefit not only as a measure of initial distress and disability and of outcome, but also heuristically, in discussion and psychoeducation with the patient. In research, an instrument derived from CAT to measure psychotherapeutic competence, the Competence in Cognitive Analytic Therapy (CCAT; Bennett & Parry, 2004), may be used to evaluate treatment integrity and fidelity. The CCAT has demonstrated and confirmed the importance of adherence to the model in achieving positive outcomes. It has been also used more generally in evaluating other treatment approaches.

Evidence base for CAT in borderline personality disorder

Cognitive analytic therapy conforms almost entirely to generic features of effective therapies for borderline personality disorder (Roth & Fonagy, 2004; National Collaborating Centre for Mental Health, 2009). Therefore, a key research question for the future is the extent to which CAT overlaps with other approaches and/or complements and extends them. Much of the formal evidence for the effectiveness of CAT has been naturalistic (Ryle & Golynkina, 2000; Ryle & Kerr, 2002) although a large randomised controlled trial demonstrating its efficacy has more recently been reported (Chanen *et al*, 2008, 2009*a,b*). Two further comparative trials of CAT for borderline personality disorder have recently been completed and should be published in the near future (personal communications: S. Clarke, 2012; G. Parry, 2012).

Given the important role of a range of professionals, from psychiatrists to social workers, in patient care, a pilot project has been run offering intensive training in CAT skills to mental health social workers and community psychiatric nurses (Thompson *et al*, 2008). This largely successful pilot demonstrates the feasibility of a whole-team approach to thinking about treatment.

Therapy in practice

The following fictionalised case vignette illustrates some of the points that we have discussed. It involves a whole-team approach to care, highlighting contextual and social factors, both formative and current, along with the challenges implicit to our ways of working.

Case vignette: Anna

Anna was a young woman in her mid-20s with a long history of difficulties of a borderline personality disorder type complicated by anorexia nervosa. She had had multiple hospital admissions for emergency treatment of anorexia and for incidents of serious self-harm (including overdoses and cutting). At one point, she had spent several months in a residential therapeutic community but was discharged home to local services after self-harming following the suicide of her best friend Susan (also a community resident) and interpersonal difficulties with a member of staff. A despairing local psychiatrist and the community mental health team referred her for assessment for psychotherapy. She lived alone in modest flat funded by her parents in a small town in a socioeconomically deprived area. She felt very isolated and rarely went out, partly because of social anxiety.

Anna's family background was characterised by an atmosphere of tension between her parents. Her father (an accountant and an aggressive man dependent on alcohol) was preoccupied with material wealth and 'succeeding' in life. Her mother tried to keep the peace and not offend or upset her husband. Anna's father had forced her to attend a distant school with a good academic reputation. She hated school and sometimes claimed sickness to avoid going. She 'couldn't' tell anyone about this. Her younger sister Mary was less pressured and somehow more 'thick-skinned', but has also had problems with anxiety.

At presentation, Anna stated that she saw no future for herself and no point in living and that only a small part of her wished to think about any further attempts at treatment. Part of her would rather join her dead friend Susan, whom she envied. She appeared very wary and rather hostile towards her therapist. She refused to contact the local eating disorder service, saying that the staff there did not listen to her or take her seriously and that she did not trust them. However, she agreed to see a community psychiatric nurse intermittently and attend a (different) psychiatrist for occasional review.

In the absence of a more specialist intensive treatment service locally she was offered, and agreed to, an initially time-limited (24 sessions with subsequent review) course of CAT. She remained worryingly underweight although she continued to feel overweight and to believe that this would be disgusting to everybody, including her therapist. There was serious concern about her cognitive ability (concentration and memory) to make use of therapy. During the initial months of CAT, she remained mostly very gloomy and hopeless about change or about any future. She attended regularly, apart from two periods when she was re-admitted to hospital following episodes of self-harm. One of these occurred while the therapist was away and the community psychiatric nurse was off ill with no replacement.

During the course of CAT, Anna was supported by regular contact with her mother, from whom she received some (mostly practical) support. She had worried about contact with her father, whom she rarely saw. She clearly had strong feelings about him, but was very reluctant to talk about him. She was, however, able to engage with the work of reformulation, which she described as illuminating and helpful. This appeared to firm up the therapeutic alliance considerably and to provide an agreed joint understanding that could be referred to. During this early period, the therapist received repeated calls from colleagues (e.g. Anna's psychiatrist) about 'dealing' with her and whether therapy was 'working'.

Together, Anna and her therapist explored formative reciprocal roles in Anna's life (Fig. 18.2) and created a self states diagram (Fig. 18.3). The following extracts are from the therapist's reformulation letter, written after the first eight sessions of CAT.

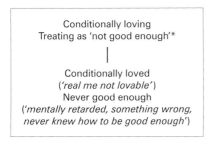

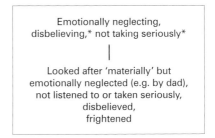

Conditionally loving
Treating as 'not good enough'*

|

Conditionally loved
('real me not lovable')
Never good enough
('mentally retarded, something wrong,
never knew how to be good enough')

Emotionally neglecting,
disbelieving,* not taking seriously*

|

Looked after 'materially' but
emotionally neglected (e.g. by dad),
not listened to or taken seriously,
disbelieved,
frightened

Fig. 18.2 Formative reciprocal roles for Anna; *internalised dialogical voices.

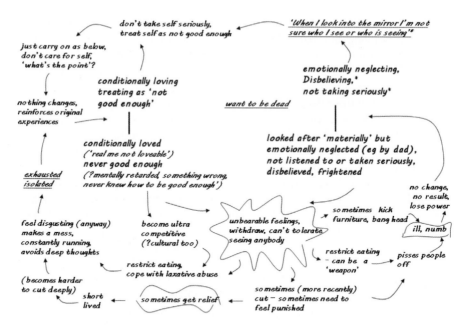

Fig. 18.3 Extended multiple self-states diagram for Anna showing different self states and maladaptive procedures; *internalised dialogical voices.

Dear Anna,

This is a letter attempting to summarise some of the key issues which seem to have emerged in the course of our initial work together and to try to think about how they are affecting your life at present as well as to think about what might historically lie behind them, as we have been doing. I hope that this will ultimately help you to move on to a more rewarding future. We have already attempted to sketch some of this in a diagrammatic form, which I think by your account seemed quite useful, although I think it seemed also quite disturbing and upsetting in some ways as well. This will only be my version of what we have been talking about and is very much open to your feedback or modification. [...]

In looking back over some of the things I have jotted down over the past few months I am very struck by the importance for you of not having other people's versions of events or their expectations imposed upon you, which does seem to have been your experience very frequently throughout your life, both in childhood and more recently. In fact, looking back at our very first meeting, one of the first things you said to me was that you felt that you had not really ever been listened to. In looking back over some of my notes, I am also struck by just how painfully difficult life must seem to you day to day and this was also reinforced by looking through your psychotherapy file again, where you highlighted some very extreme and difficult states. [...]

As well as the unbearable feelings, I have been very struck by how hard day-to-day life must be with little to do and few real social contacts, your difficulties with sleep and the terrible dreams which you sometimes describe, and just generally with the panicky feelings which seem to accompany you most of the time. We have talked about various ways you have coped with these unbearable feelings over the years by doing controlled overdoses, laxative misuse and other forms of self-harm, such as cutting, although this seems to have become more difficult for you recently. It did seem very striking both from our chats and the diagram we did that the consequences of these ways of coping unfortunately on the whole still leave you, even if numbed out for a while, ultimately on your own, unappreciated and often pressurised and rejected by people again. All of which, of course, in a vicious cycle seems to reinforce your original experiences and keep them going. These cycles do seem to have acquired quite a life of their own. [...]

I would like to emphasise, however, how impressed I have been at you sticking with the work we have been able to do, even if it has been interrupted by your trips to the ward occasionally or our other difficulties in getting together (sometimes mine). If the small part of you which is holding on can continue to keep thinking together with me about these issues, reflecting on them and considering jointly ways of addressing and challenging them, then it is perfectly possible that you will be able to move on to a more fulfilling and meaningful life – although the path I am sure will not be easy or straightforward. [...]

With best wishes

In subsequent sessions, key issues (important reciprocal role procedures) were highlighted and articulated, along with therapeutic aims.

Key issues/target problem procedures (TPPs)

TPP1: Because of your experience of being frequently criticised, pressurised and only ever conditionally loved, you have finished up assuming that there is something wrong with you (e.g. missing some chromosome!) and have finished up frequently enacting these criticising roles towards yourself. This leads you to never feeling good about yourself and never trying to do good things for yourself – which reinforces your original experiences.

Aim: To try to watch out for that self-criticising and self-pressurising 'voice' and identify it as we have been doing and to try to consider whether you really accept its validity.

TPP2: Because of your experiences of never feeling properly listened to or respected, you finish up feeling abandoned and alone and often full of desperate feelings which you have coped with in various ways, including self-harm and dietary restriction – as well as sometimes, perhaps, behaviour towards other people that they may have experienced as apparently 'difficult'. This all tends to lead you to be again rejected and misunderstood and leaves you still unappreciated and with your emotional needs unmet, so reinforcing your original experiences.

Aim: To try to bear in mind when you are feeling desperate how it is that these feelings have come about and the consequences of your traditional ways of coping and try to consider alternatives such as communicating calmly to trusted people (as we have begun perhaps to do in therapy) how you are feeling and what your needs are.

Progress

Anna continued to attend therapy, with apparently increasing commitment and less wariness and hostility. Continued collaborative use of diagrams in therapy appeared to assist in containing 'unbearable feelings' and to reflect on her habitual patterns of feeling, thinking and coping. She seemed more willing and able to discuss feelings in relation to her therapist. Towards the end of the initial contract, she finally agreed to discuss her feelings about her father and to address him using an empty chair approach. Through this, she expressed powerful, unresolved and angry feelings about the effects of his behaviour on her and her wish that he could be able to appreciate this. This appears to be an important moment which seems to considerably 'loosen up' her thoughts and feelings overall. Despite this progress, patterns (reciprocal role procedures) of restricted eating and misuse of laxatives and medications remained major problems, with little apparent change. However, the frequency of self-harm episodes reduced considerably. Anna complained of always being tired, finding concentration difficult and experiencing frequent palpitations. However, she stated that she was now keen to remain in therapy and a further 24-session course was agreed. She reluctantly agreed to consider seeing a member of the local eating disorder team to address nutritional concerns. She agreed that reduction of various psychotropic and other medications was also a long-term aim but was reluctant to countenance this at the time. With Anna's enthusiastic permission, her diagram was shared usefully with other team members, to enable understanding and communication. During one admission, she requested that a copy be sent for this purpose to the ward. However, Anna remained socially isolated and lonely and felt stigmatised by family and others. She recurrently talked of wishing to be 'out of it all' and appeared still at considerable risk of serious self-harm.

Background problems

In terms of case conceptualisation, Anna's problems appeared to be due to a mix of factors: temperamental vulnerability (a possible tendency to obsessional perfectionism and dissociation); dysfunctional, intense (nuclear) family dynamics (criticising, conditional love, not listening to or taking seriously); and cultural influences (a competitive school environment, cultural preoccupation with dieting and appearance). These were apparently exacerbated and perpetuated contextually by the 'doing to', authoritarian approach of many mental health services, which apparently colluded with her historic reciprocal roles. No collective meaningful attempt at social therapy or rehabilitation was possible in these circumstances.

Reflections on treatment outcome

Overall, the cognitive–analytic approach appears to have been successful in collaboratively and empathically engaging Anna in therapy and in generating insight and understandings of her difficulties and their origins.

In turn, this improved the integrity of her self, partly through the joint creation of the collaborative tools of reformulation. The improvement was reflected in significant reductions in her PSQ and CORE-OM scores. However, some issues remained problematic and refractory, including her long-standing patterns of dietary restriction, occasional (although greatly reduced) self-harm because of intense, unmanageable feelings, and difficult and disturbing memories and emotions surrounding her experiences of her father. These may require further active processing, perhaps using the empty chair method that has already been of help. Major contextual issues relating to the absence of social support and active rehabilitation and the absence for Anna of a sense of common social purpose, identity and meaning remain obstacles to further therapeutic improvement. However, these appear to be beyond the reach or remit of psychotherapy services within the National Health Service (whatever its working model) as presently constituted.

Future perspectives

There is good evidence that CAT is an effective, conceptually coherent and robust approach to the treatment of borderline personality disorder in individual and group therapy, as well as an effective common language to inform and improve collective team and/or systemic function. Further extended formal studies are required to determine its comparative effectiveness for a range of patients and types of problem – as is the case for all therapeutic models in the field. Large controlled studies must be complemented by much more comparative and 'dismantling' research, especially of a qualitative nature (e.g. the hermeneutic single-case efficacy design (HSCED) described by Elliott, 2001), that moves beyond the simplistic pre- and post-treatment group-mean type of controlled trial currently employed as the benchmark of clinical research – and recognised to be seriously limited in this respect (Elliott, 2001; Roth & Fonagy, 2004). Practitioners of CAT have been active in these areas with, for example: the randomised controlled trial reported by Chanen et al (2008) in Australia; an extended multiple case series being undertaken by Ryle and his team in the UK (Kellet et al, 2011); and a naturalistic study of a multicomponent CAT-based programme in Spain (Mirapeix et al, 2006). The partly CAT-based technique of dialogical sequence analysis (Leiman, 2004) is a further powerful tool for conceptualising and exploring research into the process of change in borderline personality disorder. It will also be important to evaluate effectiveness in terms of cost and resources (Bartak et al, 2007; Arnevik et al, 2009). It appears that many patients with less severe disorder can be treated on an individual, short-term basis (as in the case of Anna above). However, those with more severe disorder may require more intensive, longer-term multidisciplinary programmes, in line with the emerging consensus (National Collaborating Centre for Mental Health, 2009).

The sociocultural dimension of borderline personality disorder remains poorly conceptualised and studied, despite the demonstrable partial effectiveness of many relational approaches (Roth & Fonagy, 2004; National Collaborating Centre for Mental Health, 2009). We see this as an urgent challenge for the future. We are currently studying the possible importance of internalised social conditions and values from a CAT-informed perspective, through assessment of what we have described as a patient's sense of 'subjective communality' (Kerr, 2009) and through approaches involving the active participation of a broader community. This we see as complementing but extending the demonstrable significance of phenomena such as social capital (Whitley & Mackenzie, 2005). It is clear that socioeconomic and political interventions will ultimately be necessary to improve all aspects of mental health, but especially borderline personality disorder. This is implied and argued by authors such as Wilkinson & Pickett (2009), James (2007) and Marmot (Marmot & Wilkinson, 2006). Clearly, these initiatives are beyond the immediate scope or remit of mental health professionals, but we argue that our models need to reflect these realities and that, along with colleagues in sociology and medical epidemiology, we have a duty and responsibility to articulate and publicise them. A CAT-based perspective can offer a helpful framework within which to discuss and articulate these issues and on which to base effective treatments, be they one-to-one therapy or multidisciplinary team-based interventions.

References

American Psychiatric Association (1994) *Diagnostic and Statistical Manual of Mental Disorders (4th edn) (DSM-IV)*. APA.

Arnevik, E., Wilberg, T., Urnes, Ï., *et al* (2009) Psychotherapy for personality disorders: short-term day hospital psychotherapy versus outpatient individual therapy: a randomized controlled study. *European Psychiatry*, **24**, 71–78.

Bartak, A., Soeteman, D., Verheul, R., *et al* (2007) Strengthening the status of psychotherapy for personality disorders: an integrated perspective on effects and costs. *Canadian Journal of Psychiatry*, **52**, 803–810.

Bateman, A. & Fonagy, F. (2004) *Psychotherapy for Borderline Personality Disorder: Mentalization-Based Treatment*. Oxford University Press.

Bedford, A., Davies, F. & Tibbles, J. (2009) the Personality Structure Questionnaire (PSQ): a cross-validation with a large clinical sample. *Clinical Psychology & Psychotherapy*, **16**, 77–81.

Bennett, D. & Parry, G. (2004) A measure of psychotherapeutic competence derived from cognitive analytic therapy (CCAT). *Psychotherapy Research*, **4**, 176–192.

Bennett, D. & Ryle, A. (2005) The characteristic features of common borderline states: a pilot study using the States Description Procedure. *Clinical Psychology & Psychotherapy*, **12**, 58–66.

Bennett, D., Pollock, P. & Ryle, A. (2005) The States Description Procedure: the use of guided self-reflection in the case formulation of patients with borderline personality disorder. *Clinical Psychology & Psychotherapy*, **12**, 50–57.

Chanen, A. M., Jackson, H. J., McCutcheon, L. K., *et al* (2008) Early intervention for adolescents with borderline personality disorder using cognitive analytic therapy: randomised controlled trial. *British Journal of Psychiatry*, **193**, 477–484.

Chanen, A. M., Jackson, H. J., McCutcheon, L. K., *et al* (2009*a*) Early intervention for adolescents with borderline personality disorder: quasi-experimental comparison with treatment as usual. *Australian and New Zealand Journal of Psychiatry*, **43**, 397–408.

Chanen, A. M., McCutcheon, L. K. & Germans, D. (2009*b*) The HYPE Clinic: an early intervention service for borderline personality disorder. *Journal of Psychiatric Practice*, **15**, 163–172.

Cox, B. D. & Lightfoot, C. (eds) (1997) *Sociogenetic Perspectives on Internalisation*. Lawrence Erlbaum Associates.

Dimaggio, G., Carcione, A., Petrilli, D., *et al* (2005) State of mind organisation in personality disorders: typical states and the triggering of inter-state shifts. *Clinical Psychology & Psychotherapy*, **12**, 346–359.

Dimaggio, G., Semerari, A., Carcione, A., *et al* (2006) Toward a model of self pathology underlying personality disorders: narratives, metacognition, interpersonal cycles and decision making processes. *Journal of Personality Disorder*, **20**, 597–617.

Elliott, R. (2001) Hermeneutic single case efficacy design (HSCED): an overview. In *Handbook of Humanistic Psychology* (eds K. J. Schneider, J. F. T. Bugental & J. F. Fraser), pp. 315–324. Sage.

Evans, C., Connell, J., Barkham, M., *et al* (2002) Towards a standardised brief outcome measure: psychometric properties and utility of the CORE–OM. *British Journal of Psychiatry*, **180**, 51–60.

Golynkina, K. & Ryle, A. (1999) The identification and characteristics of the partially dissociated states of patients with borderline personality disorder. *British Journal of Medical Psychology*, **72**, 429–445.

Gunderson, J. G. (2003) *Borderline Personality Disorder: A Clinical Guide* (2nd edn). American Psychiatric Press.

Hagan, T. & Smail, D. (1997) Power-mapping: 1 Background and basic methodology. *Journal of Community and Applied Social Psychology*, **7**, 257–267.

Hubbuck, J. (2008) The States Description Procedure: some clinical implications for the CAT Self-States Sequential Diagram [SSSD]. *Reformulation* (Summer), 46–53 (http://www.acat.me.uk/reformulation.php?issue_id=7&article_id=111).

James, O. (2007) *Affluenza*. Vermilion.

Kellett, S., Bennett, D., Ryle, A., *et al* (2011) Cognitive analytic therapy for borderline personality disorder: therapeutic competence and effectiveness in routine practice. *Clinical Psychology and Psychotherapy*, doi:10.1002/cpp.796 (Epub ahead of print).

Kennard, D. (1999) *An Introduction to Therapeutic Communities*. Jessica Kingsley.

Kerr, I. B. (1999) Cognitive-analytic therapy for borderline personality disorder in the context of a community mental health team: individual and organizational psycho-dynamic implications. *British Journal of Psychotherapy*, **15**, 425–438.

Kerr, I. B. (2009) Addressing the socially-constituted self through a common language for mental health and social services: a cognitive-analytic perspective. In *Confluences of Identity, Knowledge and Practice: Building Interprofessional Social Capital* (eds J. Forbes & C. Watson). ESRC Seminar 4 Proceedings, Research Paper 20, pp. 21–38. University of Aberdeen.

Kerr, I. B. & Leighton, T. (2008) Dual challenge: a cognitive analytic therapy approach to substance abuse. *Healthcare Counselling and Psychotherapy Journal*, **8**, 3–7.

Kerr, I. B. & Ryle, A. (2005) Cognitive analytic therapy. In *Introduction to the Psychotherapies* (ed. S, Bloch), pp. 268–286. Oxford University Press.

Kerr, I. B., Dent-Brown, K. & Parry, G. D. (2007) Psychotherapy and mental health teams. *International Review of Psychiatry*, **19**, 63–80.

Leiman, M. (1992) The concept of sign in the work of Vygotsky, Winnicott and Bakhtin: further integration of object relations theory and activity theory. *British Journal of Medical Psychology*, **65**, 209–221.

Leiman, M. (2004) Dialogical sequence analysis. In *The Dialogical Self in Psychotherapy* (eds H. J. M. Hermans & G. Dimaggio), pp. 255–270. Brunner-Routledge.

Linehan, M. M. (1993) *The Skills Training Manual for Treating Borderline Personality Disorder*. Guilford Press.

Marmot, M & Wilkinson, R. G. (2006) *Social Determinants of Health* (2nd edn). Oxford University Press.

Mirapeix, C. (2008) Desarrollo del self, múltiples estados mentales y metodología de evaluación desde la psicoterapia cognitivo analítica [Self development, multiple self states and evaluation methodology from cognitive analytic therapy]. *Revista de la Asociación de Psicoterapia de la República Argentina*, September (http://www.revistadeapra. org.ar/pdf/Mirapeix_APRA_2008.pdf).

Mirapeix, C., Uríszar-Aldaca, M., Landin, S., *et al* (2006) Tratamiento multicomponente, de orientación cognitivo analítica del TLP [Cognitive analytic oriented, multicomponent treatment of TLP]. *Psiquiatria.com*, **10** (1) (http://www.psiquiatria.com/revistas/index. php/psiquiatriacom/article/view/271).

National Collaborating Centre for Mental Health (2009) *Borderline Personality Disorder: Treatment and Management (NICE Clinical Guideline 78)*. National Institute for Health and Clinical Excellence.

Ogden, P., Minton, K. & Pain, C. (2006) *Trauma and the Body: A Sensorimotor Approach to Psychotherapy*. W. W. Norton.

Pollock, P. H., Broadbent, M., Clarke, S., *et al* (2001) The Personality Structure Questionnaire (PSQ): a measure of the multiple self states model of identity disturbance in cognitive analytic therapy. *Clinical Psychology & Psychotherapy*, **8**, 59–72.

Reddy, V. (2008) *How Infants Know Minds*. Harvard University Press.

Roth, A. & Fonagy, P. (2004) *What Works for Whom? A Critical Review of Psychotherapy Research* (2nd edn). Guilford Press.

Ryle, A. (1997) The structure and development of borderline personality disorder: a proposed model. *British Journal of Psychiatry*, **170**, 82–87.

Ryle, A. (2004) The contribution of cognitive analytic therapy to the treatment of borderline personality disorder. *Journal of Personality Disorders*, **18**, 3–12.

Ryle, A. & Fawkes, L. (2007) Multiplicity of selves and others: cognitive analytic therapy. *Clinical Psychology & Psychotherapy*, **63**, 165–174.

Ryle, A. & Golynkina, K. (2000) Effectiveness of time-limited cognitive analytic therapy of borderline personality disorder: factors associated with outcome. *British Journal of Medical Psychology*, **73**, 169–177.

Ryle, A. & Kerr, I. B. (2002) *Introducing Cognitive Analytic Therapy: Principles and Practice*. John Wiley & Sons.

Sheard, T., Evans, J., Cash, D., *et al* (2000) A CAT-derived one to three session intervention for repeated deliberate self-harm: a description of the model and initial experience of trainee psychiatrists in using it. *British Journal of Medical Psychology*, **73**, 179–196.

Stern, D. N. (2000) *The Interpersonal World of the Infant: A View from Psychoanalysis and Developmental Psychology* (2nd edn). Basic Books.

Thompson, A. R., Donnison, J., Warnock-Parkes, E., *et al* (2008) A multidisciplinary community mental health team (CMHT) staff's experience of a 'skills' level training course in cognitive analytic therapy (CAT). *International Journal of Mental Health Nursing*, **17**, 131–137.

Trevarthen, C. & Aitken K. J. (2001) Infant intersubjectivity: research, theory and clinical applications. *Journal of Child Psychology and Psychiatry*, **42**, 3–48.

Whitley, R. & Mackenzie, K. (2005) Social capital and psychiatry: review of the literature. Harvard Review of Psychiatry, 13, 71–84.

Wilkinson, R. & Pickett, K. (2009) *The Spirit Level: Why More Equal Societies Almost Always Do Better*. Allen Lane.

CHAPTER 19

Contemporary therapeutic communities: complex treatment for complex needs

Rex Haigh and Helen den Hartog

Summary   In this chapter, we describe the principles of therapeutic communities and how they work. We discuss some of the challenges for both policy and research in relation to therapeutic community services for personality disorder. We emphasise the importance of listening to the voices of those who use therapeutic community services, as well as to professional voices, when evaluating such services.

Therapeutic communities are not a 'brand' of therapy, with a manual and an uncomplicated evidence base. Rather, they are a treatment culture and structure into which other therapies are incorporated as intensive programmes of integrated sociotherapy. They have long and far-reaching historical roots, and share features with numerous psychological, social and educational approaches and movements (Box 19.1). Whichever specific therapies are integrated (Box 19.2), the predominant focus is the supportive and challenging network of relationships that exists between the members, both staff and service users. This is what Foulkes (1964), the founder of group analytic psychotherapy, termed the dynamic matrix.

The diffuse and complex nature of this core concept presents some difficulties for a mental health system that requires treatments to be managed with a degree of precision and predictability, to be measurable and auditable, and to be described in a straightforward, learnable way as in a manual. This is as true for the day-to-day hurly-burly of interpersonal interaction as it is for setting up a service, and it can cause therapeutic communities to be repeatedly pressured to 'justify' their therapeutic value.

However, new techniques, processes and guidelines are now available that help to deal with these necessary complexities, and this account will draw attention to them. It focuses on therapeutic communities for personality disorder, but it also considers their use for psychosis, addictions, offending behaviour, and emotional and conduct disorders in children and

Box 19.1   Allied movements and approaches

Geel, Flanders	1300s	Worship at the shrine of St Dymphna for 'mentally afflicted' pilgrims
Moral treatment	Late 1800s	William Tuke: The Retreat in York (1796); Philippe Pinel: Salpêtrière in Paris ('treatment through the emotions')
Quakerism	1800s	Many therapeutic community pioneers have been Quakers. Quaker hospital in Pennsylvania (1751); several contemporary 'mini-therapeutic communities' are held in Friends meeting houses
Progressive education	Late 1800s onwards	Homer Lane, A. S. Neill, George Lyward, Marjorie Franklin, David Wills, Maurice Bridgeland
Anthroposophy	Early 1900s	Rudolf Steiner; common roots with Montessori; now Camphill and L'Arche 'intentional communities' for intellectual disability
Psychoanalysis	1940s	Wilfred Bion, John Rickman, Thomas Forrest Main, Harold Bridger, S. H. Foulkes: the Northfield experiments
Social psychiatry	1950s	Maxwell Jones, David Clarke, others: 'unlocking the asylums'
Synanon organisation	1958	Charles Dederich; led to 'concept houses' and worldwide modern addiction therapeutic communities (mostly in USA). Contemporary theory and research: George De Leon
Antipsychiatry	1960s	R. D. Laing and David Cooper. Arbours and Philadelphia organisations survive as psychoanalytic training and therapeutic housing charities
Forgiving justice	1962	HM Prison Grendon (England), Chino prison (USA)
Group analysis	1970s	S. H. Foulkes: psychotherapeutic training and practice networks (mostly UK and Europe)
Systems theory, chaos theory, uncertainty theory	1950s	Complex interconnectivity, impossibility of prediction, interdependency
Service user involvement	1990s	Partnership in clinical decisions; empowerment; critical psychology
Pedagogy	1990s	Orthopedagogy (Belgium); critical theory in education
Greencare	2000s	Sustainabilty, holism, spirituality, value base (Sempik *et al*, 2010)

Box 19.2 Recognised therapies used in therapeutic communities

Group analytic psychotherapy	Small, medium and large groups: improves prosocial functioning and perspective-taking
Psychodrama	Specific exploration and mutual understanding
Creative arts	Experiential and reflective: specialist regular groups or occasional workshops
Art therapy	More interpretative and analytic: specialist regular groups or occasional workshops
Transactional analysis (TA)	With teaching of its methods: specialist regular groups or occasional workshops
Cognitive–behavioural therapy (CBT)	Contracts, diaries, aims – all frequently used; also specialist regular groups
Dialectical behaviour therapy (DBT)	Can form specialist regular groups, particularly promotes mindfulness and emotion regulation
Interpersonal therapy (IPT)	Most groups have interpersonal focus
Cognitive analytic therapy (CAT)	Can be used in specific groups, e.g. diagrammatic reformulations can be discussed in community meetings and other therapy groups
Mentalisation-based treatment (MBT)	Empathic processes and 'mind of others': both individual and group therapy
Gestalt	Specialist regular groups or occasional workshops
Music therapy	Specialist regular groups or occasional workshops
Dance and movement therapy	Specialist regular groups or occasional workshops
Systemic therapy	Positive involvement of, for example, family and friends often helpful
Individual case management	Should aim to avoid a close one-to-one relationship that conflicts with group therapy process
Individual psychoanalysis	Requires careful integration; usually not recommended in group-based programmes

---

adolescents. Treatment cultures and structural features of different services are being increasingly recognised to be more alike than different (Haigh & Lees, 2008).

Standardisation and quality

In response to the perceived isolation of individual therapeutic community services, and uncertainty about what are the common and essential elements of good practice, the Community of Communities was established in 2002 as a standards-based quality network at what is now the Royal

College of Psychiatrists' Centre for Quality Improvement (CCQI). Existing practice standards were used as a starting point, with a democratic process of editing and refining them. The standards are reviewed and revised regularly, and are now in their fifth edition. With growing membership and sophistication, there are now several subsections: a values-based set of core standards (which are necessary and sufficient for a service to call itself a therapeutic community – see Box 19.3), several specialist sections for different contexts (to achieve, maintain and improve standards of practice), and accreditation standards (for units to periodically undergo a rigorous process of scrutiny and inspection). The standards are all accompanied by clear and measurable criteria, which need to be fulfilled for the standard itself to be considered met. Information about the Community of Communities and the most recent versions of the different sets of standards can all be found on the CCQI website (www.rcpsych.ac.uk/quality/qualityandaccreditation.aspx).

Box 19.3 Community of Communities core standards

1 The community meets regularly
2 The community acknowledges a connection between emotional health and the quality of relationships
3 The community has clear boundaries, limits or rules, and mechanisms to hold them in place which are open to review
4 The community enables risks to be taken to encourage positive change
5 Community members create an emotionally safe environment for the work of the community
6 Community members consider and discuss their attitudes and feelings towards each other
7 Power and authority in relationships is used responsibly and is open to question
8 Community members take a variety of roles and levels of responsibility
9 Community members spend formal and informal time together
10 Relationships between staff members and client members are characterised by informality and mutual respect
11 Community members make collective decisions that affect the functioning of the community
12 The community has effective leadership which supports its democratic processes
13 All aspects of life are open to discussion within the community
14 All behaviour and emotional expression is open to discussion within the community
15 Community members share responsibility for one another

(College Centre for Quality Improvement, 2008)

As important as external standards is the annual process of self- and peer review. For the self-review, all in the community (service users and staff) consider, debate and mark how they are performing on the core and specialist standards. The specialist standards for personality disorder communities, for example, consists of five sections: the physical environment; staff and training; joining and leaving; the therapeutic environment; and external relations (Keenan & Paget, 2006). This information is collated and used for the peer review. As part of this process, a nominated neutral lead reviewer convenes a visit on which members from one therapeutic community (ideally two staff and two service users) visit another, to discuss their performance against the standards. A report is compiled, which highlights areas of achievement and recommendations. This report is then used to benchmark the community against the aggregated achievement of all therapeutic communities in an annual report. Nearly 100 therapeutic communities in the UK, and about a dozen overseas, now participate in this process, and most send delegates to an annual forum held in London.

Complex treatment needs complex evidence

As therapeutic communities are not a single treatment modality, they are not easily subjected to the type of experimental comparison trials that form the basis of the meta-analyses used to inform clinical guideline development groups for the National Institute for Health and Clinical Excellence (NICE). However, NICE guidelines for the treatment of borderline personality disorder (National Collaborating Centre for Mental Health, 2009) recommend many general features of care that are also covered by the practice standards set for members of the Community of Communities quality network (College Centre for Quality Improvement, 2011). Box 19.4 shows examples summarised from the NICE guidelines that match many therapeutic community principles.

Outcomes in therapeutic community services

There are differences in emphasis between different therapeutic communities as to what constitutes a 'worthwhile' outcome. There are also real differences in therapeutic priorities between those involved: service users; family, friends and carers; clinicians; academic researchers; and service commissioners. Commonly agreed service outcomes are:

- reduction of acute distress
- less chaotic help-seeking behaviour
- more integrated sense of personal identity
- improved interpersonal relationships and greater fulfilment in life
- increased chances of settled engagement in education or work.

Box 19.4   Principles of care for people with borderline personality disorder recommended by the NICE guidelines

- Build an optimistic and trusting relationship
- Work in an open, engaging and non-judgemental manner
- Be consistent and reliable
- Use an atmosphere of hope and optimism
- Explain that recovery is possible and attainable
- Bear in mind that many people will have experienced rejection, abuse and trauma
- Use an explicit and integrated theoretical approach, which is shared with the service user
- Provide therapist supervision
- Adapt the frequency of sessions to the person's needs and context of living
- Do not use brief psychotherapeutic interventions (of less than 3 months' duration)

At times of crisis:

- explore the person's reasons for distress
- try to understand the crisis from the person's point of view
- avoid minimising the person's stated reasons for the crisis
- stimulate reflection about solutions
- do not offer solutions before receiving full clarification of the problems
- maintain a calm and non-threatening attitude

(After National Collaborating Centre for Mental Health, 2009)

These are generally realistic outcomes following good engagement in a well-run programme.

Since 2006, a number of therapeutic communities for personality disorder have joined a coordinated practice-based research network (the Therapeutic Community Research Network) to collect outcome data. Each community uses standardised measures, including: the Standardised Assessment of Personality – Abbreviated Scale (SAPAS; Moran et al, 2003); Axis I, functioning and risk items on the Clinical Outcomes in Routine Evaluation – Outcome Measure (CORE-OM; CORE Information Management Systems, 2012); the Social Functioning Questionnaire (SFQ; Tyrer et al, 2005); the Service Use Questionnaire (SUQ), on the use of health and social services; the Self-Harm Questionnaire (SHQ); and a questionnaire developed for the network on medication use (the last three are unpublished). Support is being sought to collate and analyse the data as an extra service from the Community of Communities network. In the medium term, the project may result in a multicentre experimental outcome study based on a pilot project currently collecting data in Oxford.

A more fruitful approach may be to conduct long-term cohort studies, with economic and quality-of-life analyses. Some cost-offset studies (e.g., Dolan *et al*, 1997) have shown considerably reduced health service expenditure following treatment in a therapeutic community. Extrapolation of these ideas over the course of a person's life could result in the cost of treatment being very easily justified using the normal criteria applied by health economists (Haigh, 2012). Unfortunately, no robust long-term studies have yet been attempted, and it seems unlikely that they will be supported in a medically led research climate of short-termism, with no cross-budget collaboration and little cross-disciplinary cooperation.

Modern delivery formats and lower doses

Although there was widespread national regret at the closure of nearly all the residential therapeutic community beds in the National Health Service (Hansard, 2008), there have been welcome developments in non-residential therapeutic communities and communities experimenting with 'lower-dose' modifications of therapeutic programmes. An early example of this trend is described by Main (1990), who reports on the psychological effects on a group of moving from 'total immersion' in therapy (effectively 168 hours a week as a hospital in-patient) to a reduced weekdays-only programme (about 120 hours a week).

'Full-time day therapeutic communities' subsequently saw the value of people receiving therapy while simultaneously having to manage 'normal life' with their family and friends. These services (based on the full-time working week, Monday to Friday) provided about 30 hours of therapy a week (Knowles, 1997; Haigh, 2007*a*). This model is sometimes described as partial hospitalisation.

Further pressure on limited resources (both of staff and of physical space) has now led to 'part-time day therapeutic communities'. These offer about 18 hours of group time a week, commonly with programmes on three alternate days – such as Monday, Wednesday and Friday, with the staff undertaking other psychotherapeutic work in general services on Tuesdays and Thursdays. The government-funded community personality disorder projects, now running in the country's 14 'innovation centres' (www.personalitydisorder.org.uk/services/innovation-centres), operate on this model (Haigh, 2007*b*).

The lowest dose of therapy yet used is in the 'mini-therapeutic communities'. These may have half a day a week together as a group, with community lunch, plus a weekly group session in, for example, group analytic psychotherapy, modified dialectical behaviour therapy, psychodrama or schema-based cognitive–behavioural therapy (Pearce & Haigh, 2008). This amounts to about 8 hours a week together as a group. It is important to note that, even though the therapeutic community is not physically together for most of the time in these models, much of the culture-building psychotherapeutic work is to establish a 'therapeutic community in the head' for its members throughout the week. This can be seen as a group version of the popular mentalisation-based treatment's 'theory of mind', and it underlies a carefully structured support system in which members telephone or visit each other at times of crisis (Higgins, 1997).

In rural areas with the population spread over considerable distances, weekly meeting has been supplemented by use of specially designed and secure website-based networks for therapeutic contact (Rigby & Ashman, 2008). A virtual online community has also been developed by an active user-led group, with defined structures and rules to allow regular and *ad hoc* physical meetings in a public place (further details available from the authors). However, without professional clinical staff, and no physical premises in which to meet, it could be argued that this cannot be considered a therapeutic community. These service innovations are in the process of building their evidence base, and evidence is emerging with new efficacy data, economic analyses and the randomised controlled trial currently under way in Oxford (Lees *et al*, 2004).

Future possibilities, which are already being developed by the government and the Royal College of Psychiatrists, are 'psychologically informed planned environments' (PIPEs) for penal settings, 'psychologically informed environments' (PIEs) for homeless hostels and 'enabling environments' (EEs) for a wide range of settings. These are currently in pilot and pre-pilot stages of development (Johnson & Haigh, 2011).

Pathways and phases

In line with the recent evidence stressing the importance of engagement in services for those with extreme sensitivities, vulnerabilities and avoidance of seeking help (Crawford *et al*, 2009) it is now common to think of all 'doses' of therapeutic community programmes as having four phases (Kennard & Haigh, 2009):

1   engagement (which can take a very short time or may need years)
2   assessment and preparation (usually less than a year)
3   intensive treatment (usually a year or more)
4   recovery and rehabilitation (at least a few months, often years, sometimes indefinite).

A long-recognised problem of therapeutic communities is attrition: the experience of intensive therapy is sometimes too painful for people to bear, and they drop out. Theoretically, this happens less if the necessary therapeutic groundwork has been done in the engagement and preparation phases – but no unequivocal evidence has yet demonstrated this. Analysis of outcome data is also made more difficult by the frequent occurrence of people doing 'as much as they can' in one episode, and then dropping out of therapy. It may be some time (even years) before such people gradually realise that they need and benefit from therapy, so they return more ready to tolerate the anxiety and distress of it. In any standard analysis, these individuals would be considered 'treatment failures' or at least 'treatment drop-outs' after their first attempt. Yet they may have done enough therapeutic work to set them on a path to which they can later return and successfully complete. Or they may have done just enough to make a difference to how they are as parents to their children, or to prevent escalation of self-harm or violence, or numerous other possibilities. Conventional quantitative analysis of treatment efficacy, which compares just two time points and one follow-up (usually in terms of months), will struggle to make sense of so many intermediate and long-term outcome variables.

A complementary problem for therapeutic community members is that of endings, and their avoidance of any form of ending or distance because of the feelings of fear and abandonment that these generate. Avoidance of these feelings can make people with personality disorders avoid endings by cutting off relationships before the planned ending is experienced, effectively leaving the relationship before the relationship can leave them. This translates into all aspects of their lives, including work, friendships, romantic attachments and (inevitably) professional therapeutic arrangements, often much to the frustration of professionals. These feelings of fear and distress are experienced in the therapeutic community, while preparing for the transition and ending of a therapeutic relationship, and may be difficult to manage, especially with an open therapy group. Many people announce their premature departure rather than wanting to stay for the period of the entire programme and experience a planned ending.

A programme with scheduled reviews during community meetings and group sessions can feel as though it is peppered with hurdles that members have to jump, and it gives rise to predictable time points for 'wanting to run away': at 3 months (with the 'settling in' review); at 9 months (half way through), at 1 year (anniversary of joining) and at 15 months (getting ready to leave) – in fact, whenever the prospect of the transition and leaving start to loom:

'I started the journey full of hope and expectation about reaching a promised land of "Recovery", yet had no idea what that would feel like, and whether I would even like myself when or if I ever reached it. Instead I have come to realise that recovery itself is a very subjective place, which changes daily and is never tangible as if to say "I have recovered". Instead it is a case of reminding myself, "I have achieved, I have coped or I have handled a situation today that I would have not handled in previous years". I have developed the ability to congratulate myself on something well done and to be kind to myself in those situations where things were not so successful. The ability to reflect on my moods and challenge the whirlwind of thinking along the lines of "wouldn't anyone be reacting to this-or-that like this?"'
(H. den Hartog)

Although 'recovery' is now a popular concept in mental health services, there has been limited consideration of how it applies to therapeutic communities. Just as there is little research about the (really) long-term outcome for therapeutic community members, there are few services, either in policy or on the ground, for the post-community, rest-of-life period. Although at this point, the service user has many of the resources in place to enable them to move forward with their journey, on occasion people do 'slip', and at that point are in real danger of falling back into what feels like the giant hole from which they have spent so much time and effort climbing out:

> 'In my experience, community mental health teams have neither the resources nor the knowledge to support service users who have come out of therapeutic communities (who usually have more knowledge about PD [personality disorder] themselves than the CMHT staff have). I was offered pills within months of leaving a TC [therapeutic community], having worked really hard to rid myself of all psychiatric medication. It was incredibly difficult to turn away from the seemingly easy option of resorting back to the drug induced haze of avoidance and denial. But instead of accepting it, I reminded myself of how I had fought to eliminate my need for the medication when I was in the TC, and the disappointment I would feel for both myself and all the others who supported me during that time.
>
> At certain times during the rest of your life you inevitably hit the walls that everyone can hit – but the danger for someone with PD, or at least remembers how it felt to be really distressed with PD, is that you allow yourself to dive headlong into the crazy, irrational but somehow familiar place again, in a human moment of weakness.' (H. den Hartog)

Boundaries and security

Many of the terms and concepts used in therapeutic communities, alongside the commonly used 'jargon' for them, are listed in Table 19.1. One of the most important to highlight is 'boundaries'. A common maxim in group therapy training is that 'a group lives or dies by its boundaries'. This is even more accentuated in groups for people with borderline or other personality disorders, as problems with the boundary between self and other people is one of the symptoms and signs of their diagnosis. These problems range on a spectrum from having no respect for boundaries whatsoever, through to a rigid adherence that can be obsessive. In almost every case, the difficulties stem from the lack of adherence to or even formation of appropriate boundaries in childhood, which leaves the developing child with an insecure environment in which to grow up. The common result of this is the re-creation of insecurity in adulthood. This is manifest as inability to create and maintain healthy boundaries in adult life, which creates chaos in every kind of relationship they encounter.

One of the common bonds that all people with personality disorder share is an inherent need for boundaries to be held firmly in place, in order to establish a basic level of emotional safety. Much of this need is outside

Table 19.1 Therapeutic community concepts and methods

	Description	Relation to previously described themes
Concepts		
Service user partnership	Close, mutual understanding between staff and service users	Democratisation Relationship focus Agency
Agreed boundaries	Discussion of guidelines/rules and consequences of not keeping to them Effective processes for dealing with them	Reality confrontation Containment
Shared responsibilities	Service users are able to work well with each other at various tasks, including those with serious responsibility attached, such as offering support in crisis	Communalism Living-learning experience
Empowerment	Service users feel progressively more able to take certain roles (e.g. community chair) and conduct more equal relationships with staff	Permissiveness Agency
Emotional development	Basic requirements are to feel belonging and to feel safe; then to be able to say what is needed; then to find place among others and establish solid sense of self	Developmental model – based on unconscious attachment and containment
Methods		
Community meetings	All staff and service users meet to discuss all practical and emotional issues of immediate importance	Culture of enquiry and openness Involvement Reality confrontation
Mutual support systems	Encourages service users to offer each other out-of-hours support and advice, by telephone or in person; run with detailed protocols and safety mechanisms	Containment Agency
Peer learning	Recognises that 'those who have been there themselves' often have more to offer than trained professionals	Democratisation Culture of openness
Integrated supervision	Different therapeutic modalities and an overall understanding of what is happening in the milieu cannot be understood in isolated or conflicting ways – understanding must be shared through joint supervision	Culture of enquiry Democratisation
Deliberate informality	Interpersonal transactions between all participants are conducted without any formal barriers (e.g. first names are usually used)	Permissiveness Culture of openness
Diminished hierarchy	All contributions are received as equal: participants earn respect through their contributions, not through role or rank	Democratisation

of conscious awareness – like the dependable experiences of starting and finishing groups on time, whatever is happening, of knowing which staff will be around when, and of having a solid shared understanding of what to do when rules are broken. The only way that therapeutic community members will trust that this boundaries are in place is to test them, and test them hard, to destruction if possible. Like a toddler that pushes against the first restrictions put in place by their parents, members will often push against and test any group rules and norms, just to see whether the system has the capacity to withstand their assault. When rules, routines and boundaries are in place, the individual's trust in the system and the people in it can start to develop:

'The one thing that persuaded me that a TC might finally be the place for me to address my long-standing issues was the boundaries that were so tightly held in place by both the staff and the client members of the TC. Boundaries were one thing that my parents never really enforced – and the knowledge that whatever happened within the group sessions, above all, certain boundaries could and would be held in place gave me the trust I needed.

The staff in particular were rock solid, and conveyed with a quiet determination that enabled me to be assured that the splitting, conflict and chaotic behaviour that was exhibited at times would not shake the cohesive safety of the group as a whole. If the "mummies and daddies" were okay, everything else seemed okay too. Though at first the almost obsessive adherence to timekeeping, agendas and petty formalities seemed cruel and uncaring in the face of so much pain and suffering of the members. In fact, I soon learned that these rigid expectations were what enabled the other therapeutic sessions to feel safe, that there were times and places for work and play, for formality and informality, and for laughing and tears. For people who have led lifestyle of chaos and unpredictability, the set agendas and respect for the needs of others taught valuable lessons in how to live reasonably and comfortably amongst others, sometimes for the first time in years.' (H. den Hartog)

Conclusion

There is good evidence that the therapeutic community model is effective in reducing some of the most challenging aspects of living with a personality disorder. This is probably achieved via a mechanism of enhanced mentalisation and metacognition, so that community members can take their own minds, and the minds of others, seriously. Some of this reflection is evident in Box 19.5. As we have described above, there is not one therapeutic community model but many. But what they share is a commitment to respect for the person, both as an individual and among others, and a belief in the possibility of transformation – things that many people with personality disorders will not previously have experienced from mental health services.

Box 19.5 Reflections of service users

'We mustn't take the personality out of personality disorder. After all, everybody has a personality and nobody is perfect. It's all relative.'

'A service user told me in group, as a response to my challenge about their behaviour, that I was the only person that they would have accepted the challenge from – because I had been there myself and they therefore believed I was the only one really "qualified" to make the comment.'

'To understand someone suffering with personality disorder is really like trying to learn a new language, the language of PD. Once you learn the semantics and pragmatics of their communication, the understanding of the reasoning behind behaviours becomes much more simple, logical, dare I say even predictable.'

'It's a path to discovery or emergence, rather than a "recovery", for how can you "recover" to somewhere you have never previously been?'

'After three years of post-therapeutic community living I have come to the point where strategies and coping mechanisms have settled down into a more comfortable routine. I still have to work incredibly hard to stay well and sometimes, to be honest, I wish I could be unhappily unaware again, but once you learn something, it's very difficult to turn your back on it. I call it being therapised.'

'I now wake up in the mornings with a bubble-like feeling sitting within my chest – a bubble of anticipation for what the day might bring, and a knowledge that I will be able to cope with whatever is set before me. In all my 38 years I have never woken up with a bubble like this, gratitude about being alive for another day, and it feels great.'

References

Crawford, M. J., Price, K., Gordon, F., et al (2009) Engagement and retention in specialist services for people with personality disorder. *Acta Psychiatrica Scandinavica*, **119**, 304–311.

College Centre for Quality Improvement (2008) *The Development of Core Standards and Core Values for Therapeutic Communities*. Royal College of Psychiatrists (http://www.rcpsych. ac.uk/pdf/CSCV%20Final%20Briefing_Paper.pdf).

College Centre for Quality Improvement (2011) Community of Communities: Values and Standards. Royal College of Psychiatrists (http://www.rcpsych.ac.uk/quality/quality,accreditationaudit/communityofcommunities/valuesandstandards.aspx).

CORE Information Management Systems (2012) The CORE Outcome Measure (CORE-OM). CORE IMS (http://www.coreims.co.uk/About_Core_System_Outcome_Measure.html).

Dolan, B., Warren, F. & Norton, K. (1997) Change in borderline symptoms one year after therapeutic community treatment for severe personality disorder. *British Journal of Psychiatry*, **171**, 274–279.

Foulkes, S. H. (1964) *Therapeutic Group Analysis*. Allen and Unwin.

Haigh R (2007a) The new day TCs: five radical features. *Therapeutic Communities*, **28**, 111–126.

Haigh, R. (2007*b*) New kids on the block: the Government-funded English personality disorder services. *Therapeutic Communities*, **28**, 3, 300–310.

Haigh, R. (2012) Being economical with the evidence. *Group Analysis*, **45**, 73–86.

Haigh, R. & Lees, J. (2008) Fusion TCs: divergent histories, converging challenges. *Therapeutic Communities*, **29**, 347–374.

Hansard (2008) Column 308WH (http://www.publications.parliament.uk/pa/cm200708/cmhansrd/cm080116/halltext/80116h0009.htm).

Higgins, B. (1997) Does anyone feel they need support tonight? 24 hour care in a day unit. *Therapeutic Communities*, **18**, 55–61.

Johnson, R. & Haigh, R. (2011) Social psychiatry and social policy for the 21st century: new concepts for new needs – the 'Enabling Environments' initiative. *Mental Health and Social Inclusion*, **15**, 17–23.

Keenan S. & Paget, P. (2006) *Service Standards for Therapeutic Communities* (5th Edn) (CRTU037). Royal College of Psychiatrists' Research and Training Unit.

Kennard, D. & Haigh, R. (2009) Therapeutic communities. In *The New Oxford Textbook of Psychiatry* (2nd edn) (ed. M. Gelder), 142–148. Oxford University Press.

Knowles, J. (1997) 'The Reading model': an integrated psychotherapy service. *Psychiatric Bulletin*, **21**, 84–87.

Lees, J., Manning, N. & Rawlings, B. (2004) A culture of enquiry: research evidence and the therapeutic community. *Psychiatric Quarterly*, **75**, 279–294.

Main, T. F. (1990) Knowledge, learning and freedom from thought. *Psychoanalytic Psychotherapy*, **5**, 59–78.

Moran, P., Leese, M., Lee, T., *et al* (2003) Standardised Assessment of Personality – Abbreviated Scale (SAPAS): preliminary validation of a brief screen for personality disorder. *British Journal of Psychiatry*, **183**, 228–232.

National Collaborating Centre for Mental Health (2009) *Borderline Personality Disorder: Treatment and Management (NICE Clinical Guideline 78)*. National Institute for Health and Clinical Excellence.

Pearce, S. & Haigh, R. (2008) Mini therapeutic communities – a new development in the United Kingdom. *Therapeutic Communities*, **29**, 111–124.

Rigby, M. & Ashman, D. (2008) Service innovation: a virtual informal network of care to support a 'lean' therapeutic community in a new rural personality disorder service. *Psychiatric Bulletin*, **32**, 64–67.

Sempik, J., Hine, R. & Wilcox, D. (eds) (2010) *Green Care: A Conceptual Framework: A Report of the Working Group on the Health Benefits of Green Care. COST 866, Green Care in Agriculture*. Centre for Child and Family Research, Loughborough University.

Tyrer, P., Nur, U., Crawford, M., *et al* (2005) The Social Functioning Questionnaire: a rapid and robust measure of perceived functioning. *International Journal of Social Psychiatry*, **51**, 265–275.

CHAPTER 20

Nidotherapy: making the environment do the therapeutic work

Peter Tyrer and Priya Bajaj

Summary Nidotherapy is the formal term introduced to describe the systematic manipulation of the physical and social environment to help achieve a better fit for a person with a persistent or permanent mental disorder. This approach is described in detail and its merits are compared with more conventional ways of dealing with such problems. This involves the creation of a certain number of terms that may be viewed as unnecessary jargon but help to shorten communication in an area where systematic monitored interventions are relatively uncommon.

Nidotherapy (the 'i' is long) has come about from the frustrations of exercising evidence-based treatment options with a minority of patients who despise them all with equal fervour. It is a treatment that systematically adjusts the environment to suit the needs of a person with a chronic mental illness, personality disorder or similar long-term disability. The name is derived from the Latin *nidus*, or nest, as a nest, particularly a bird's nest, represents one of the best natural examples of an environment adjusted to an organism (Tyrer, 2002). Although taking the environment into account is part and parcel of clinical management, the systematic manipulation of the environment, often in a subtle way to include both physical and social environments, has not been formalised before. Many reading this chapter will regard such action as the exercise of common sense rather than any special type of intervention and will be sceptical about formalising it under a fancy title such as nidotherapy. They may be right, but we would like all to suspend judgement until they have further evidence of the value of this approach expressed in a more formalised manner.

Principles of nidotherapy

There are five essential principles of nidotherapy: collateral collocation; the formulation of realistic environmental targets; the improvement of

---

Box 20.1   Principles of nidotherapy

Collateral collocation
Seeing the environment from the patient's point of view

Formulation of realistic environmental targets
Setting clear goals for environmental change

Improvement of social function
If the targets are right, social function will improve; if it does not improve, the targets need to be reassessed

Personal adaptation and control
Throughout nidotherapy the patient takes prime responsibility for the programme

Wider environmental integration and arbitrage
Involving others, particularly a trusted arbiter, in resolving change that others may not desire

---

social function; personal adaptation and control; and wider environmental integration involving arbitrage (Tyrer *et al*, 2003*a*) (Box 20.1). These need amplification.

Collateral collocation

This alliterative couplet describes the task of seeing the environment through the eyes of the patient, a combination of 'standing side by side' and 'standing in each other's shoes'. The first task in nidotherapy is to try to interpret the environment as seen by the patient in a way that gives greater understanding of perceived priorities. Although we do this in clinical practice repeatedly, there is a tendency to be paternalistic in proposing what seems a reasonable environmental adjustment (i.e. usually one that we agree with) and rejecting others that seem to us to be unsatisfactory or unrealistic. In collateral collocation, all external judgement is suspended in the first instance and a full environmental analysis of the patient's current situation is made and potential areas of change outlined. Clearly, such an activity is focused to some extent on those needs that are judged to be relevant to mental health; others are usually presumed to be of lesser importance but always need to be considered, as they may be much more important than originally thought.

In the second phase of analysis, the potential environmental changes identified by others involved in care (an individual therapist or joint workers, or indeed the whole clinical team) are also defined in detail. This list may be very different from that provided by the patient but both need to be spelled out initially. The lists for one patient, a refugee from a Muslim country, and his nidotherapist, are shown in the first two columns of Table 20.1.

The formulation of realistic environmental targets

Once an environmental analysis has been completed, it is necessary to put the environmental needs into order of importance and merge the patient's and therapist's lists in a realistic way. Some desired outcomes have to be rejected immediately, even when they are considered to be highly relevant and important. For example, in central London it would be unreasonable to expect the patient to be accommodated in a quiet detached house completely free of noise pollution or for a homeless indigent patient to be provided with an unearned income of £30 000 a year. However, this part of nidotherapy needs to be pursued in an open spirit, as apparently unattainable goals can sometimes be achieved with sufficient determination.

Table 20.1 Environmental analysis and subsequent compromise action

Environmental area	Patient's first environmental analysis	Clinical team's environmental analysis	Agreed compromise
Comfort: warmth	Complete draught exclusion in flat and better heating	Serious deficiencies in heating arrangements in flat	Patient agrees to be moved to a smaller, centrally heated flat
Finance	Every day to have enough money for his needs	Poor personal control over finances: friends borrow his money without returning it, manipulate and exploit him	Clinical team act as patient's appointee and give him money three times a week, always keeping some in reserve
Leisure	To be close to his friends and late-night café culture	The friends he meets are not thought to be a good influence on him so this wish is not regarded as very important	Compromise solution: moved closer to social network (see comfort above) but encouraged to have more activities elsewhere during the day
Security	To feel safe when alone at home	Is vulnerable and unable to deal with potential conflict	Extra locks fitted at main door of building
Status: self-esteem	To live in surroundings where he can be taken seriously by friends, relatives and professionals	No special opinion: he appears to have good self-esteem already	Money reserved from appointeeship to furnish new flat to higher standard than might normally be expected

Case example: formulating environmental targets

The patient described in Table 20.1 has a recurrent psychotic disorder and a history of non-adherence to treatment (to protect his identity no other clinical information is given here). The environmental needs he presented (in no particular order) concern the common areas of comfort, finance, leisure activities and social contacts. Some of these are clearly objective environmental requirements. Others, such as the desire for improved self-esteem, might be regarded more as personal needs related to attitudes and thoughts and best dealt with by problem-solving or cognitive–behavioural interventions. However, the only question to be asked is 'Can this problem be addressed by an environmental change?'. If it can, then it is appropriate for nidotherapy. Each of these needs was considered by his carers and nidotherapist and, despite some reservations, all were regarded as sufficiently important to try to change them.

In examining the process of nidotherapy in this example, we will describe two of these environmental areas and what was involved in their change. The first is the management of the patient's finances through appointeeship. You may think that this is such a common exercise with those who show poor budgetary control that it cannot be looked upon as a new approach. However, the pathway to appointeeship in nidotherapy is usually different from that in other types of practice. The patient wanted environmental change but could not achieve it because of poor financial control. When asked for ways of, for example, making his flat a more inviting place when his friends visited, all options required more money for furnishings and design, and it was the patient who initiated the discussions about appointeeship by asking for help to use his income more wisely. Use of this approach also helped his self-esteem when his flat became more welcoming.

The leisure activity of staying out late at night drinking caffeine-containing drinks (never alcohol) is also not usually addressed in normal practice, except in a peremptory way under 'cultural needs' in care programme review meetings. Nidotherapy established that this social contact, regarded by the clinical team as a relatively insignificant part of the patient's daily routine (Table 20.1), was of fundamental importance and needed fostering. In discussing the eventual placement of the patient (part of the answers to the 'comfort' component of the environmental analysis) the need to be close to the late-night drinking area was recognised as being very important and it featured high on the list of essentials. Eventually a new flat was obtained less than a kilometre from the cafés.

It is often useful, but not essential, to quantify the progress made towards achieving the environmental goals set by patient and therapist. Our patient's progress in achieving each of the targets over a period of 1 year is shown in Fig. 20.1. One advantage of this system is that when one target stubbornly remains below the rest in terms of achievement it is recognised and can be separately addressed. Thus, the value of appointeeship and relocation have helped the patient in some respects, but he still has limited self-esteem and some uncertainty about his status.

The improvement of social function

Nidotherapy could be regarded as a misnomer in that the therapeutic endeavour is indirect. There is no specific attempt to change the person but, by changing the environment, improvement may take place secondarily. However, the primary improvement should be in social functioning. Social

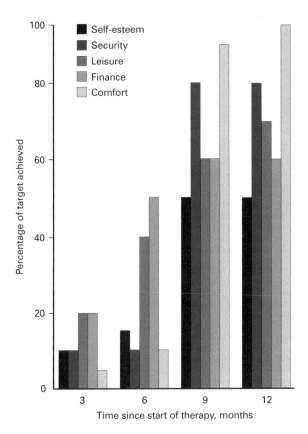

Fig. 20.1 Progress towards targets outlined in Table 20.1 over 12 months (the targets and the extent to which they were achieved were agreed jointly by therapist and patient).

function is a direct measure of the fit between person and environment, and even if psychiatric symptomatology remains unchanged, better adjustment of the environment should lead to improved social functioning.

It is perhaps not surprising that the elements of good social functioning – ability to cope with tasks with adequate performance and little perceived stress, good financial management, secure and settled relationships with friends, family and wider society, and enjoyment of spare time (Remington & Tyrer, 1979; Weissman & Bothwell, 1979) – often figure so highly in the environmental needs of patients in nidotherapy. It is even less surprising, therefore, that when they are resolved or alleviated, social function improves. However, the converse is important too. When a nidotherapy programme fails to lead to improved social function, the environmental targets need to be re-examined. They may have been inappropriately chosen, or circumstances may have changed so that some or all are no longer appropriate. In a randomised trial of nidotherapy added to conventional assertive outreach treatment (Tyrer *et al*, 2011), social function was the only

---

Box 20.2 Reasons for personal control in nidotherapy

- To prevent patronising and paternalistic decisions
- To ensure that any environmental change is more likely to be maintained after treatment
- To avoid clinicians taking control of matters that are very personal to the patient

---

clinical outcome to show significant superiority for the nidotherapy group, and this was also accompanied by marked cost savings.

Personal adaptation and control

The notion that the patient is in control of a nidotherapy programme, particularly someone who has a severe psychotic illness or lacks capacity, may at first seem strange. But there are good reasons for it (Box 20.2). By constantly going back to a plan that has been devised with the patient at its core, the errors that are so common if senior figures in authority decide, without proper consultation, what is best for others are avoided. Even when a disability is pronounced and there may be doubts about the patient's capacity to contribute to solutions for care (as, for example, in chronic schizophrenia with very little motivation, severe intellectual disability or dementia), it is important to at least try to gauge the person's wishes no matter how difficult this task becomes or how apparently inappropriate the responses. Thus, the wish of someone with a severe intellectual disability to have a certain carer (or type of care) involved in their daily life cannot be roughly cast aside in favour of something different without proper inquiry. Similarly, a recurrent sex offender who asks to be kept in secure institutional care because he feels he is no longer capable of adequate control of all aspects of his life, not just his sex drive, should not be bundled onto a complex treatment programme allegedly to change something that, in his judgement, will remain for ever unchanged.

It is also important to note that nidotherapy can still be appropriate in the management of less severe forms of mental illness than those described here, where the options of controlled environmental change to a great extent need to be coordinated by health professionals. Chronic stress in those whose lifestyle is often the cause of their difficulties can also be approached by systematically tackling environmental needs rather than by changing symptoms (Tyrer, 2003).

Wider environmental integration and arbitrage

The main aim in nidotherapy is to achieve a good personal fit between individual and environment. This cannot be done in isolation and has to take account of wider environmental needs, including those of society. For example, it may suit an individual to have loud music playing all day in his flat because this suppresses the impact of auditory hallucinations, but if it creates great distress for neighbours it would be counterproductive. It is therefore quite common for the patient's and therapist's environmental analysis to be discordant and one of the key tasks in nidotherapy is to match up these lists in a way that is acceptable to both patient and therapist. Since this can be particularly contentious, it is often necessary to have an arbiter whose authority is respected by both patient and therapist (or clinical team), so that any judgement the arbiter makes will be accepted by both parties. The phase of arbitrage is therefore often an important one in nidotherapy, and early in the treatment plan it is useful to identify a potential arbiter who will be acceptable to all involved in the programme.

The arbiter may be a relative, another independent professional, a friend or a carer. The important prerequisite is that he or she must be trusted by both patient and therapist and given authority to make decisions that will be accepted by all parties.

The arbiter is needed at the time of matching the two sections of the environmental analysis (Table 20.1) if it is impossible to reach agreement on views that appear to be opposing. This can be a particularly sticky phase in a nidotherapy programme as, without an active and trusted arbiter, opposing views on which environmental changes are needed can cause an impasse.

Phases of nidotherapy

Nidotherapy can be given in one-to-one treatment, with the nidotherapist acting as a combined therapist and advocate on behalf of the patient, or to groups of patients or groups of staff. One-to-one treatment is the format originally adopted (Tyrer, 2009), in which a number of sessions (usually over 10 in our current work) are given. Group therapy is better for people who live together in residential settings, in which all the staff know all the patients and any changes that are recommended for an individual are going to affect others. In such settings, nidotherapy operates by consensus, with compromise often being necessary to accommodate the environmental needs of others. With both treatments we adopt a five-phase approach (Box 20.3).

Box 20.3 Phases of nidotherapy

1 Selection of the patients as suitable for nidotherapy
2 Full environmental analysis
3 Implementation of a common nidopathway
4 Monitoring of progress
5 Resetting of the nidopathway and completion

Phase 1: Identification of the boundaries of nidotherapy

Nidotherapy is usually chosen for a patient who has been treated extensively and has achieved all the gains that are possible from the range of interventions available. In some instances, these gains may be very low indeed; in others, they may be substantial but with considerable residual disability. In many patients suitable for nidotherapy, there has been a long battle between therapists wishing to try interventions and patients desperate to resist them.

The nidotherapist, in introducing the treatment to the patient, emphasises that there is no intention to change the patient and that the whole focus of treatment is on examining the environment to see what environmental changes are most suited. In this early stage of treatment, there is often a gratifying improvement in collaboration and communication with the patient. After years of being battered by demands to partake in interventions that they regard as of no value, it is a welcome change for the patient to have their disability acknowledged more formally and, instead of being required to change the disability, to participate in changing the environment. This acceptance, which could be regarded as validation of disability, allows further treatment to be pursued along a consensual pathway.

By defining what can be given for the disorder and what can be done to change the environment, there is less chance of conflict and a greater chance that collaboration will be established for other interventions such as drug treatment (Tasman *et al*, 2000).

Phase 2: Full environmental analysis

This is carried out as described in the case example above. All aspects of the patient's wishes are noted, for even if they are subsequently discarded as fanciful or unattainable they can still be of value. It is often necessary to visit the patient at home or in other environments, and it is essential to embrace the ideas behind collateral collocation, so that presumptive conclusions are not reached (Box 20.4).

The therapist's environmental analysis follows that of the patient and is informed by it. It can be done with the patient or independently, but it is unlikely exactly to mirror the patient's. Once completed, the sometimes

---

Box 20.4 Things that go bump in the night

A man with paranoia complained to his community psychiatric nurse that he could hear everything going on in the flat next door and that a large machine was being moved in the middle of the night. He was shown to be correct when it was found that the flat next door was being used as business premises and the machine being moved was a photocopier.

---

difficult task of joining the two in an agreed way has to be tackled. This is when the involvement of an arbiter may be necessary (Boxes 20.5 and 20.6).

Phase 3: Implementation of a common route (the nidopathway)

Phase 2 may take several hours to complete, but if it is done successfully the next phases will be negotiated much more quickly. The different elements of the nidopathway are identified and each is planned. Obviously, many will need very careful thought and will have to take place in clearly defined steps (e.g. moving to new accommodation). An appropriate timescale for these changes needs to be set to avoid disappointment later.

Phase 4: Monitoring of progress

The phase of monitoring is not an onerous one for the nidotherapist, as although it often takes considerable time to achieve the targets, they should remain clear, with a transparent procedure for completing them. This transparency is important for patients: full feedback on the progress towards achieving targets emphasises that they have not been forgotten, and they can often offer useful ideas on how to overcome barriers. Despite this, it is highly unlikely that all targets will be achieved successfully (Fig. 20.1). Whether or not further efforts are made to finish the task depends on the patient and the degree of improvement in social functioning that has been attained.

Phase 5: Resetting the nidopathway

There may be times when targets thought to be appropriate and attainable turn out not to be. In these instances it is necessary to return and revise the pathway with different targets, usually less ambitious, but sometimes more so. The patient's role in this task is very important, as their agreement to what is decided has to be genuine.

How does nidotherapy fit in with other treatment?

Nidotherapy as a treatment package involves the five-phase approach outlined above, but the actual therapeutic input is extremely variable. It is governed by the patient's physical and social environment and may range from purely structural change (e.g. installation of a boiler) to measures to assist socialising (e.g. enrolment in clubs) or even long-term goals such as moving to alternative accommodation.

Most clients receive other treatments during the course of nidotherapy. The important questions are whether nidotherapy fits in with existing treatments and whether it offers any additional therapeutic gain(s) for the patient beyond those of just achieving a better environmental fit.

We believe it does. To begin with, nidotherapy concentrates on 'environment change' rather than 'patient change'. This has a major bearing on the pace of the therapy and also on the parameters used to judge improvement. However, this does not imply that it is mutually exclusive and unaffected by other treatments. For instance, an individual may be less depressed after a course of cognitive–behavioural therapy and this would affect the way she perceives her environment. The time at which nidotherapy is chosen in treatment is critical; it should be selected only for those aspects of symptoms or behaviour that are stable and unlikely to change in the short term.

Nidotherapy may work synchronously with existing therapies but at the same time remain independent of them. Helping the patient to focus on an environmental change might enhance adaptation to the outside world. This may manifest as better engagement or positive outcomes with other treatments. The targets set and the adjustments made to incorporate changes would be part and parcel of the nidotherapy, irrespective of the progress made with other therapies.

Who should practise nidotherapy?

Many psychiatrists reading this would regard most of the tasks described here as sufficiently basic as to be deskilling, in that they do not require any of the special skills necessary for consultant practice. Some, however, would welcome the fresh approach to engaging with the 'difficult' patients, especially when conventional approaches and therapies have failed. Focusing on a goal that is literally more 'close to home' for the patient may enhance the therapeutic relationship and help in the delivery of care.

The targets set during nidotherapy often encroach on the arena of other members of the multidisciplinary team, such as the social worker, psychologist, occupational therapist, creative therapist and support worker. We have worked with many disciplines and have found, for example, that music therapy or structured occupational therapy are particularly well placed to help many individuals, not only through any direct effects, but by altering environmental needs, which can then be addressed separately. One could well argue that each discipline has the necessary skills and expertise required to work towards one or more goals of nidotherapy, and these can be harnessed as required. The question is not who is best suited to practise nidotherapy but when is it needed?

From a patient's perspective, a nidotherapist detached from the clinical team could be viewed as 'neutral' in the event of a stormy therapeutic relationship – and these are common with individuals who have persistent disability and an alternative view of the world from their carers. A separate, consistent and collaborative environmental therapy may serve as an anchor for patients drifting between opposition and despair when receiving other unwanted treatments. As mental illness is often chronic and enduring, the focus on working towards a stable and healthy environment may offer a ray of hope.

We have generally found that a nidotherapist separate from the clinical team, but working closely with it, is the best solution. The exception to this is when the patient is living in a residential setting with other patients, when the group approach, preferably combining both staff and patients, may be preferable. For an individual trying to achieve greater autonomy – one of the strongest held and most common aims identified by patients in nidotherapy – the combined therapist–advocate model working within a therapeutic setting, allows nidotherapy to proceed in parallel with other forms of care without coming into conflict with them.

We are in the process of manualising nidotherapy for wider use in clinical teams and have a set of annual workshops where further training is provided. Details of these are on the nidotherapy website (www.nidotherapy.com) and additional training is also being provided in Sweden and Australia. The main focus of treatment to date has been on patients with personality disorder, severe mental illness and substance misuse (Ranger *et al*, 2009; Tyrer *et al*, 2011), but it is now being extended to people with intellectual disability, autism spectrum disorders and chronic depression, where many of the problems are linked to personality function. One great advantage of nidotherapy compared with many other psychological treatments is that most of the patients who prefer it do not want to change their personalities. They have Type R (treatment-resisting) personalities as opposed to Type S (treatment-seeking) ones (Tyrer *et al*, 2003b; Ranger *et al*, 2004) and currently there are very few treatments available for these. Almost all evidence-based treatments are for borderline personality disorder (Bateman & Zanarini, 2011), which accounts for only 20% of all people with this group of conditions. Those with the externalising antisocial and impulsive personalities do not like psychological treatments focused on changing their behaviour but do respond when the input is given in an environmental context (Spencer *et al*, 2010).

We would appreciate feedback from colleagues who are motivated to try this approach for themselves. For those patients for whom it seems necessary to 'go that extra mile' beyond the bounds of standard evidence-based psychiatry, nidotherapy may be a suitable option.

References

Bateman, A. & Zanarini, M. (2011) Personality disorder. In *Effective Treatments in Psychiatry* (eds P. Tyrer & K. R. Silk), pp. 293–303. Cambridge University Press.

Ranger, M., Methuen, C., Rutter, D., *et al* (2004) Prevalence of personality disorder in the case load of an inner-city assertive outreach team. *Psychiatric Bulletin*, **28**, 441–443.

Ranger, M., Tyrer, P., Miloseska, K., *et al* (2009) Cost-effectiveness of nidotherapy for comorbid personality disorder and severe mental illness: randomized controlled trial. *Epidemiologia Psichiatria Sociale*, **18**, 128–136.

Remington, M. & Tyrer, P. (1979) The Social Functioning Schedule – a brief semi-structured interview. *Social Psychiatry*, **14**, 151–157.

Spencer, S. J., Rutter, D. & Tyrer, P. (2010) Integration of nidotherapy into the management of mental illness and antisocial personality: a qualitative study. *International Journal of Social Psychiatry*, **56**, 50–59.

Tasman, A., Riba, M. B. & Silk, K. R. (2000) *The Doctor–Patient Relationship in Pharmacotherapy: Improving Treatment Effectiveness*. Guilford Press.

Tyrer, P. (2002) Nidotherapy: a new approach to the treatment of personality disorder. *Acta Psychiatrica Scandinavica*, **105**, 469–471.

Tyrer, P. (2003) *How to Cope with Stress* (2nd edn). Sheldon Press.

Tyrer, P. (2009) *Nidotherapy: Harmonising the Environment with the Patient*. RCPsych Publications.

Tyrer, P., Sensky, T. & Mitchard, S. (2003a) The principles of nidotherapy in the treatment of persistent mental and personality disorders. *Psychotherapy and Psychosomatics*, **72**, 350–356.

Tyrer, P., Mitchard, S., Methuen, C., *et al* (2003b) Treatment-rejecting and treatment-seeking personality disorders: Type R and Type S. *Journal of Personality Disorders*, **17**, 265–270.

Tyrer, P., Miloseska, K., Whittington, C., *et al* (2011) Nidotherapy in the treatment of substance misuse, psychosis and personality disorder: secondary analysis of a controlled trial. *Psychiatrist*, **35**, 9–14.

Weissman, M. M. & Bothwell, S. (1979) Assessment of social adjustment by patient self-report. *Archives of General Psychiatry*, **33**, 1111–1115.

Index

Compiled by Linda English